AF565110

Atlas of Coronary Balloon Angioplasty

FUNDAMENTAL AND CLINICAL CARDIOLOGY

1. *Drug Treatment of Hyperlipidemia*, edited by Basil M. Rifkind
2. *Cardiotonic Drugs: A Clinical Review, Second Edition, Revised and Expanded*, edited by Carl V. Leier
3. *Complications of Coronary Angioplasty*, edited by Alexander J. R. Black, H. Vernon Anderson, and Stephen G. Ellis
4. *Unstable Angina*, edited by John D. Rutherford
5. *Beta-Blockers and Cardiac Arrhythmias*, edited by Prakash C. Deedwania
6. *Exercise and the Heart in Health and Disease*, edited by Roy J. Shephard and Henry S. Miller, Jr.
7. *Cardiopulmonary Physiology in Critical Care*, edited by Steven M. Scharf
8. *Atherosclerotic Cardiovascular Disease, Hemostasis, and Endothelial Function*, edited by Robert Boyer Francis, Jr.
9. *Coronary Heart Disease Prevention*, edited by Frank G. Yanowitz
10. *Thrombolysis and Adjunctive Therapy for Acute Myocardial Infarction*, edited by Eric R. Bates
11. *Stunned Myocardium: Properties, Mechanisms, and Clinical Manifestations*, edited by Robert A. Kloner and Karin Przyklenk
12. *Prevention of Venous Thromboembolism*, edited by Samuel Z. Goldhaber
13. *Silent Myocardial Ischemia and Infarction: Third Edition*, Peter F. Cohn
14. *Congestive Cardiac Failure: Pathophysiology and Treatment*, edited by David B. Barnett, Hubert Pouleur, and Gary S. Francis
15. *Heart Failure: Basic Science and Clinical Aspects*, edited by Judith K. Gwathmey, G. Maurice Briggs, and Paul D. Allen
16. *Coronary Thrombolysis in Perspective: Principles Underlying Conjunctive and Adjunctive Therapy*, edited by Burton E. Sobel and Désiré Collen
17. *Cardiovascular Disease in the Elderly Patient*, edited by Donald D. Tresch and Wilbert S. Aronow
18. *Systemic Cardiac Embolism*, edited by Michael D. Ezekowitz
19. *Low-Molecular-Weight Heparins in Prophylaxis and Therapy of Thromboembolic Diseases,* edited by Henri Bounameaux
20. *Valvular Heart Diseases*, edited by Muayed Al Zaibag and Carlos M. G. Duran
21. *Implantable Cardioverter-Defibrillators: A Comprehensive Textbook*, edited by N. A. Mark Estes III, Antonis S. Manolis, and Paul J. Wang
22. *Individualized Therapy of Hypertension*, edited by Norman M. Kaplan and C. Venkata S. Ram
23. *Atlas of Coronary Balloon Angioplasty*, Bernhard Meier and Vivek K. Mehan

ADDITIONAL VOLUMES IN PREPARATION

Cholesterol Lowering: Clinical and Population Aspects, edited by Basil Rifkind

Interventional Cardiology: New Techniques and Strategies for Diagnosis and Treatment, edited by Christopher J. White and Stephen Ramee

Atlas of Coronary Balloon Angioplasty

Bernhard Meier
University Hospital
Bern, Switzerland

Vivek K. Mehan
Jaslok Hospital and Research Center
Bombay, India

formerly:
University Hospital
Bern, Switzerland

Marcel Dekker, Inc.

New York • Basel • Hong Kong

Library of Congress Cataloging-in-Publication Data

Meier, Bernhard.
Atlas of coronary balloon angioplasty / Bernhard Meier, Vivek K. Mehan.
p. cm. — (Fundamental and clinical cardiology ; v. 23)
Includes index.
ISBN 0-8247-9407-9
1. Transluminal angioplasty—Atlases. 2. Coronary heart disease--Surgery—Atlases. I. Mehan, V. K. II. Title. III. Series.
RD598.35.A53M45 1994
617.4'13—dc20 94-30841
CIP

The publisher offers discounts on this book when ordered in bulk quantities. For more information, write to Special Sales/Professional Marketing at the address below.

This book is printed on acid-free paper.

MARCEL DEKKER, INC.
270 Madison Avenue, New York, New York 10016

Current printing (last digit):
10 9 8 7 6 5 4 3 2 1

PRINTED IN THE UNITED STATES OF AMERICA

To our wives
Monika Meier
Archana Mehan

Series Introduction

Marcel Dekker, Inc., has focused on the development of various series of beautifully produced books in different branches of medicine. These series have facilitated the integration of rapidly advancing information for both the clinical specialist and the researcher.

My goal as editor-in-chief of the Fundamental and Clinical Cardiology series is to assemble the talents of world-renowned authorities to discuss virtually every area of cardiovascular medicine. In the current monograph Drs. Meier and Mehan have drawn on their considerable experience to create a much-needed and timely book. Future contributions to this series will include books on molecular biology, interventional cardiology, and clinical management of such problems as coronary artery disease and ventricular arrhythmias.

Samuel Z. Goldhaber

Preface

"A picture is worth a thousand words." An atlas builds on the fact that knowledge is better assimilated and recollected if visual images are presented. This atlas aims to achieve this goal by presenting a series of pictorially illustrated examples describing the procedure and pitfalls of coronary angioplasty. The examples speak eloquently for themselves, guiding the reader along the case as it unfolded in real life.

The atlas is intended for both the invasive and non-invasive cardiologist. Typical, illustrative examples are described, along with a few uncommon ones which, notwithstanding, anyone can come across in the catheterization laboratory. The book can be utilized by the less experienced as a textbook or a guide when faced with an unfamiliar situation in regard to approach and choice of angioplasty material. More experienced colleagues can enjoy comparing the handling of a case with their own way.

The atlas is devoted to balloon coronary angioplasty, which represents more than 95% of all angioplasty procedures worldwide. Stenting has to be considered an integral part of balloon angioplasty and is mentioned liberally in the book. Other techniques, however, such as atherectomy, Rotablation, and laser, form a very small proportion of coronary angioplasty procedures. They are not discussed, to avoid deviation of focus and space from balloon angioplasty.

The examples in this atlas were selected from over 5000 angioplasty cases performed by the authors, one of whose personal experience dates back to the first angioplasty ever performed, by Andreas Gruentzig in Zurich, Switzerland. Typical cases, as well as some of the rare situations encountered with PTCA, are discussed. The intent is to convey a humble but positive attitude toward the potential of angioplasty. Moreover, a plea is made to keep PTCA simple, because simplicity is its prime asset. Besides, simplicity is of paramount importance for the sake of the patient, as is cost containment, for financial restraint, precipitated by a worldwide economic recession, dictates that health costs be cut back where feasible.

The book reflects the authors' way of performing angioplasty. The emphasis lies in the approach to a case and the strategy adopted. Procedural details are left to the discretion of the reader.

Coronary balloon angioplasty has continued to grow in importance. Progress has been made in materials and techniques. However, coronary angioplasty remains a fascinating but rather primitive way of performing "heart surgery by remote control." This must prompt us to be reasonable in what we attempt and be ready to accept failures and setbacks. If one sticks to judicious indications, the downside of the procedure is more than compensated for by the daily triumphs of resolving a patient's problems with minimal invasiveness and suffering. The authors are indebted to Susi Buerki for her photographic assistance.

Bernhard Meier
Vivek K. Mehan

Contents

Abbreviations

AL 2 catheter: Amplatz left catheter with a 2-cm curve
CABG: coronary artery bypass grafting
CPK: creatine phosphokinase
ECG: electrocardiogram
F: French size of catheters (1F = 0.33 mm diameter)
JL 4 catheter: Judkins left catheter with a 4-cm curve
LAD: left anterior descending coronary artery
LAO: left anterior oblique view
LCx: left circumflex coronary artery
LIMA: left internal mammary artery
PE: polyethylene
PET: polyethylene terephthalate
PM: polymer
POC: polyolefin copolymer
PTCA: percutaneous transluminal coronary angioplasty
RAO: right anterior oblique view
RCA: right coronary artery

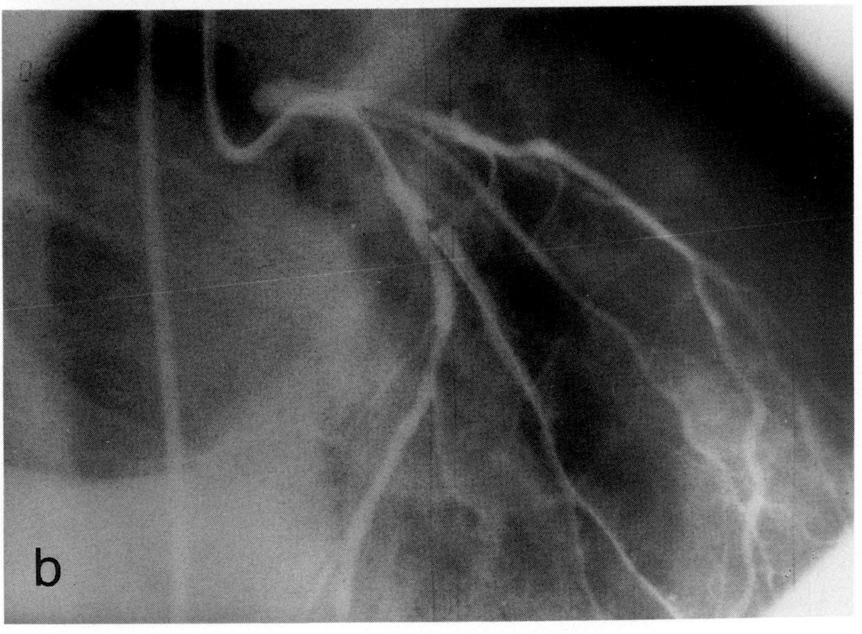

Figure 1

1
Basic Technique

1.1
STARTING OFF

A discussion of indications for angioplasty is beyond the scope of this book. A general examination with appropriate laboratory investigations for medical conditions that may influence the course of the intervention (e.g., renal failure, bleeding disorders, electrolyte imbalance, etc.) is important. A baseline ECG and CPK value are recommended for comparison in case of problems. Surgical standby is necessary only for selected cases, but it is a safety feature welcome for all. Only local shaving of the groin is required. Several views of the coronary arteries are mandatory, to define the stenosis precisely and rule out stenoses of other vessels which may not be evident in some views. Old films may give important information about collaterals not visible on the present film, disease progression in the various regions of interest, and prior technical problems regarding catheterization or angioplasty. Previous reports should also be studied diligently for the same reasons.

Careful review of the current angiographic study is imperative, especially when performing ad hoc angioplasty (angioplasty at the same sitting as the diagnostic study). Occasionally, mistakes may lead to unnecessary interventions. Angiography was performed in a 65-year-old man with angina. A decision was made based on video images to attempt what appeared to be a high-grade stenosis of the marginal branch of the LCx (Fig. 1a). Attempts to cross the stenosis were unsuccessful, but the wire easily passed distally into the marginal branch at a site lower than expected (Fig. 1b). Only at this time did the anatomy become clear. Review of the angiographic film clearly revealed an aneurysmal outpouching of the LCx proximal to the marginal branch, which itself was not narrowed significantly (Fig. 1c). This had been misinterpreted on the video image. The unexpected course of the wire unveiled the truth (Fig. 1b). False interpretation of video images can occur and was commoner with older catheterization laboratories and video systems. With modern equipment, resolution of video images is much improved and such mistakes are rare.

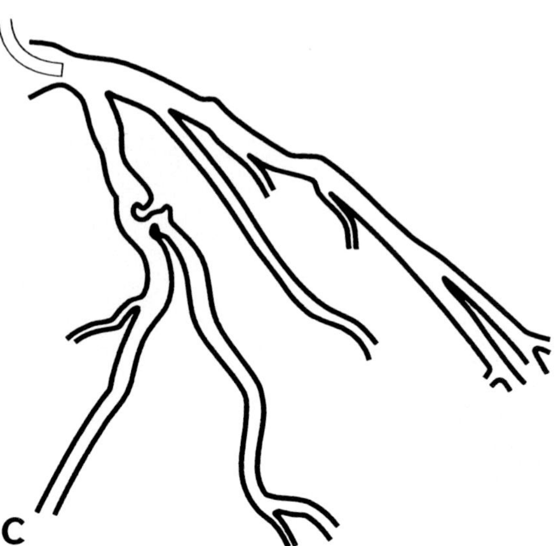

Figure 1 (Continued)

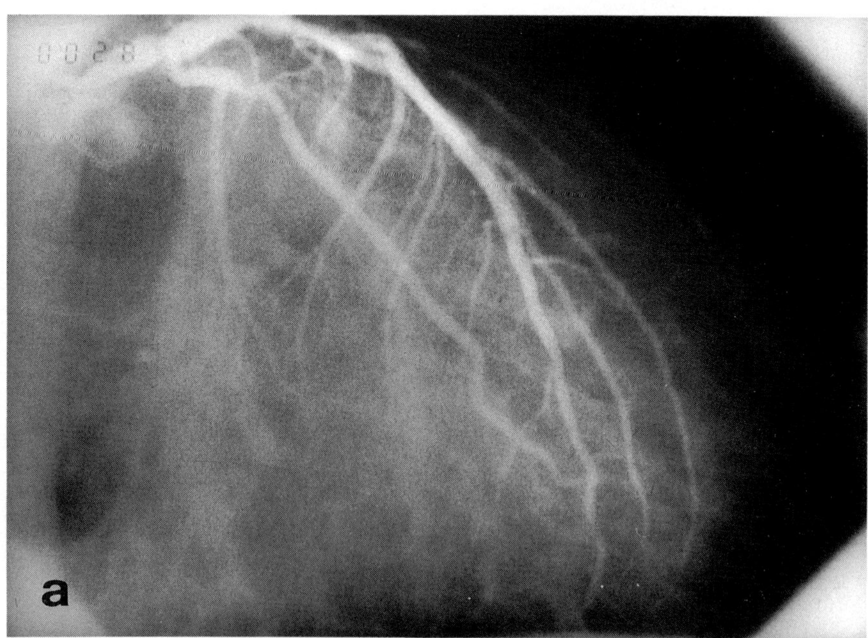

Figure 2

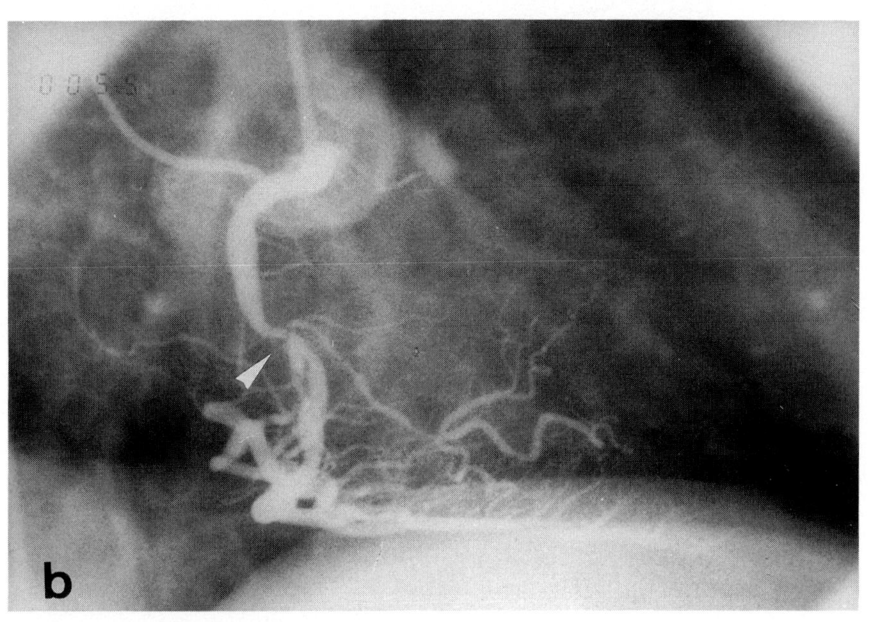

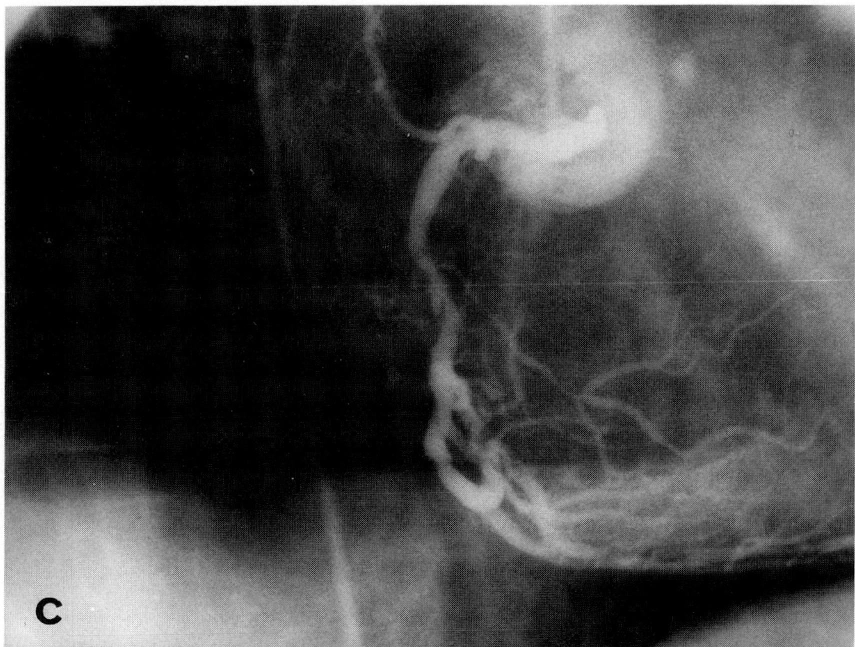

A more serious mistake is one in which a significant stenosis of an important vessel is overlooked. A 60-year-old man with unstable angina underwent urgent coronary angiography. The angiographer judged the left coronary artery to be normal (Fig. 2a). A tight stenosis of the RCA was seen (Fig. 2b), which was subjected to ad hoc angioplasty, with an acceptable result (Fig. 2c). However, the patient's unstable angina persisted unabated. A control angiogram the next morning revealed a stable RCA lesion (Fig. 2d). The cause of the problem became evident with the left coronary angiogram using different views (Fig. 2e). A tight left main stenosis had been overlooked the previous day. The patient underwent CABG the same day. Such an error should not occur in the modern catheterization laboratory, which affords a wide range of oblique projections and adequate video imaging. However, such examples remind us to review angiograms carefully before proceeding to angioplasty.

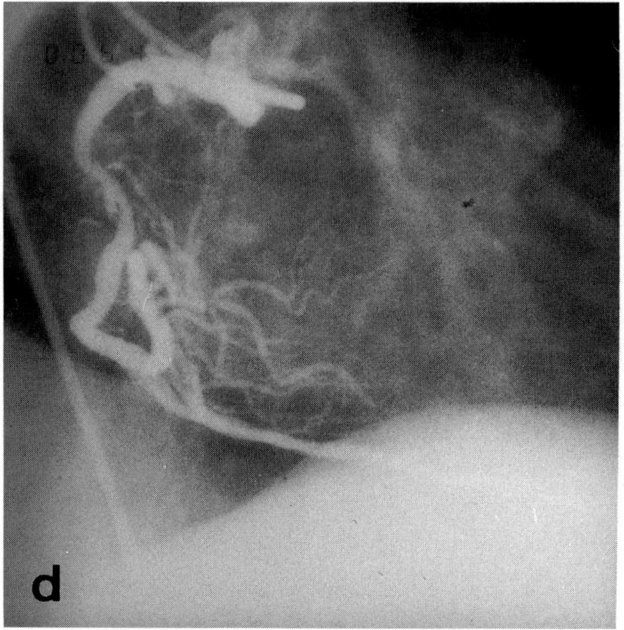

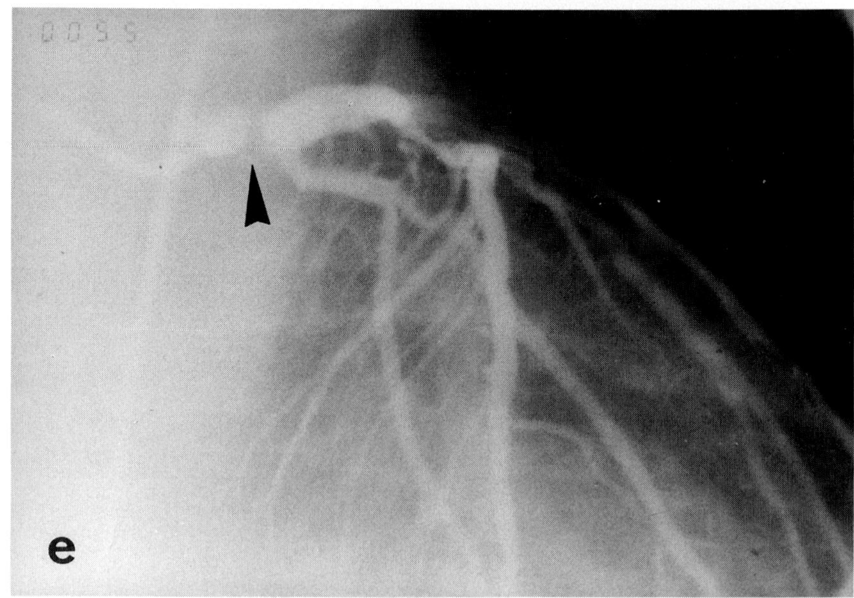

Figure 2 (Continued)

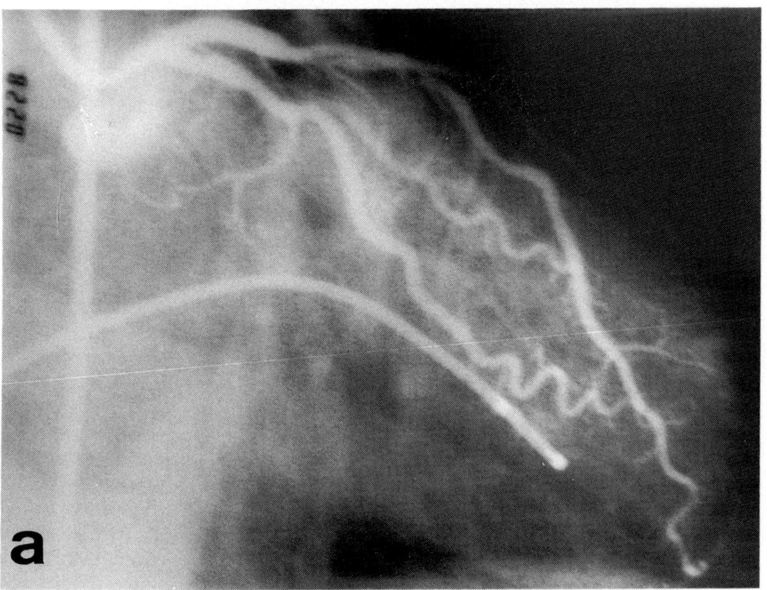

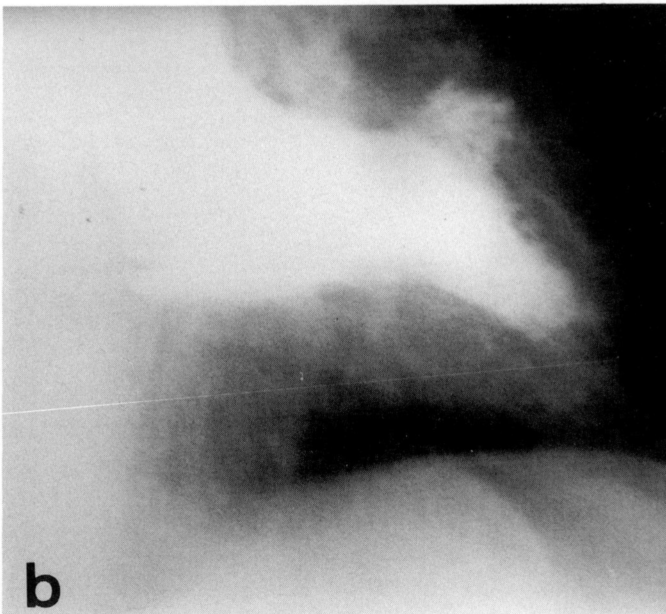

Figure 3

The practice of performing angioplasty at the same sitting as the diagnostic study (ad hoc PTCA or PTCA at first sight if no prior film is available) is convenient and economical, although occasionally it can lead to mistakes such as those described above. Such errors may be avoided if angioplasty is performed at a later date after careful interim analysis of the angiogram by several experienced people. However, the advantages of ad hoc PTCA far outweigh its disadvantages. Contrast-medium load, total radiation time, and length of hospitalization are reduced. An additional advantage is demonstrated by the case of a 58-year-old man in whom an angiogram revealed a stenosis of the proximal LAD (Fig. 3a) with a normal ventricle (Fig. 3b, systolic frame). A PTCA was planned for the following month. However, 2 weeks later the patient suffered an acute myocardial infarction (Fig. 3c, systolic frame) following closure of the LAD (Fig. 3d). This would have been prevented if angioplasty had been performed as an ad hoc procedure immediately following the diagnostic study.

It is essential to study all available old films just prior to angioplasty. This is crucial to get a clear idea about the anatomy of the coronary circulation, left ventricular function, collaterals, and so on. In case of difficulties during the procedure it is often helpful to review an old film once again. A 50-year-old man presented with post-infarction angina following an anterior wall infarction. Angiography revealed an occluded LAD (Fig. 4a). Angioplasty was attempted at the same sitting. However, it was impossible to advance the wire (Magnum wire with nonradiopaque ball tip) distally (Fig. 4b), despite the very fresh occlusion, which should have been easy to cross. In addition, a puddle of contrast medium appearing below the guidewire (Fig. 4b, arrow) worried the operator.

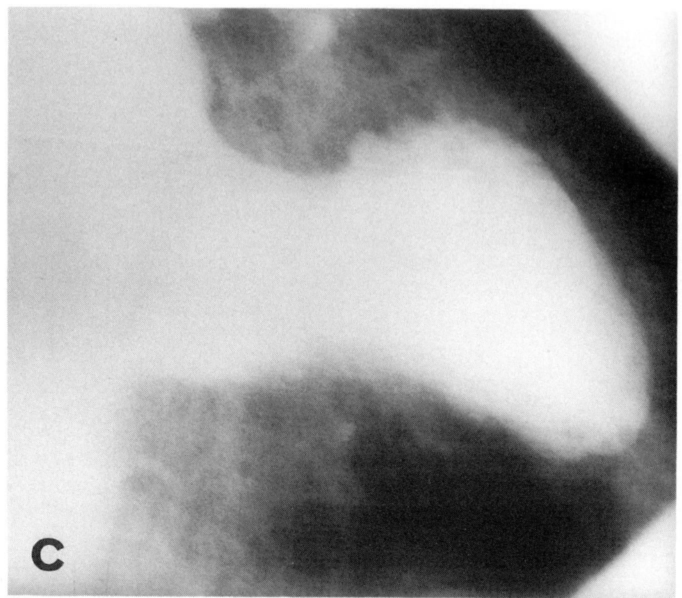

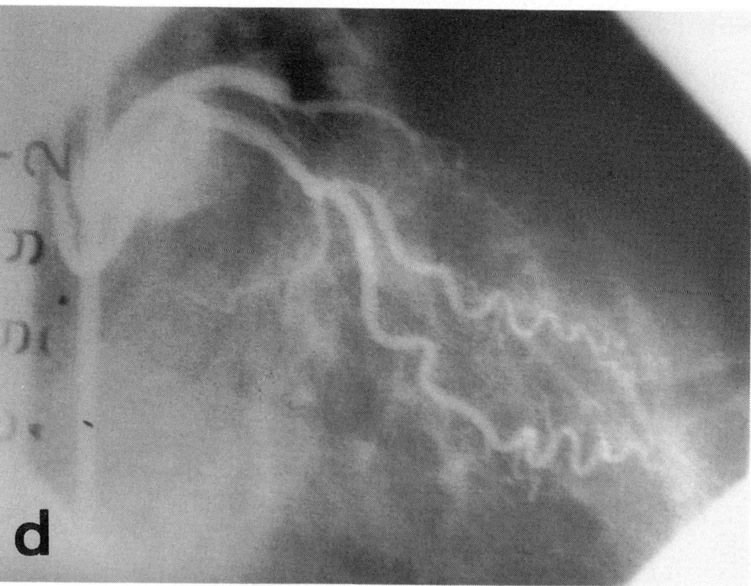

Figure 3 (Continued)

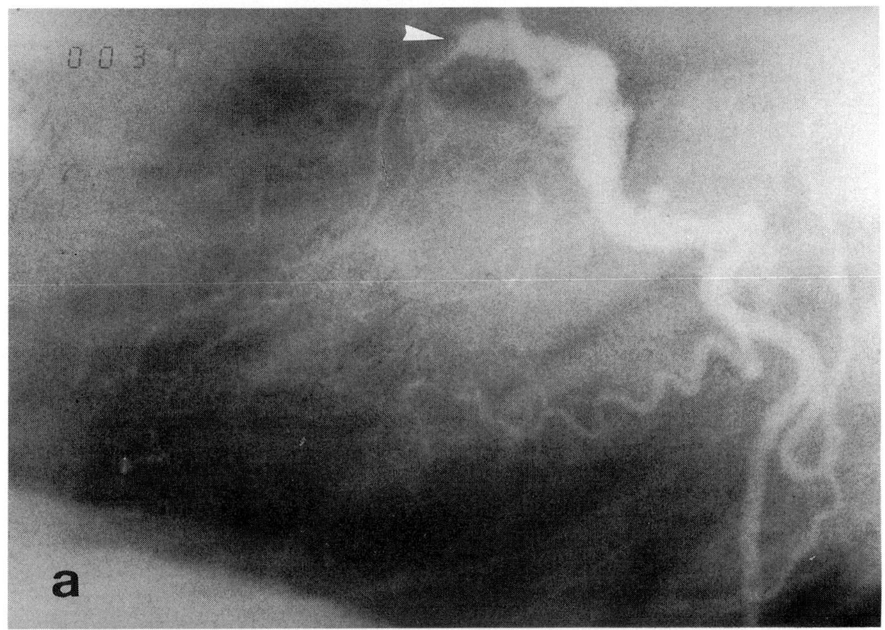

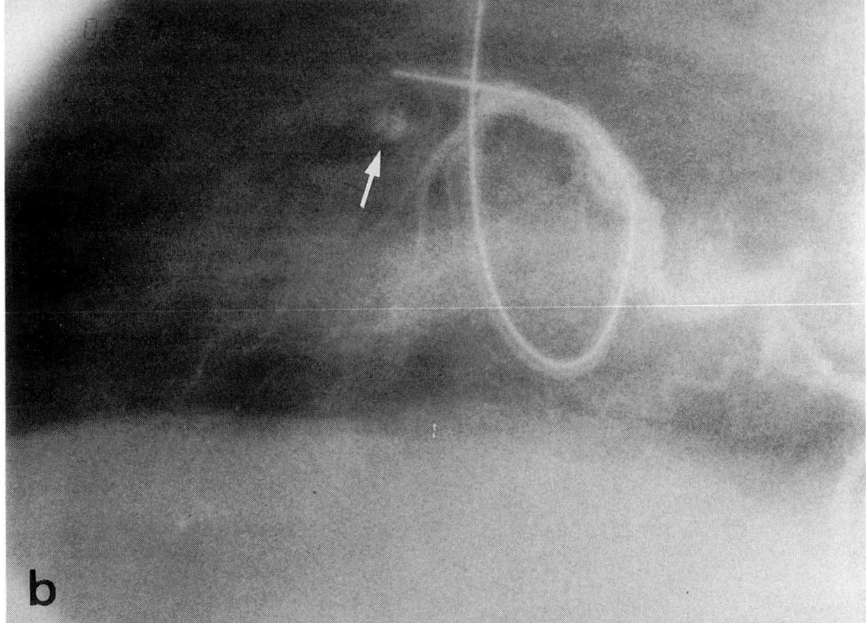

Figure 4

At this time a previous angiogram performed 6 years prior was reviewed (Fig. 4c). The cause for the inability to advance the wire, owing to an acute curve in the vessel, became clear, and the dye accumulation was identified as being within the proper lumen. With knowledge of the anatomy of the vessel, the wire could easily be negotiated across the bend in the vessel (Fig. 4d), and angioplasty was performed successfully (Fig. 4e). The final result was good (Fig. 4f).

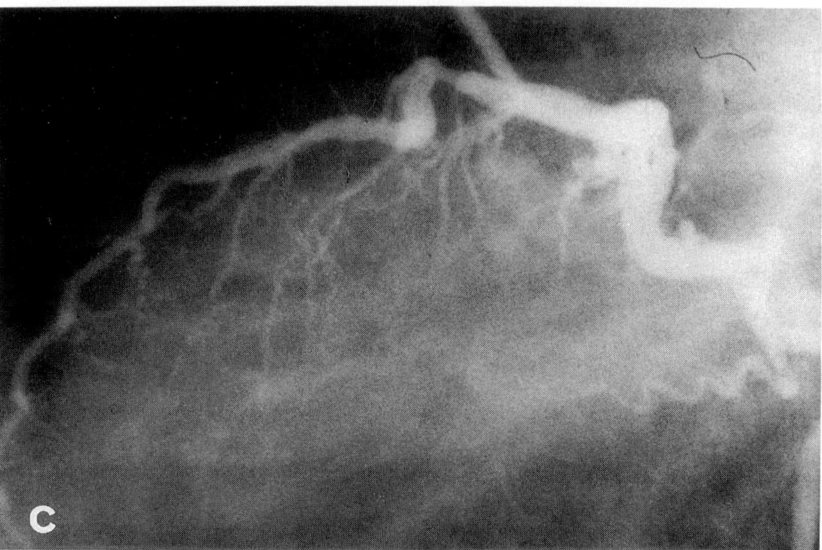

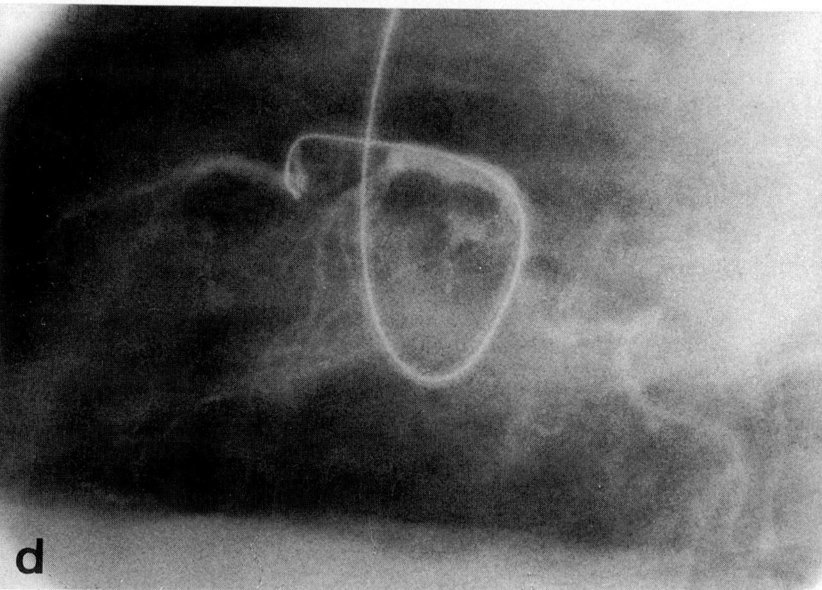

Figure 4 (Continued)

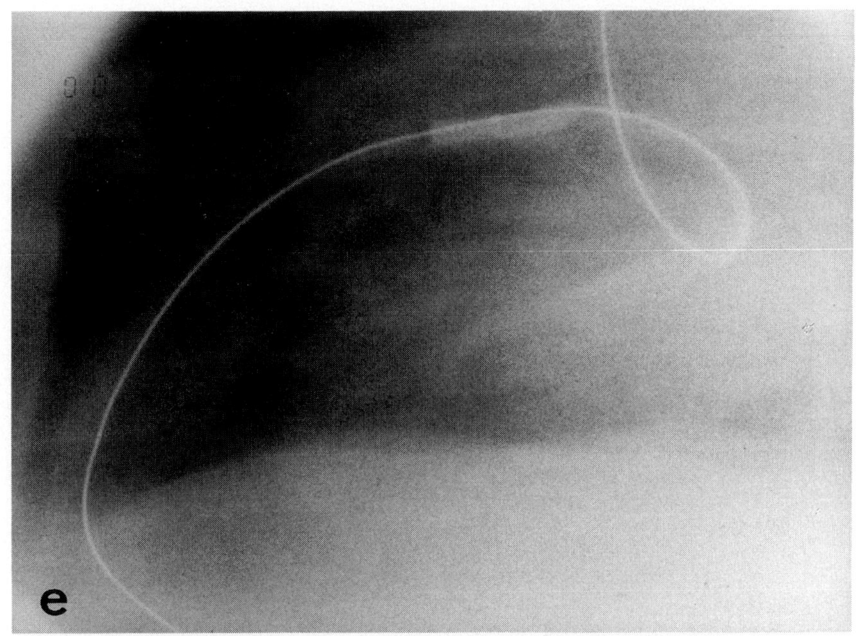
e

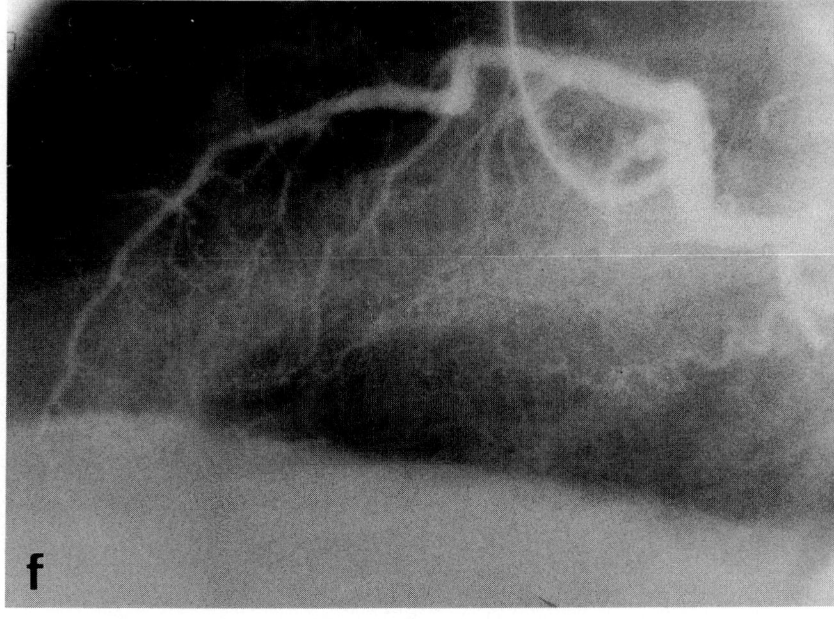
f

The importance of the administration of nitrates prior to angiography and angioplasty cannot be overemphasized. Nitrates serve to dilate the coronary arteries, resulting in better flow and opacification, this demonstrating lesions better. Moreover, the tendency to coronary spasm is reduced, avoiding diagnostic difficulties. Additionally, maximal dilatation of coronary arteries facilitates the choice of balloon size, thereby preventing suboptimal results. Spasm can affect any vessel. In this example a tight stenosis of the LCx was noticed during the diagnostic study (Fig. 5a). This narrowing disappeared following 0.2 mg intracoronary nitroglycerine (Fig. 5b). Although spasm of the left main coronary artery is rare, it can occur (Fig. 6a). In this patient, the spasm was relieved (Fig. 6b) following sublingual nitroglycerine. The importance of adequate

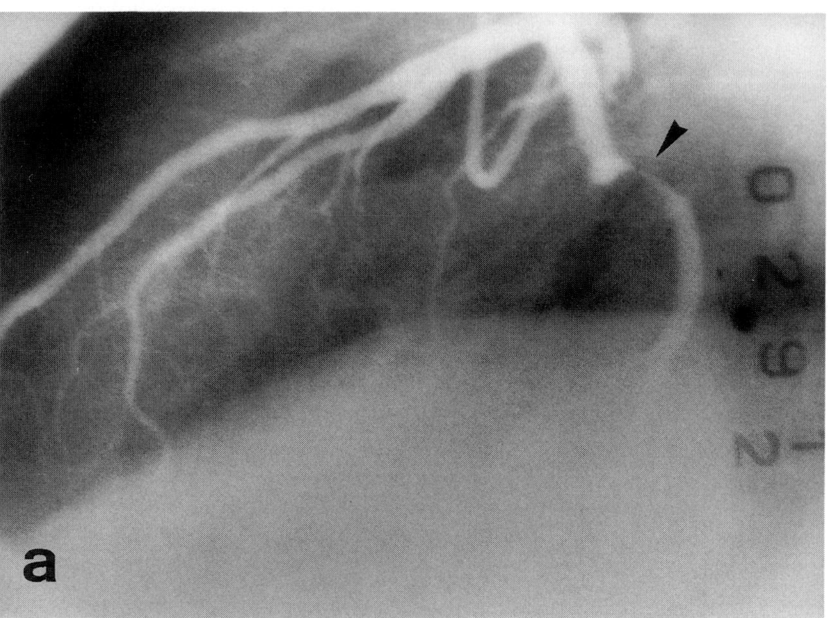

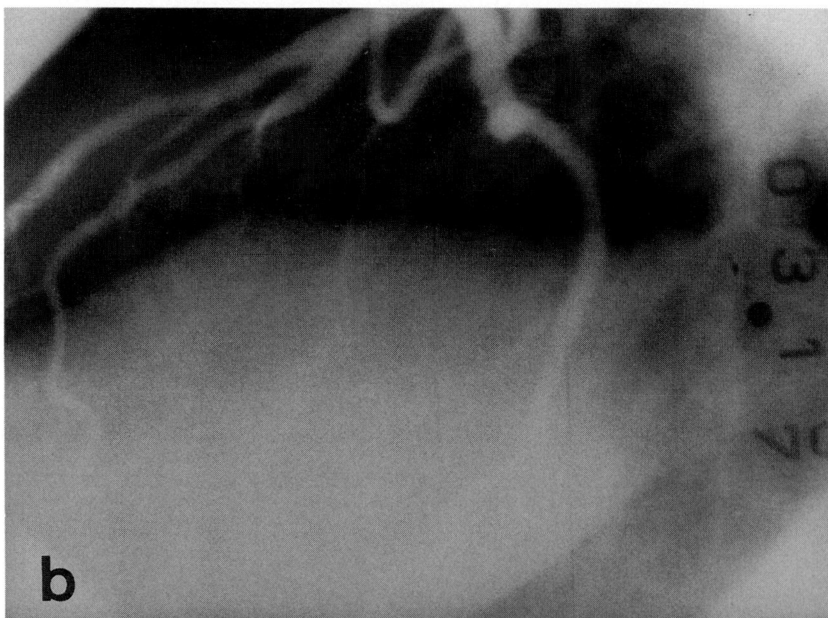

Figure 5

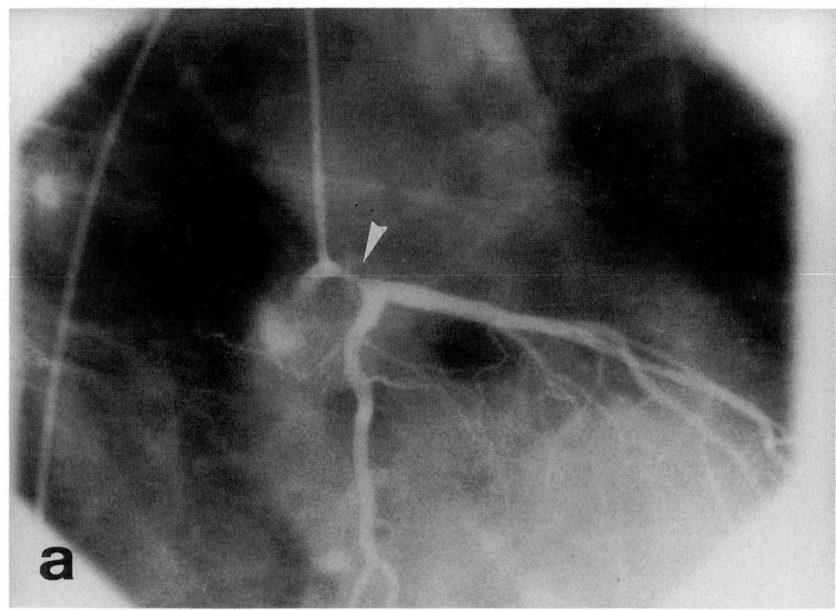

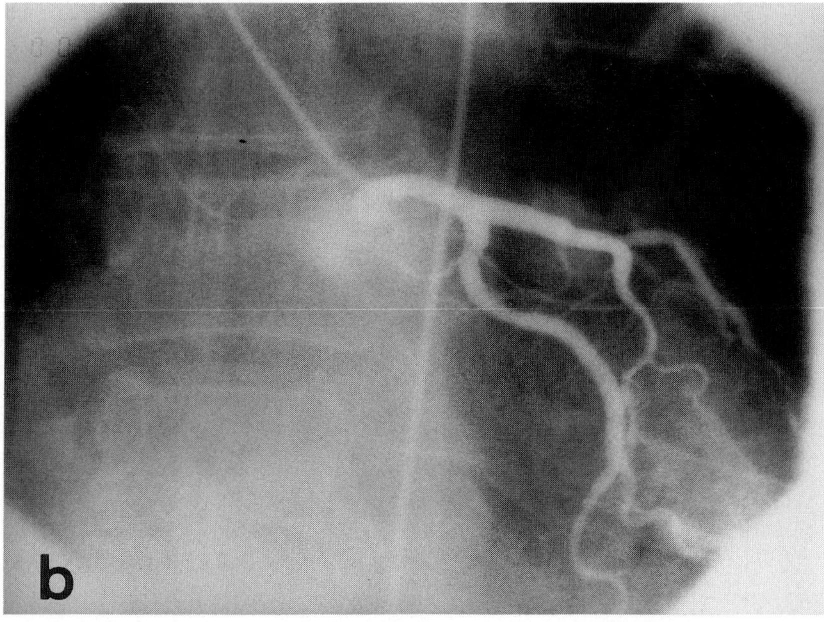

Figure 6

vasodilation is also demonstrated in this 66-year-old man with a venous graft to the LAD. A graft angiogram prior to nitrates revealed a healthy graft ending in a threadlike LAD (Fig. 7a). The angiogram was repeated following an intracoronary injection of 0.2 mg nifedipine, which revealed adequate runoff into a well-defined LAD, providing collaterals to a marginal branch of the LCx (Fig. 7b). Absence of adequate vasodilatation in such instances can lead to diagnostic errors and needless interventions.

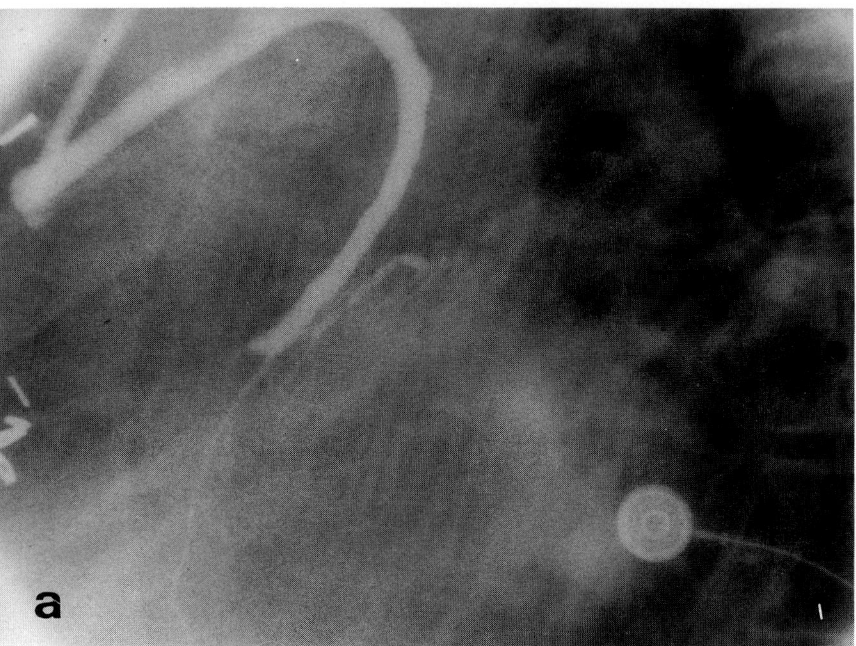

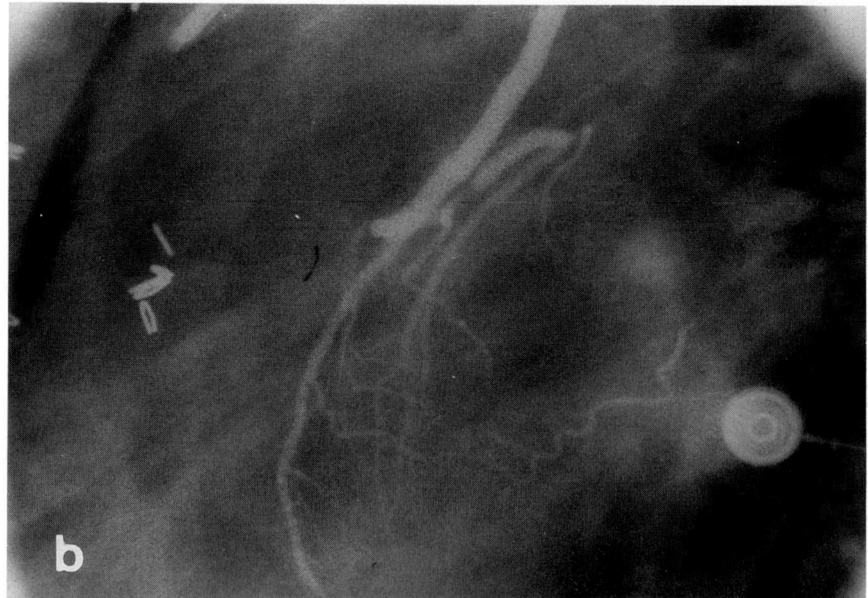

Figure 7

1.2 ANGIOPLASTY SETUP

The angioplasty setup consists of a guiding catheter introduced through an introducer sheath. A long sheath facilitates negotiation of the iliac artery and protects the vessel from dissections during catheter exchange. It also prevents inadvertent sheath expulsion after angioplasty and obviates the need for suture attachment. The guidewire and balloon catheter run within the guiding catheter, which also serves for pressure measurement and dye injection. A torquer at the proximal end of

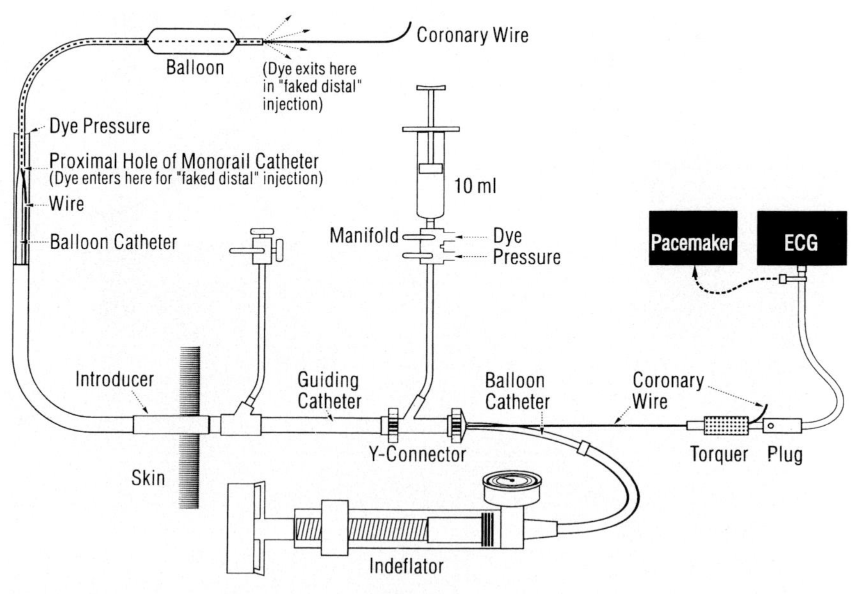

Figure 8

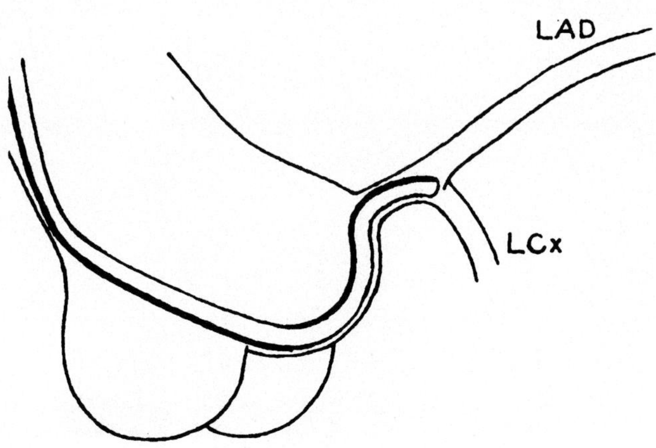

Figure 9

the coronary guide wire is used for manipulation of the wire. In addition, it permits electrical contact between the guidewire and a cable that may be used for intracoronary ECG recording or pacing. A two-spike manifold allows for convenient pressure measurement or dye injection.

1.3 GUIDING CATHETER

A coronary guiding catheter differs from a diagnostic catheter in that it:

- Does not taper distally
- Has a particularly soft tip
- Has an internal lining of Teflon to lower friction
- Has a steel braiding in its wall which allows for a larger lumen and for increased support and stability, while allowing for reduced wall thickness (several manufacturers now make diagnostic catheters similarly)
- Costs at least three times as much

Guiding catheters are available in various shapes and sizes, the smallest available commercially being 6 French. However, angioplasty can be performed through smaller catheters (5F or 4F) when using diagnostic catheters as guiding catheters.

Shape

The shape chosen will depend on the artery to be approached. For the LAD (and often for a ramus intermedius), a left Judkins guiding catheter is optimal for relatively direct access into these arteries. A Judkins catheter also permits deep intubation for increased backup support with relative ease. The more vertical the takeoff, the smaller should be the curve of the Judkins catheter selected. Curves of 3.5 or less, however, tend to fold in the ascending aorta of most adult males.

For LCx (and occasionally, ramus intermedius) lesions, a left Amplatz guiding catheter is preferable. This directs the guidewire preferentially toward the LCx (Fig. 9). Angioplasty was attempted in a 45-year-old patient with stenosis of the LCx, using a JL 4 guiding catheter and a 0.014-in. guidewire. However, during attempts to advance the balloon across the stenosis, the wire tended to buckle and prolapse into the LAD (Fig. 10a, small arrows). The lesion could not be crossed with

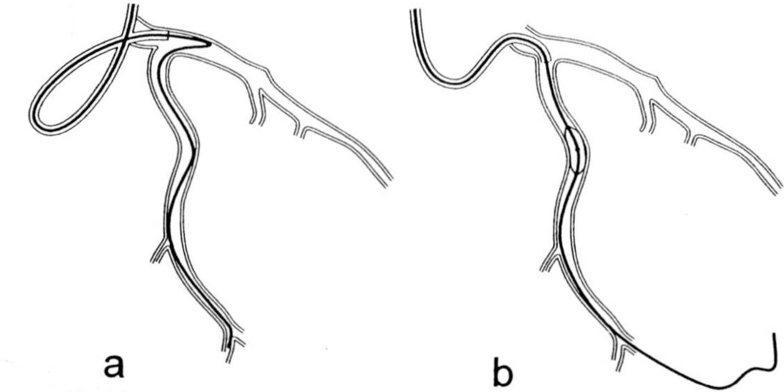

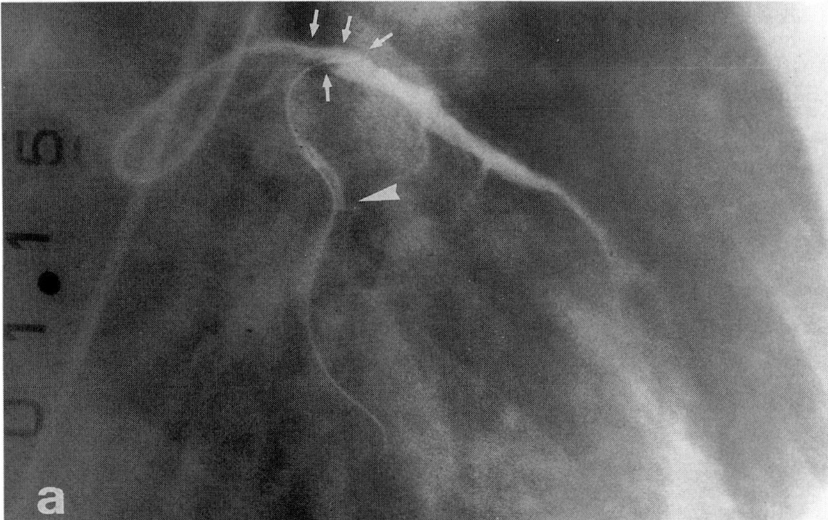

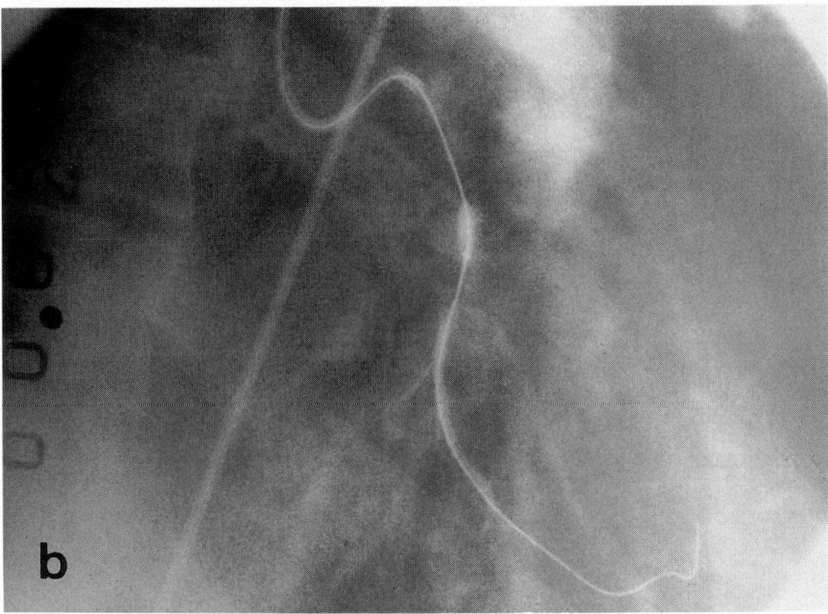

Figure 10

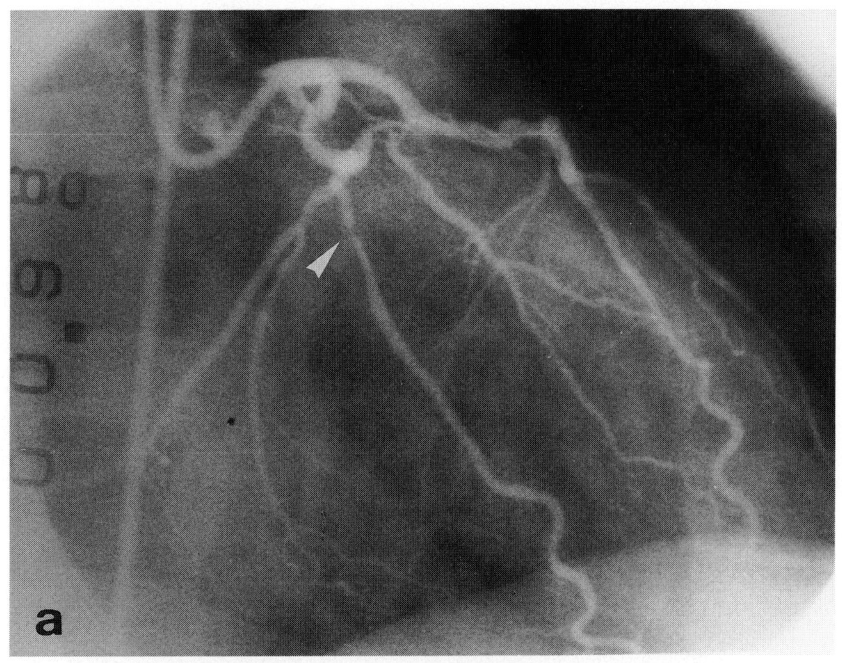

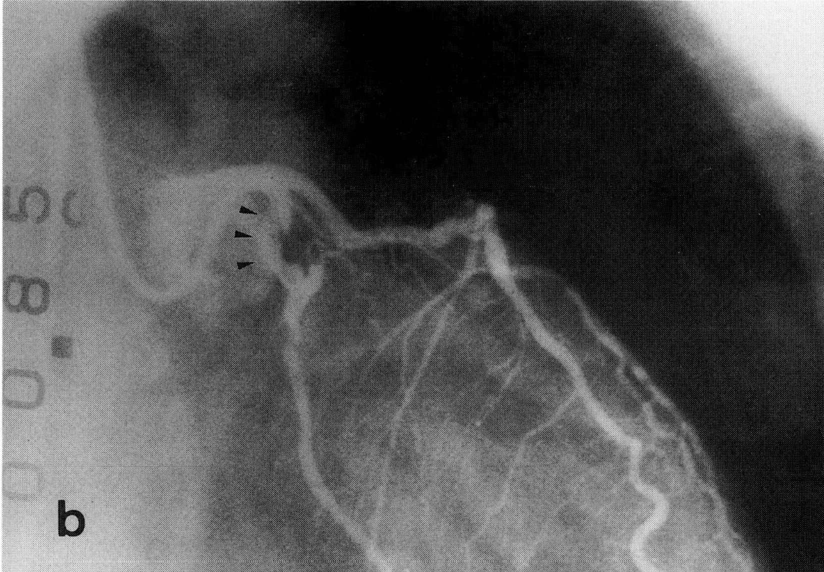

Figure 11

the balloon despite deep intubation of the Judkins guiding catheter for increased backup support. The problem was easily overcome by exchanging the Judkins catheter for an Amplatz left II guiding catheter, which directed the guidewire and balloon optimally (Fig. 10b).

The Amplatz catheter is more difficult to handle than the Judkins catheter. Owing to its tendency to engage deeply, it often results in wedging or may dissect the coronary artery. This tendency is largely eliminated with 6F or smaller versions.

A 41-year-old man underwent angioplasty for stenosis of a large marginal branch of the LCx, using an 8F AL 2 guiding catheter (Fig. 11a). However, its tip dissected the proximal LCx (Fig. 11b), which functionally occluded the artery. The dissection was stabilized with a balloon inflation, which resulted in some flow in the distal LCx (Fig. 11c, curved arrow). A control angiogram the next day revealed some improvement in distal flow, the dissection remaining stable (Fig. 11d). Angiographic evaluation 8 months later revealed a progression of stenosis at the site of dissection. It should be remembered that an Amplatz catheter operates as a hinge, with its fulcrum on the aortic cusp. Pulling back on the catheter results in its tip being deflected more deeply into the coronary artery, often resulting in wedging and sometimes causing dissections. An alternative method of removing the Amplatz catheter is by a pushing and rotating motion which disengages the catheter. This maneuver should be performed under fluoroscopic control. A third method of achieving a relatively atraumatic removal is to withdraw the Amplatz catheter over the balloon catheter and then withdraw the balloon.

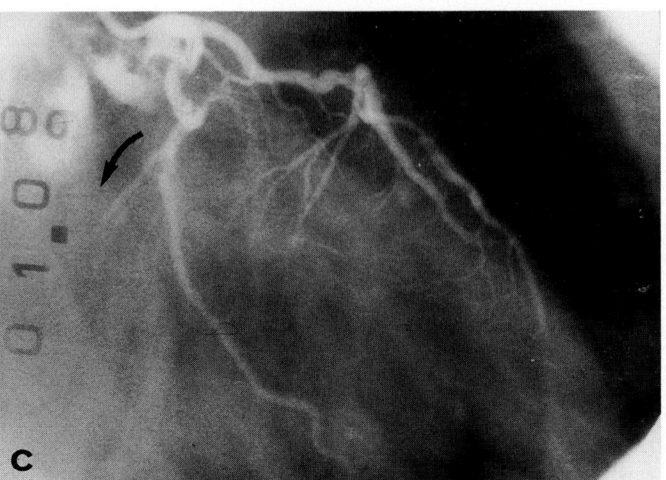

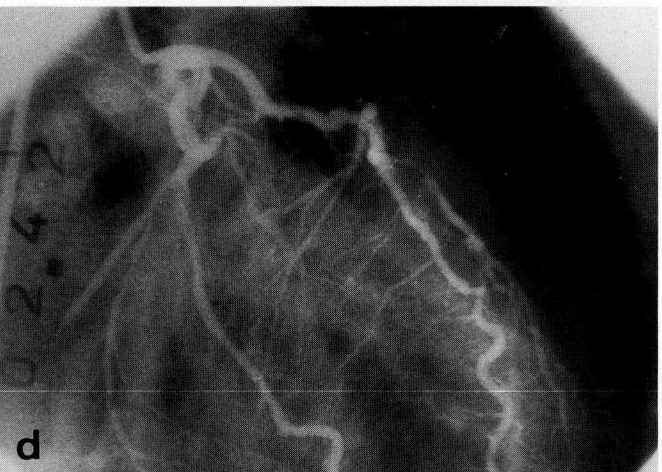

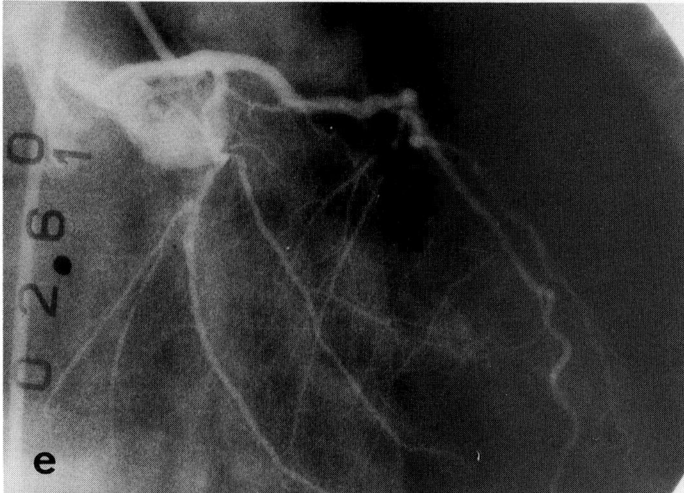

Figure 11 (Continued)

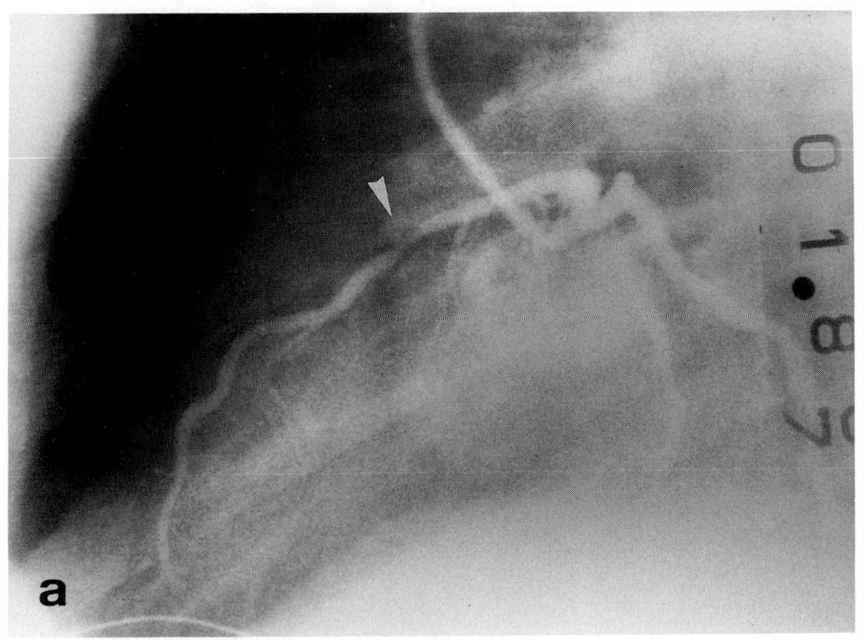

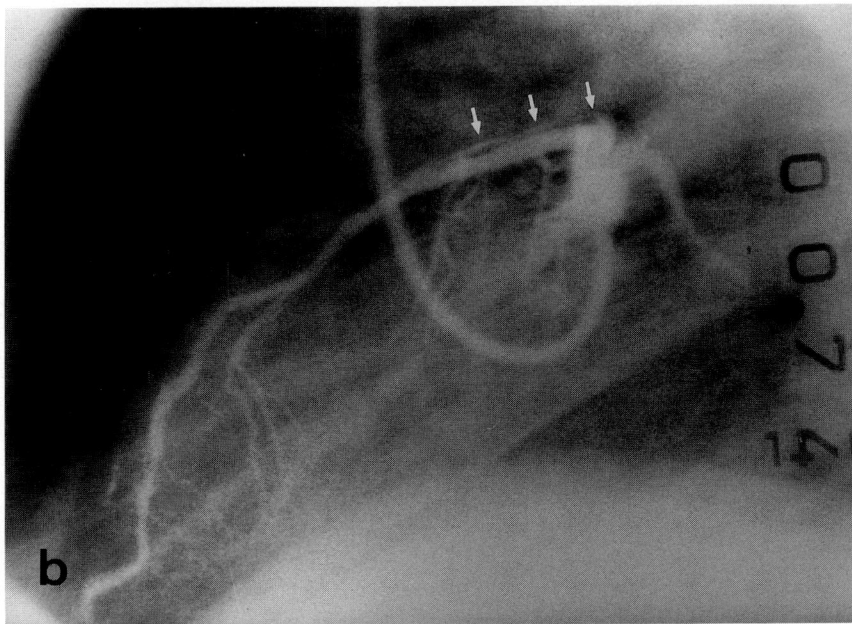

Figure 12

A Judkins catheter can also dissect important vessels. A patient with a normal proximal LAD (Fig. 12a) underwent angioplasty for a stenosis of the LAD using a JL 4 guiding catheter. During manipulation of the guiding catheter a dissection of the proximal LAD occurred (Fig. 12b). Since flow was unimpeded, conservative management was selected. An angiogram 2 weeks later revealed a stable dissection (Fig. 12c). A repeat angiogram 20 months later revealed a normal-looking LAD, with healing of the dissection and a good long-term result of the dilated site (Fig. 12d).

For RCA lesions, a Judkins right coronary guiding catheter or an Amplatz left II coronary guiding catheter (Fig. 13, especially useful when increased backup is required) is commonly utilized. However, other shapes may be required, such as a multipurpose or El Gamal shape for a vertical takeoff, or an Arani catheter for a shepherd's crook takeoff of the right coronary artery.

For any artery, several other shapes of guiding catheters are available, such as the Voda, internal mammary guiding catheter, and catheters for the brachial approach. Of note is the foreshortened internal mammary artery catheter to allow for increased reach of balloon catheters during angioplasty of distal vessels through bypass grafts, for example. Additionally, it may sometimes be necessary to custom-shape catheters, or to modify a curve slightly for optimal backup. This can be per-

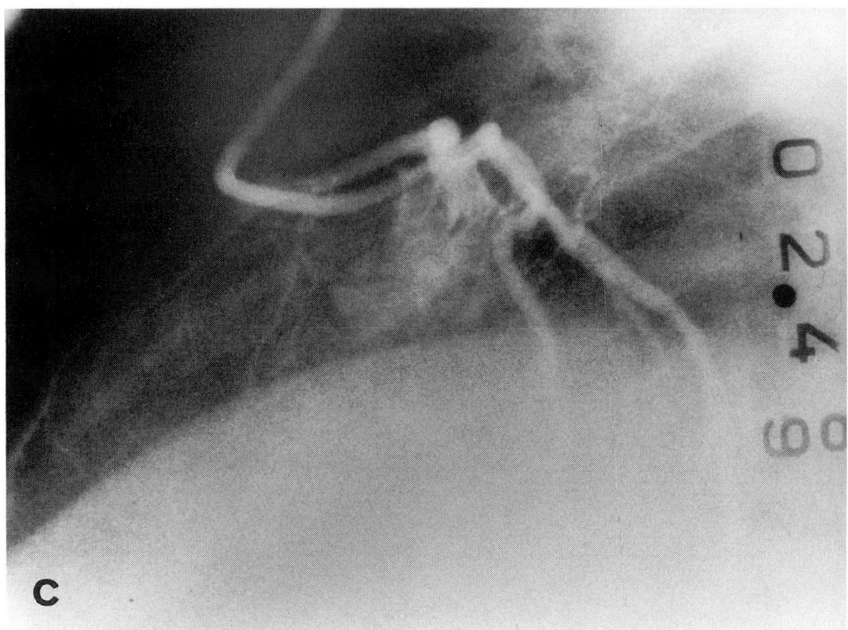

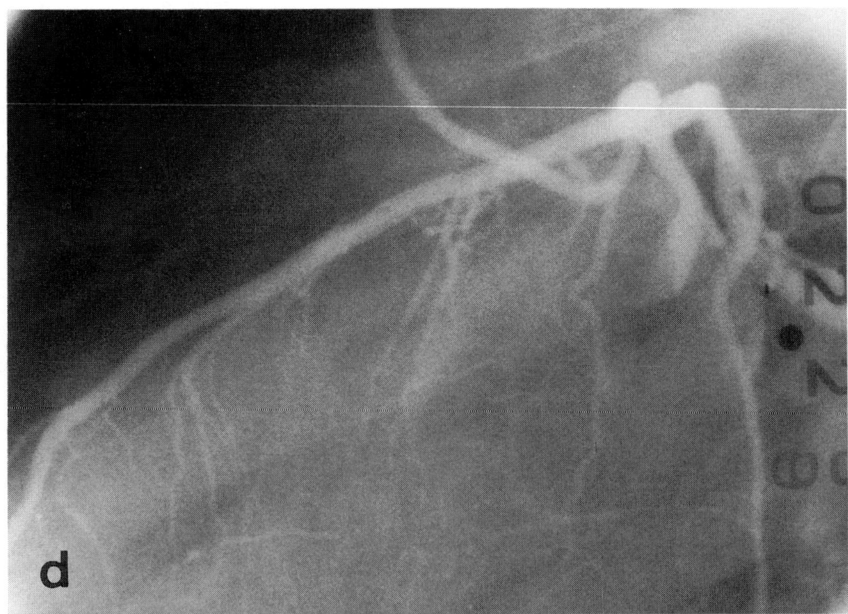

Figure 12 (Continued)

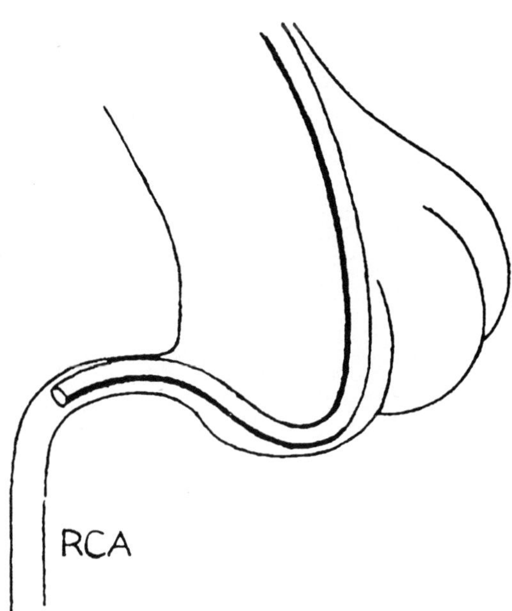

Figure 13

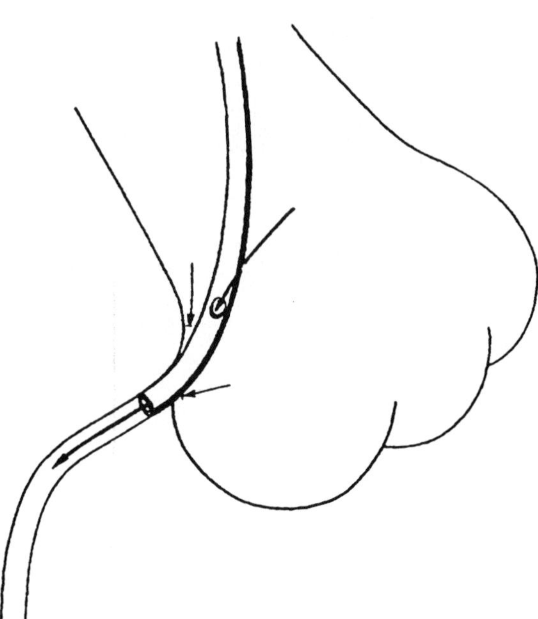

Figure 14

formed with a hot-air gun, but such a procedure is rarely necessary nowadays in light of the large number of commercially available shapes. In addition, the thin walls of the modern guiding catheters exhibit a poor memory for heat-modified shapes. When using guiding catheters larger than 6F, the need for side holes to control wedging problems arises regularly. Instead of changing to a new catheter with side holes, a single small side hole may be carved into the lateral wall of the catheter with a blade (Fig. 14). This is more economical.

The shapes of the same types of guiding catheters manufactured by different companies may vary in terms of curves and tip lengths. In addition, the stiffness and intrinsic stability of the catheters, or the ease with which they allow deep intubation of the artery, may vary. An example of this are the "Pink Power" and "Brite Tip" catheters of the Schneider and Cordis companies, respectively. The Cordis guiding catheter is stiffer and has greater intrinsic support and kink resistance, while the Schneider catheter is softer and has less intrinsic support but superior ability to be deeply introduced for improved backup support. Knowledge of the different properties of various guiding catheters is important, since sometimes one type may succeed where another with the same curve has failed. This is exemplified by a 64-year-old man with an LAD stenosis, with tortuous coronary arteries and an abnormal takeoff angle of the left main coronary artery (Fig. 15a). Cannulation of the left coronary ostium was extremely tedious during the diagnostic study, and angioplasty had to be postponed to the next day, due to the high dye load administered. The same problem was encountered during the angioplasty attempt, when different shapes and sizes of guiding catheters of different companies offered inadequate support. Finally, a Cordis JL 4 catheter (which is relatively stiff) solved the problem (Fig. 15b,c), although the same shape of another manufacturer had failed to cannulate the ostium.

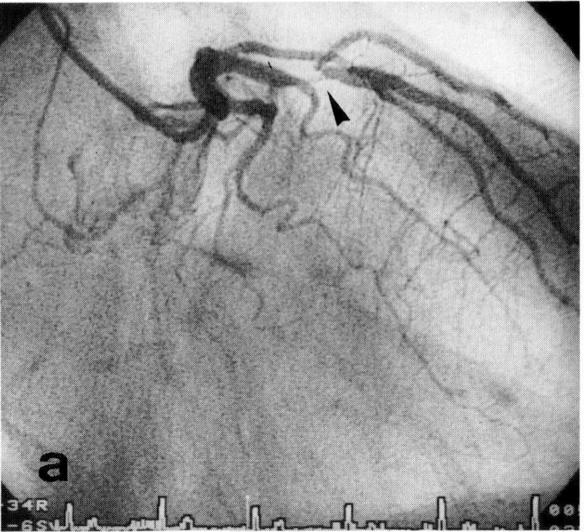

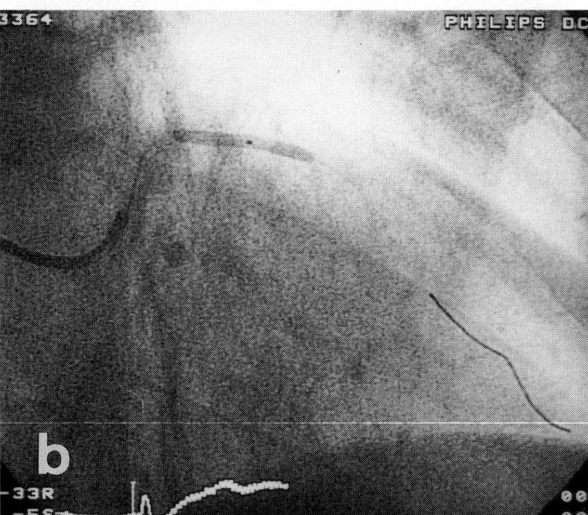

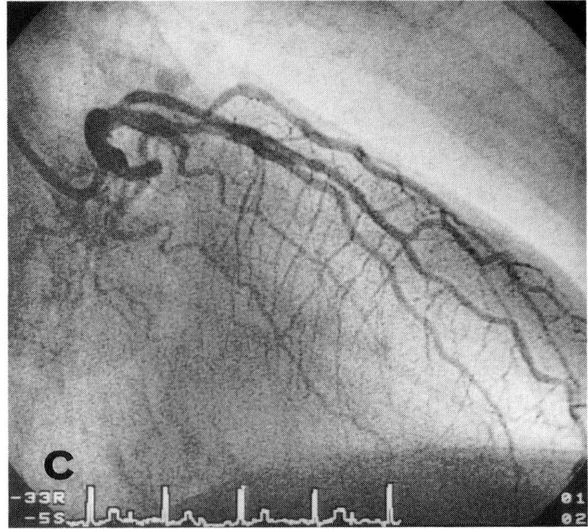

Figure 15

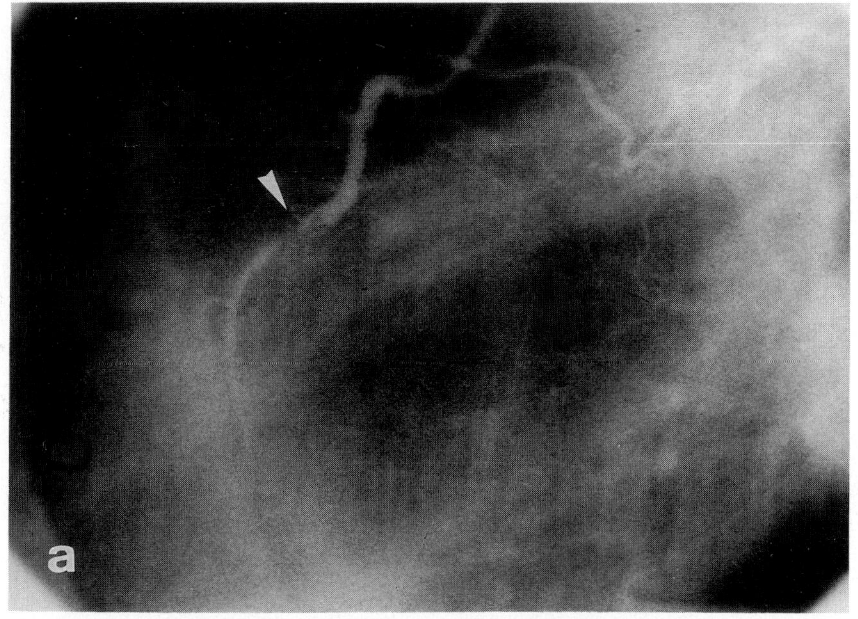

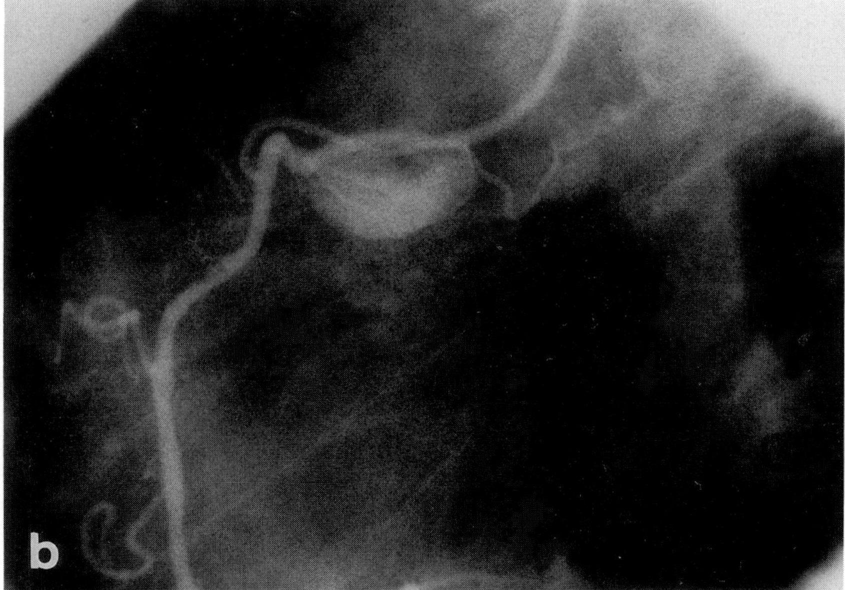

Figure 16

Size

The external diameter of guiding catheters has shrunk over the years. A typical example of this trend is a 55-year-old man who underwent angioplasty of the RCA in 1987 with an 8F guiding catheter (Fig. 16a,b). In 1989 he had angioplasty of the LAD through a 6F diagnostic catheter (Fig. 16c,d), and in 1991 of the LCx using a 4F diagnostic catheter as a "guiding" catheter (Fig. 16e,f). This example also serves to demonstrate another aspect of PTCA: how a patient can be treated over the years with a series of angioplasties for single-vessel lesions while triple-vessel disease develops. To wait for the full development of triple-vessel disease will necessitate bypass surgery at that time and carries the risk of intercurrent infarction in the interim. To perform bypass surgery earlier would result in a reintervention at the time of involvement of an additional vessel.

A 6F guiding catheter is the current standard at our institution. This drastically reduces wedging problems and has the additional advantages of a smaller arterial injury with lesser bleeding complications, shorter compression times, earlier ambulation, and reduced incidence of pseudoaneurysms and arteriovenous fistulae. The newer generation of high-flow 6F catheters with lumens up to 0.062 in. (0.16 mm)

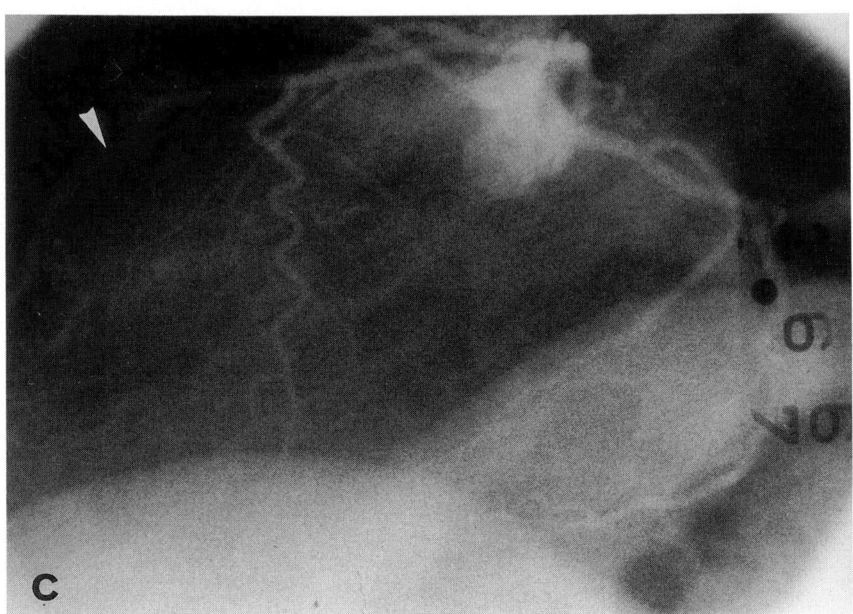

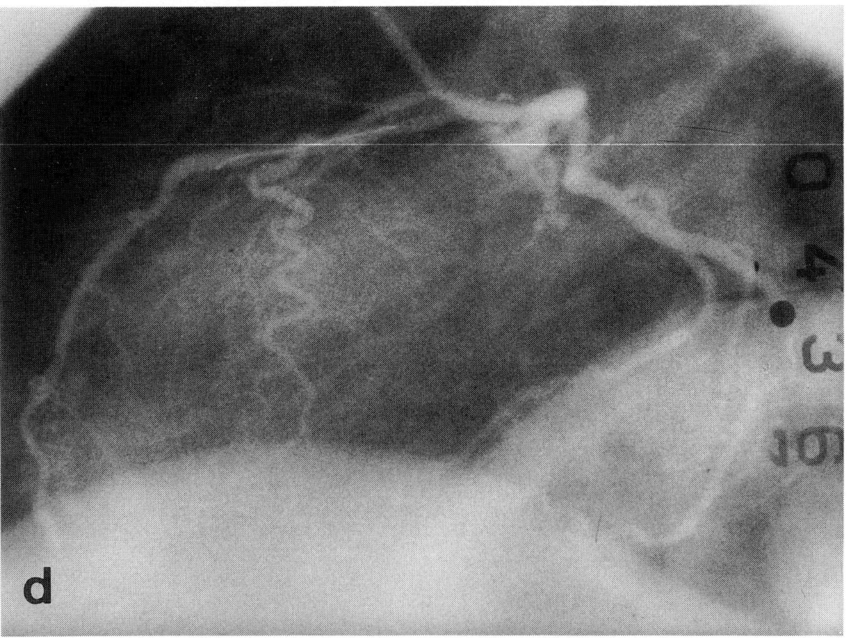

Figure 16 (Continued)

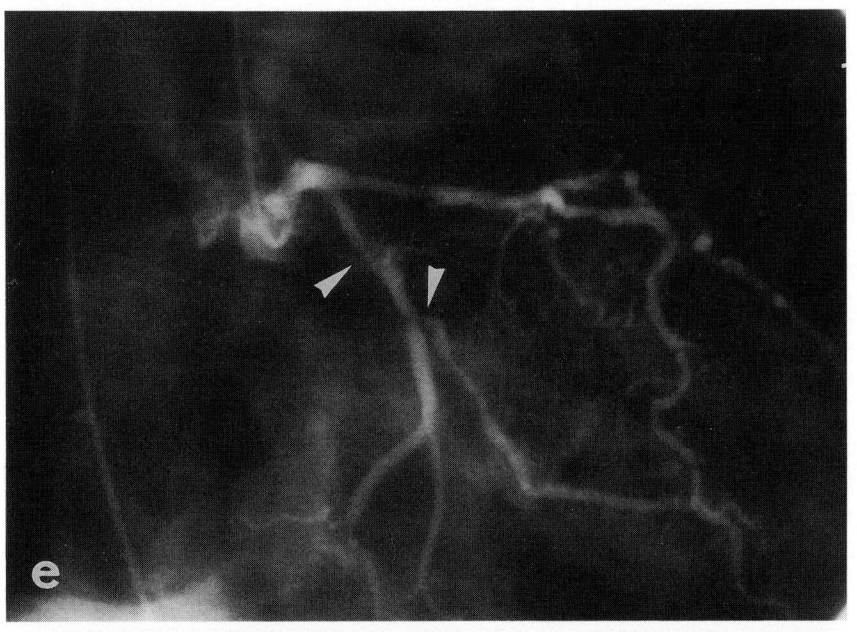

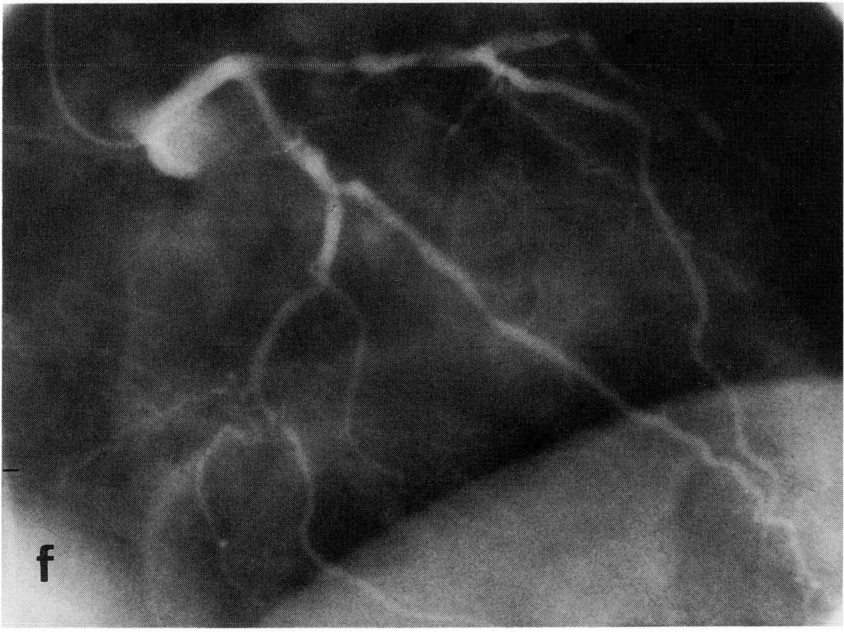

allow for stenting using crimp-on Palmaz-Schatz stents and for the use of Monorail-type perfusion balloons (e.g., Flow Track from ACS and Speedflow from Schneider). However, the use of a 0.021-in. (0.53-mm) Magnum wire with a compatible balloon and over-the-wire perfusion balloons or premounted stents is not possible with current 6F catheters. Many centers routinely use 7F or even 8F guiding catheters, but a 6F system seems preferable in most cases. For selected patients undergoing ad hoc angioplasty, the procedure may be carried out through 5F or even 4F diagnostic catheters used for angiography provided that a fixed-wire balloon is employed. Such an approach may be quite frequent (20% at our center) and economical for centers performing ad hoc angioplasty. Additionally, these smaller catheters may reduce the incidence of an infrequent but serious complication seen following angioplasty using larger catheters: that of accelerated left main stenosis. A 63-year-old man underwent angioplasty for an occluded LAD (Fig. 17a) with a 7F guiding catheter (Fig. 17b). The final result was good (Fig. 17c). The patient presented 6 months later with angina. It was assumed that he had developed restenosis. However, angiography revealed a severe stenosis of the left main stem, with a good long-term angioplasty result of the LAD (Fig. 17d).

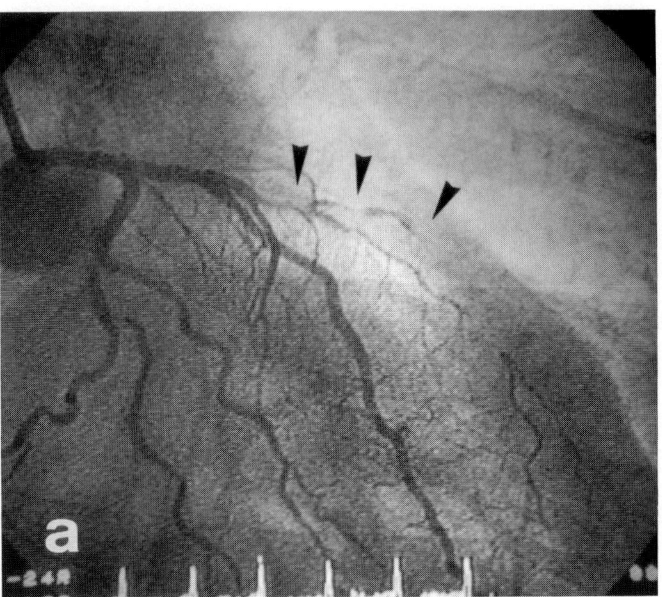

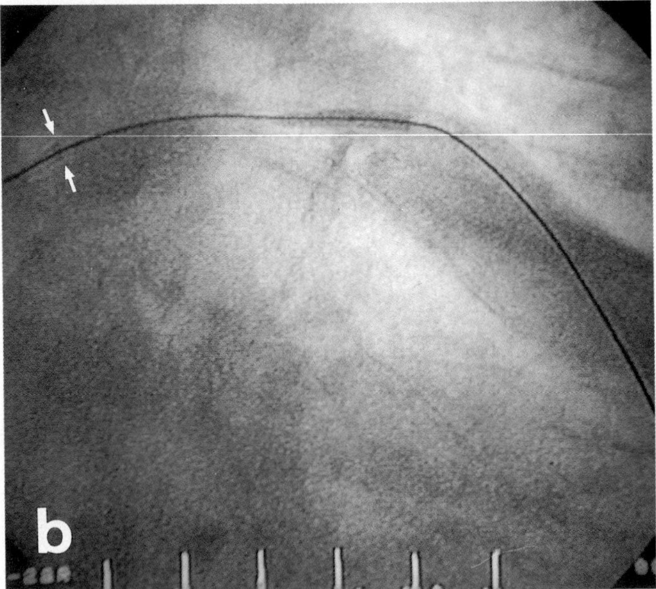

Figure 17

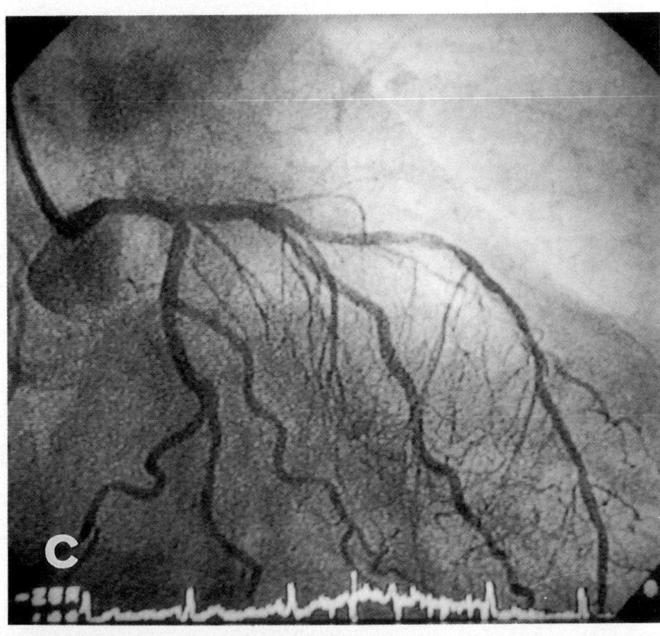
c

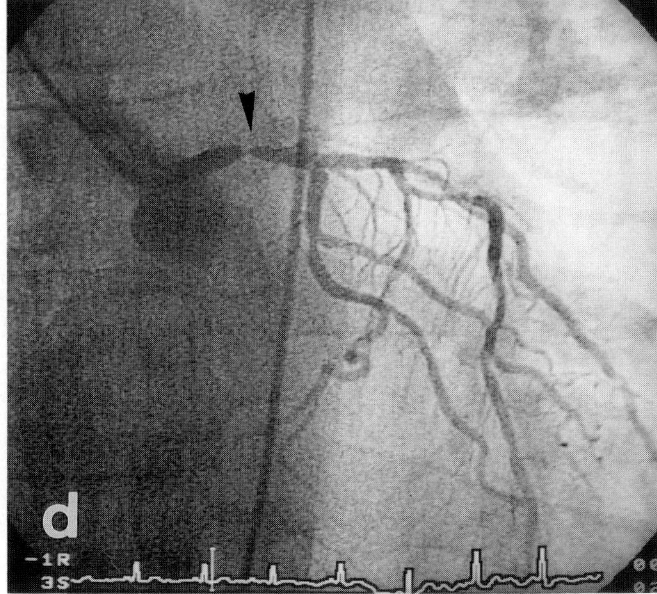
d
-1R
3S

Manipulations

It is sometimes difficult to advance, or manipulate, a guiding catheter in the presence of a tortuous iliac artery (Fig. 18a), even with a guidewire within the catheter. In such an event the problem can be solved by using an extra-stiff guidewire (e.g., 0.035-in. "backup wire" from Schneider) instead of the normal guidewire. This backup wire causes straightening of the iliac artery, thus facilitating guiding catheter introduction and manipulation (Fig. 18b). However, at times tortuosity may render a PTCA attempt impossible, as in the case of a 75-year-old man with angina. The highly tortuous aorta (Fig. 19a) and iliac artery (Fig. 19b) made cannulation of the left coronary artery extremely difficult. Cannulation of the RCA was impossible in this case despite use of a backup wire and a long arterial sheath.

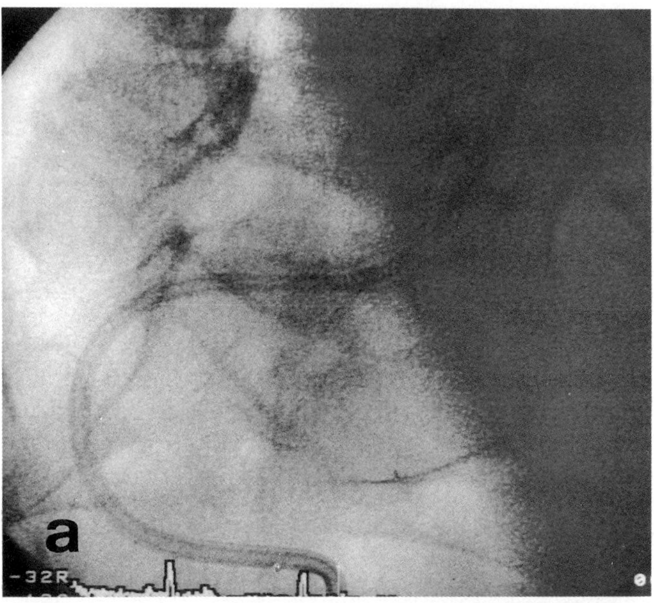

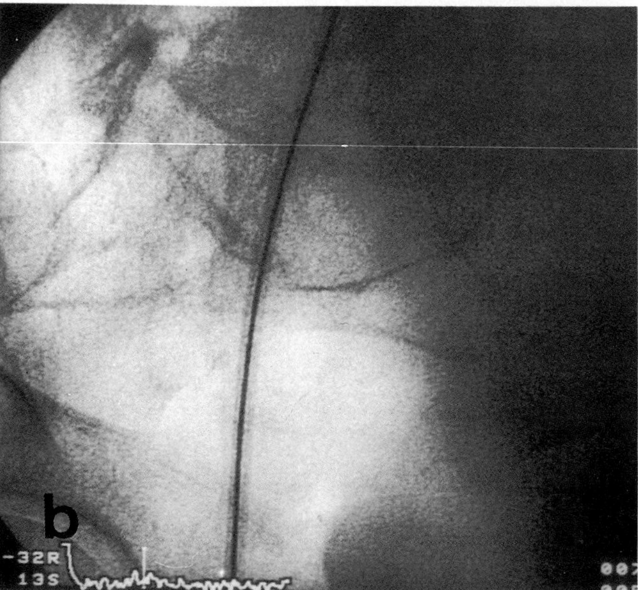

Figure 18

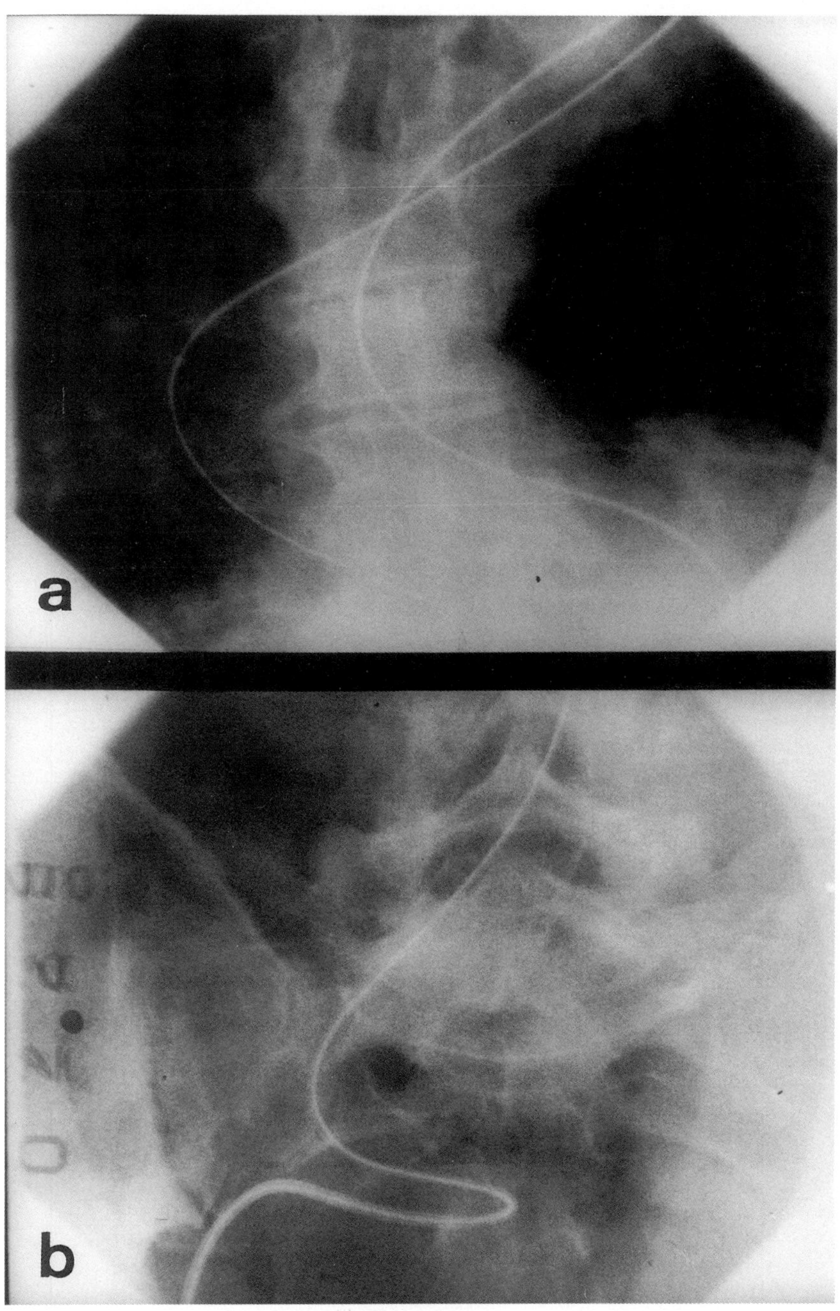

Figure 19

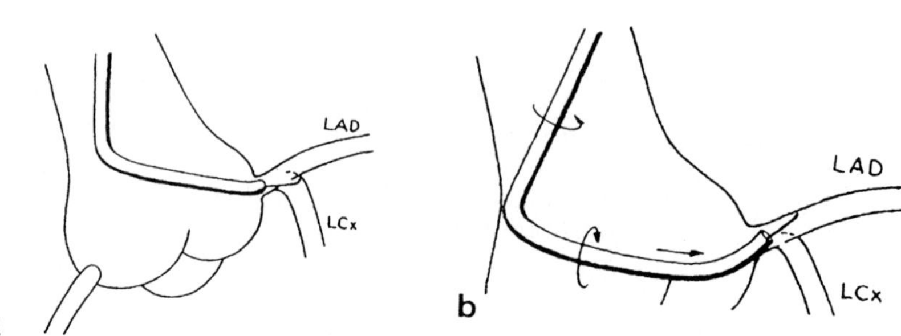

Figure 20

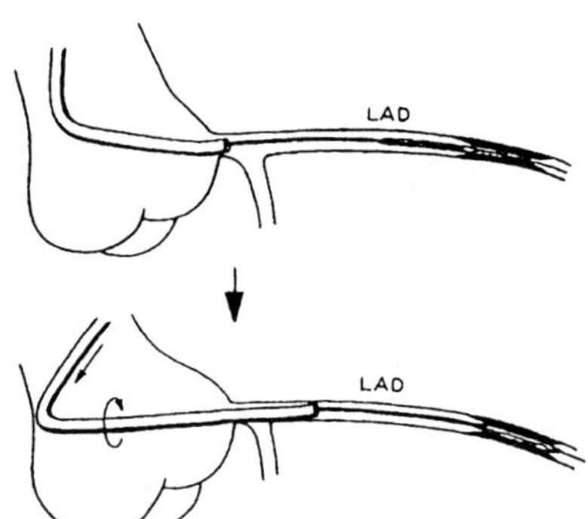

Figure 21

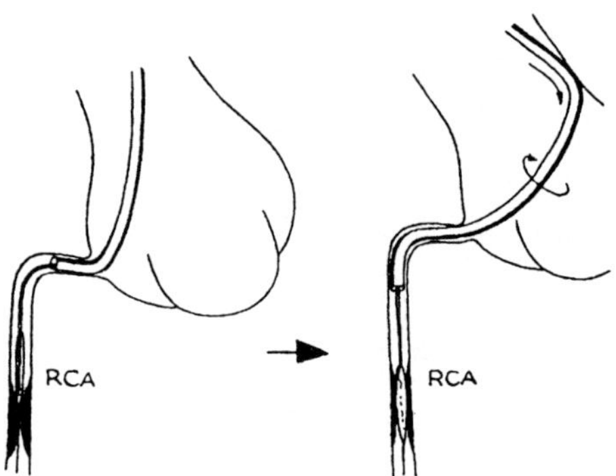

Figure 22

The direction in which the guiding catheter tip points determines how it directs the guidewire. Rotation of the guiding catheter, or pushing or pulling on it slightly, may direct its tip more preferentially into the target vessel. A guidewire that may initially have a tendency to enter the LCx (Fig. 20a) can be directed into the LAD by pushing and counterclockwise rotation of the Judkins catheter (Fig. 20b). Although a guiding catheter may be seated correctly in the coronary ostium, it may not offer optimal backup support for crossing tortuous arteries or tight stenoses. At such times the guiding catheter may be manipulated to improve backup support (Fig. 21). In case of a lesion in the LAD, the Judkins catheter may be rotated counterclockwise, at the same time advancing it. This converts the Judkins into an Amplatz-like shape, allowing it to lean against the opposite coronary sinus and in this way offer more backup support. This maneuver also leads to a deeper intubation of the artery, which further increases backup support. Similarly, for the RCA, a right Judkins catheter may be manipulated to improve support by clockwise rotation and advancement (Fig. 22). Such manipulations are best performed by first advancing the balloon catheter into the coronary artery and then manipulating the guiding catheter over the support offered by the balloon catheter shaft. Such "power positions" should be maintained only as long as required. The guiding catheter must be withdrawn to its normal position once the lesion is crossed and while the balloon catheter is still in place. Such manipulations are more often required when working with smaller guiding catheters, where lack of intrinsic backup support has to be compensated by deeper intubation. However, these smaller catheters are less likely to wedge in the coronary arteries than larger catheters, so this is a real trade-off. If deep intubation is required when working with larger catheters, the consequences of wedging can be reduced by using side hole guiding catheters or by making such holes in the catheter as mentioned above.

1.4 GUIDEWIRE

Guidewires are all constructed similarly, with a central metallic core overlaid with stainless steel coil, coated with a slippery, nonthrombogenic substance. The construction of the tip segment varies to allow for varying floppiness, rigidity, and shapeability.

Size

The size of guidewires range from the 0.009-in. Rotablator wire to the 0.021-in. Magnum wire. The commonest wire diameter is 0.014 in., which with the present technology seems to have achieved an optimal compromise between maneuverability and ease of lesion crossing, on the one hand, and rigidity and support for the balloon, on the other. The largest magnum wire has a 0.021-in. diameter and a 1-mm ball tip. This wire has superior pushability and is based on the concept of snowploughing across a lesion in a relatively atraumatic way, owing to its ball tip (rather than negotiating a stenotic lumen as with a conventional wire). It has been shown to be superior to standard guidewires for angioplasty of occlusions and some specific situations of nontotal occlusions.

Shape

Guidewires are available with straight tips or with a mild J curve 2 to 3 mm long. The shape of the tip may be altered in acuteness and length of the curve based on the anatomy of the lesion. In case the need for a greater curve is felt once the guidewire is introduced into the coronary system, this can often be achieved by causing it to buckle within a small branch. Such a maneuver increases the curve and allows the target vessel to be entered but may damage the wire if excessive buckling occurs in the attempt to curve it. Extreme curves may occasionally be necessary, to enter acute takeoffs of vessels or to negotiate branch point stenoses.

Floppiness

Guidewires come in various degrees of floppiness (or "softness"). The trackability of a floppy tip at one extreme, and better pushability of a stiff tip at the other, have to be weighed against each other for individual lesions. A floppy-tipped wire is ideal for subtotal occlusions, but a stiffer tip is necessary for total occlusions.

1.5 BALLOON CATHETER

Diameter

The diameter of the balloon is chosen based on the diameter of the vessel. Undersizing of the balloon leads to suboptimal results and to frequent need for a second balloon, with its implied additional cost. Oversizing the balloon increases the risk of dissection. While correct initial sizing of the balloon is important, it may occasionally be necessary to revert to a smaller balloon when a larger balloon cannot pass a tight stenosis. A smaller balloon with its lower deflated profile is often able to cross, and the lesion can be predilated to make way for the adequately sized balloon.

Length

Most balloons are 20 mm long. This is sufficient to adequately cover the large majority of stenoses. Longer balloons (30 to 60 mm long) are available from various companies and are useful for long or tandem lesions. Short balloons 9 to 15 mm in length are not very popular but are available commercially

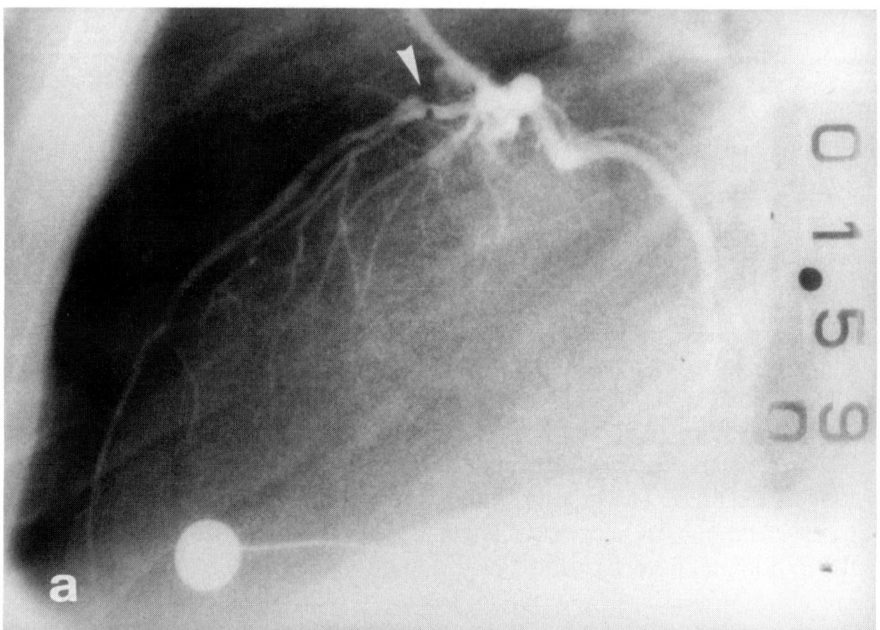

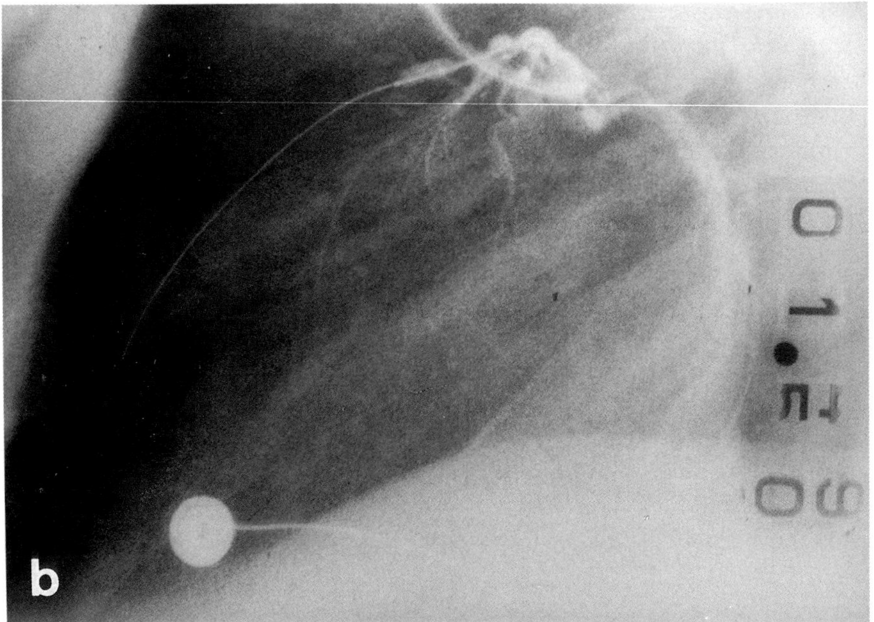

Figure 23

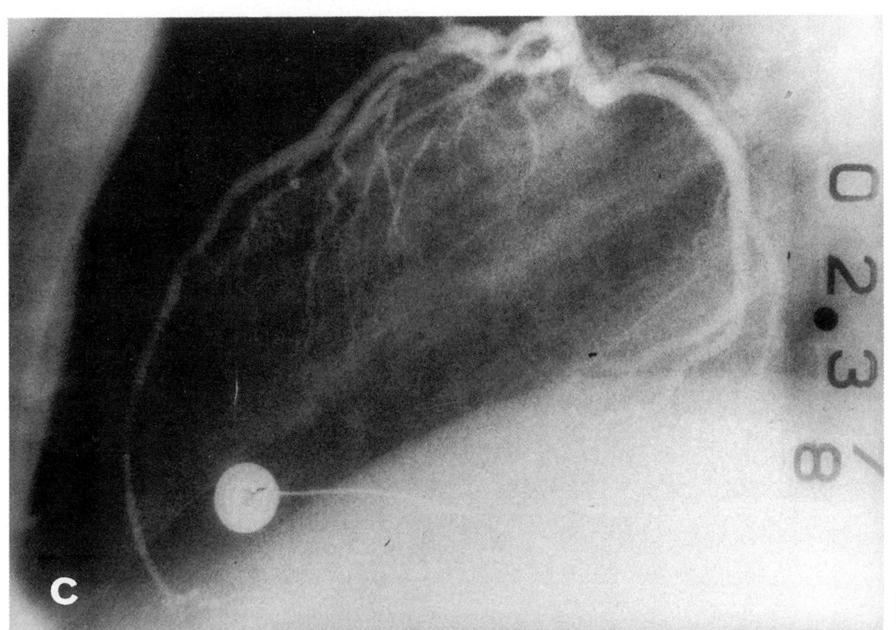

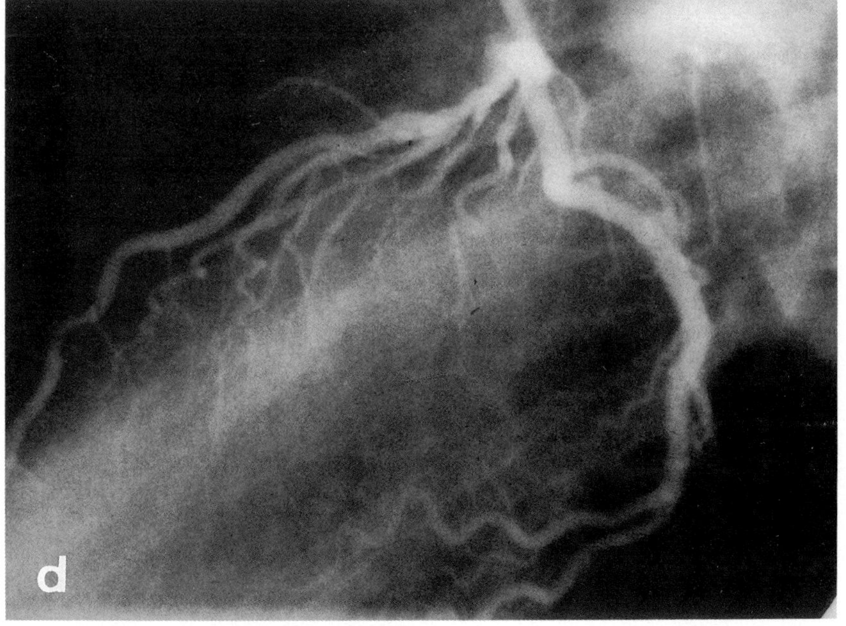

and intended for discrete stenoses. Such a lesion (Fig. 23a) was dilated with a 3.5-mm short balloon ("Shorty," Schneider) (Fig. 23b) with good immediate (Fig. 23c) and 10-month follow-up (Fig. 23d) results. Short balloons may theoretically restrict balloon-induced injury to a shorter segment of the coronary artery. However, the short balloon is relatively difficult to place, owing to its tendency to slip out of the lesion during inflation. Hence short balloons never really caught the fancy of angioplasters. Currently, their primary use is to overdilate slightly within a stent while avoiding injury to the surrounding normal vessel.

Compliance

Most balloons are constructed with materials that have some degree of compliance (i.e., they expand with pressure). This is a useful property since it allows for some degree of expansion of a balloon rather than replacement by an additional larger balloon when the need for increased balloon diameter becomes apparent during a procedure. A suboptimal result due to a slightly undersized balloon may be improved on by increasing inflation

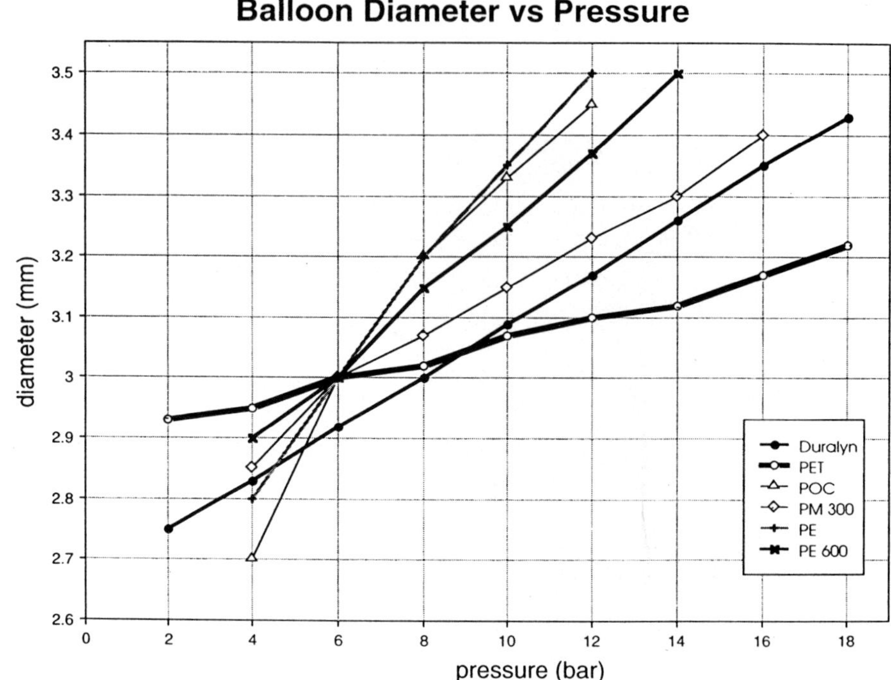

Figure 24

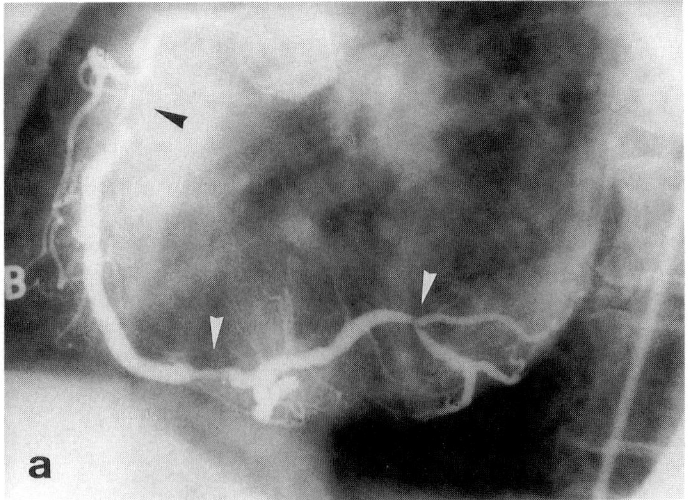

Figure 25

pressure without having to change the balloon. Noncompliant balloons, on the other hand, are useful for tough stenoses which yield only at high pressures, where the stenosis can be cracked without the risk of overdilating the adjacent vessel.

Figure 24 shows the relative compliance of commonly used balloon materials for a 3.0-mm balloon. The PET balloons are relatively noncompliant (and hence suitable for tough lesions), whereas the PE and POC balloons are compliant and would be best suited when dealing with multiple stenoses.

The choice of balloon size depends on the size of the vessel to be dilated. However, when dealing with multiple stenoses, it is cost-effective to compromise on balloon size so as to be able to address all lesions with the same balloon. In this example with multiple stenoses of the RCA (Fig. 25a), a 3.0-mm balloon was chosen to dilate all three stenoses sequentially (Fig. 25b,c,d). The final result was good (Fig. 25e). Although the sequence of dilatation in this case was proximal to distal, this was inconsequential since a noncompliant (PET) balloon was used. Using a compliant balloon (preferable for such cases), one should begin with

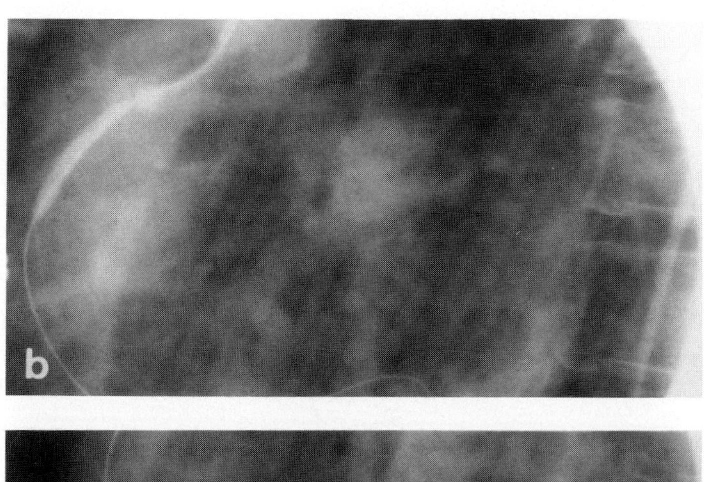

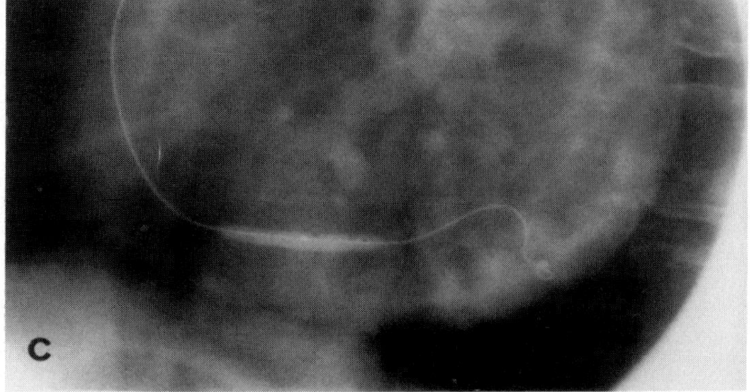

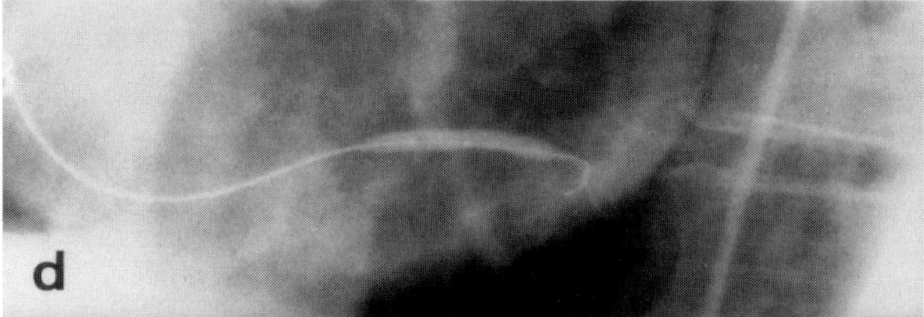

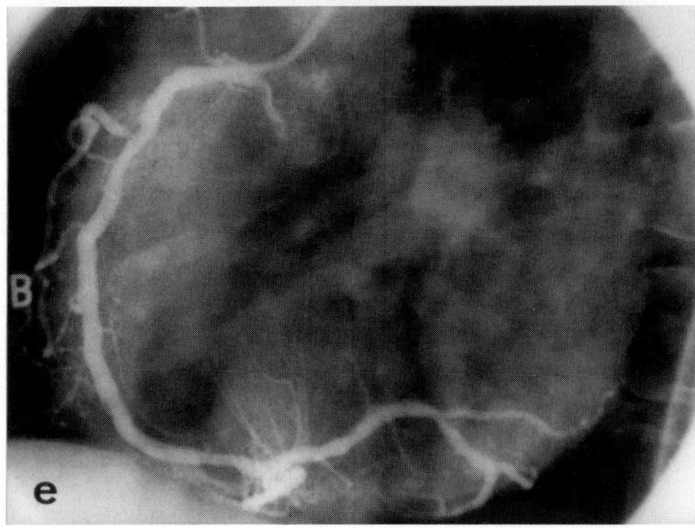

the distal-most lesion using low pressures, and progress to the more proximal stenoses with higher pressures, thereby achieving greater balloon diameters. However, if the proximal stenosis is tight and interferes with distal passage of the balloon, it should be dilated first.

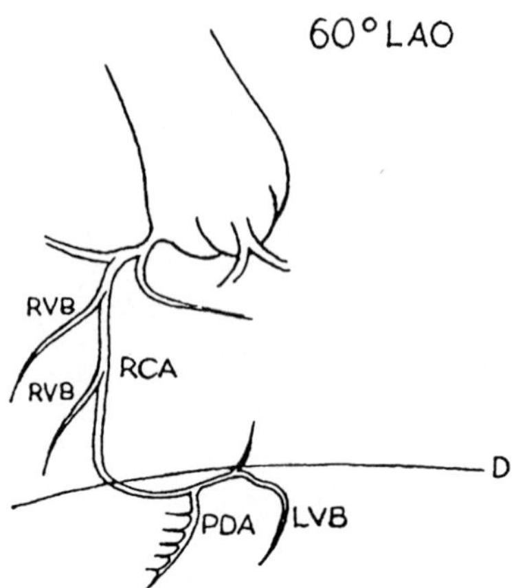

Figure 26

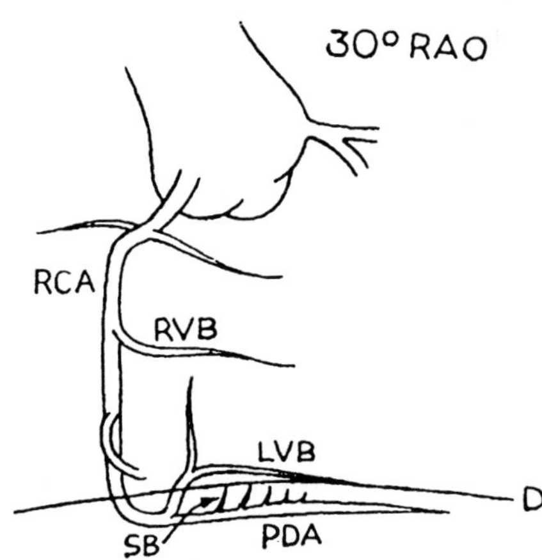

Figure 27

1.6 RIGHT CORONARY ARTERY ANGIOPLASTY

In accordance with the general rule of angioplasty, the best views for delineating the lesion should be obtained. In general, the proximal RCA is best depicted by the left anterior oblique (LAO) (Fig. 26) or the lateral views. For the middle part of the RCA, the right anterior oblique (RAO) (Fig. 27) or the anteroposterior views are best. The bifurcation of the RCA into the posterior descending and the posterolateral branches is best displayed by the LAO or anteroposterior views, both with cranial angulation. The posterior descending artery is best visualized in the RAO view.

The Judkins right coronary catheter can be utilized for most RCA stenoses. Increased backup support may be obtained by clockwise rotation and advancement of the catheter (Fig. 22). However, in the event of insufficient backup support due to a superior takeoff (Shepherd's crook), or when addressing tight stenoses or occlusions where the need for more backup is anticipated, an Amplatz left catheter (commonly a type 2 curve) is prefer-

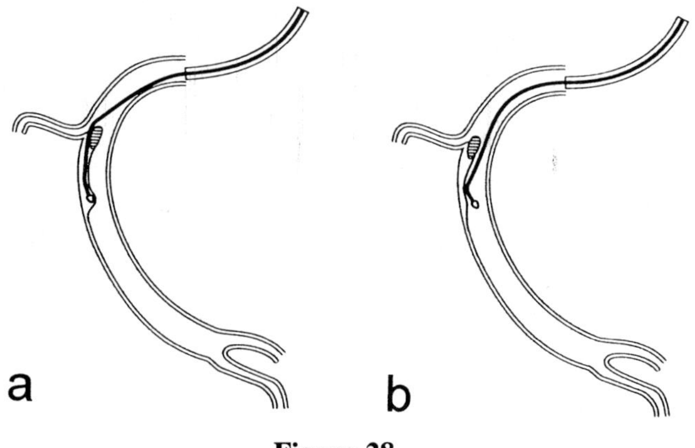

Figure 28

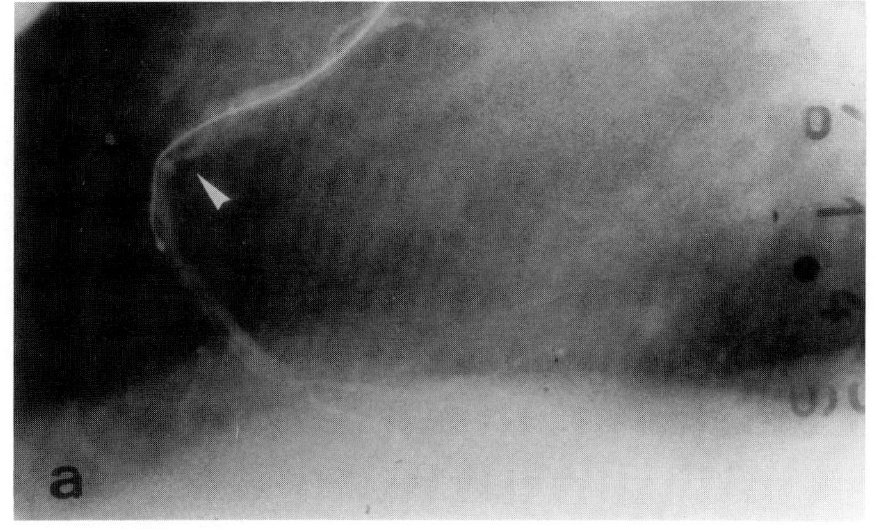

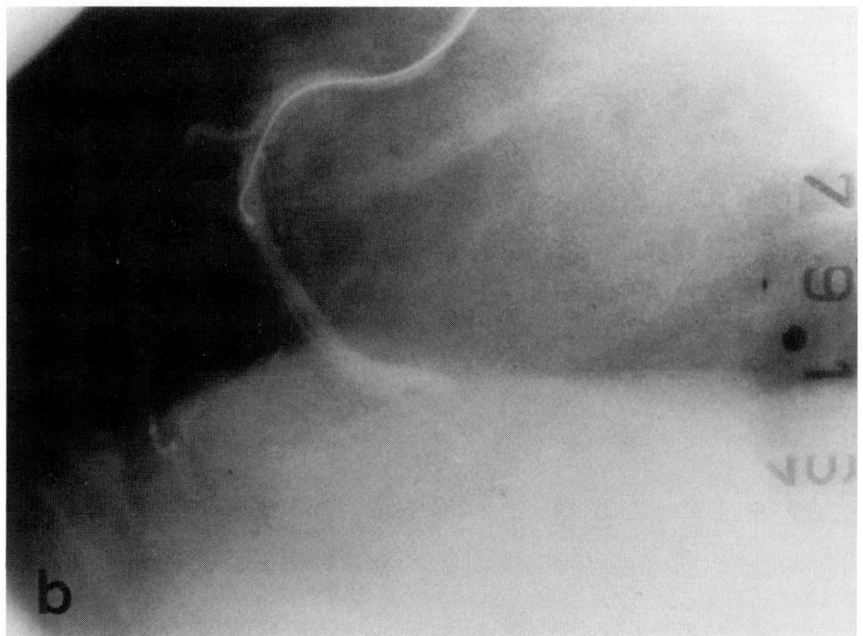

Figure 28 (Continued)

able (Fig. 13). In such cases a multipurpose, El Gamal, or Arani curve may also be useful.

It is logical that a guidewire has a tendency to hug the outer curve of the RCA. In the presence of eccentric plaques at the outer border of the RCA, it is important to keep the guidewire directed toward the inside of the curve. Failure to do so may result in a subintimal course of the wire. In one example, the Magnum wire, hugging the outside curve of the RCA, entered subintimally under an eccentric plaque (arrow) (Fig. 28a). The true lumen could be found only by withdrawing the wire and manipulating it along the inner curve of the artery across the plaque (Fig. 28b).

An interesting finding has been described to occur following successful PTCA of an RCA stenosis. Angioplasty was performed in a 55-year-old man with RCA stenosis (Fig. 29a). However, the control angiogram after removal of the balloon but with the wire in place revealed a proximal stenosis which had not been present earlier (Fig. 29b), the dilated site showing a good result (curved arrow). This stenosis was no longer seen once the wire was removed (Fig. 29c). This phenomenon occurs due to a curved vessel being straightened by the wire or the guiding catheter, resulting in artificial folds. Once the guidewire is removed and the guiding catheter position relaxed, the vessel can assume its original curves and the "pseudostenosis" disappears. This has been referred to as the *accordion* (or *concertina*) *phenomenon*.

1.7 LEFT ANTERIOR DESCENDING CORONARY ARTERY ANGIOPLASTY

The best views for delineating the origin and proximal part of the LAD are the anteroposterior or LAO view with caudal angulation ("spider view") (Fig. 30). For the middle part, and to separate the diagonal branches from the LAD, the lateral view [where the LAD runs almost horizontally whereas the diagonal branches (DB) are more vertically oriented] is best (Fig. 31). The LAO view with cranial angulation (where the LAD runs in the center of the field with the septal branches on its left side and the diagonal branches on its right) is also helpful (Fig. 32). So is

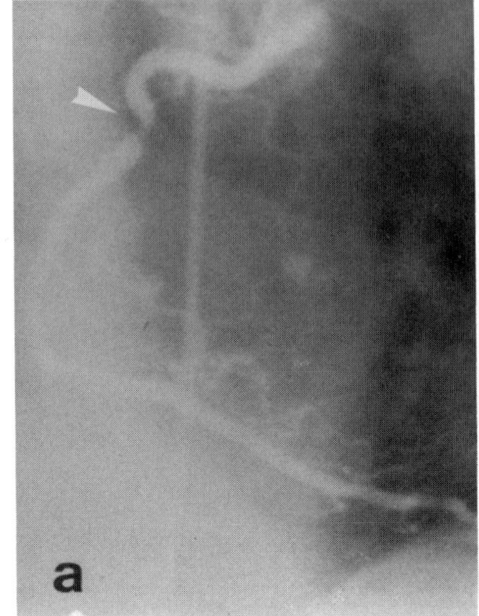

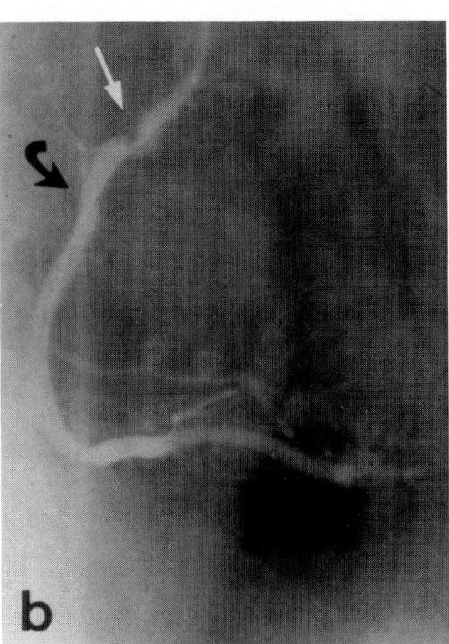

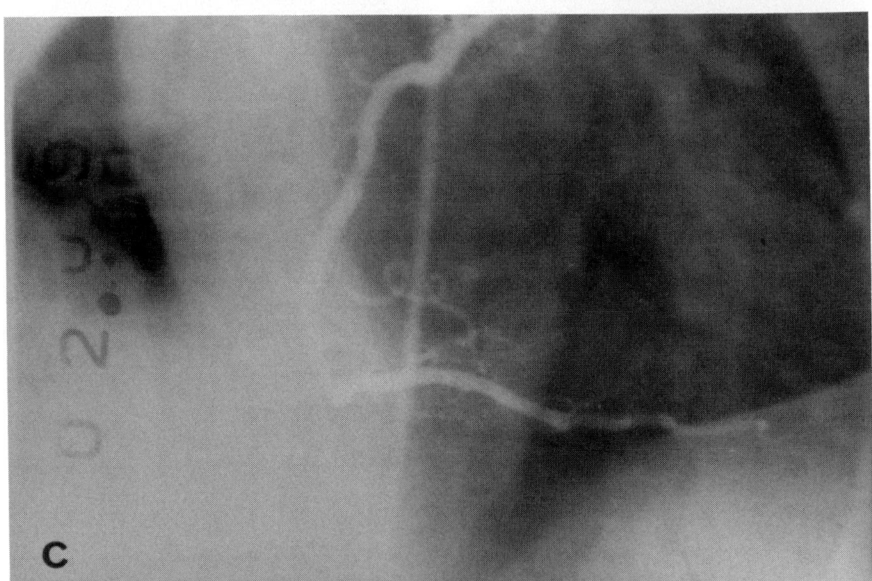

Figure 29

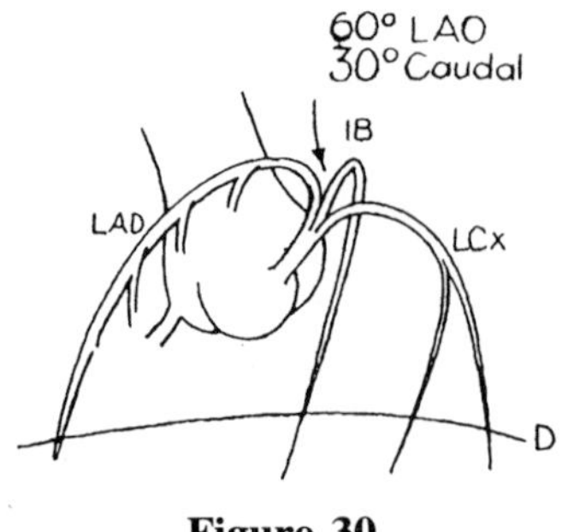

Figure 30

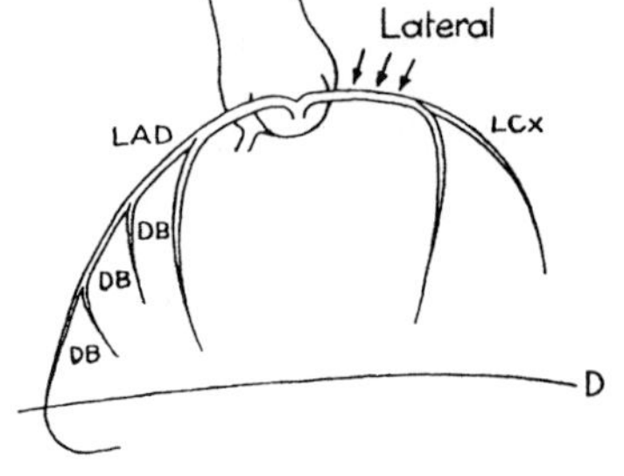

Figure 31

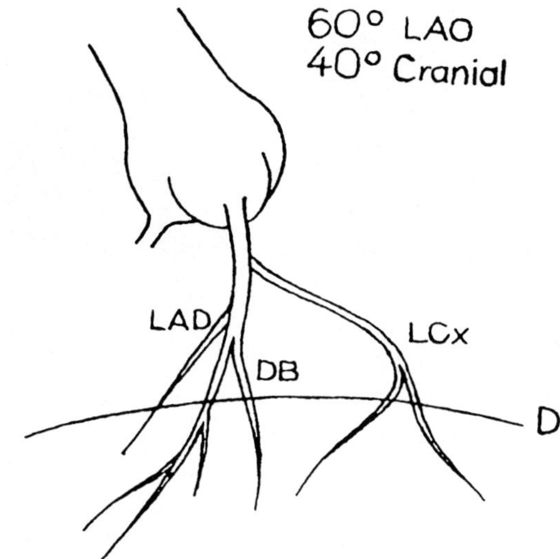

Figure 32

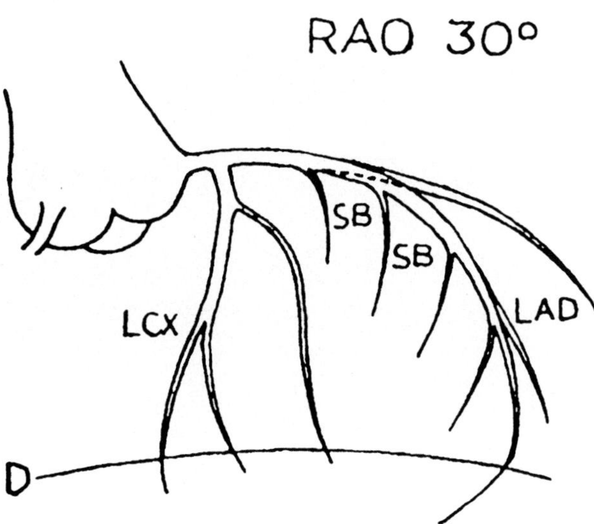

Figure 33

the RAO view with cranial (or occasionally caudal) angulation. Optimal delineation of the vessels is essential, since overlapping and foreshortening of the LAD and its branches is common (Fig. 33), and significant lesions may be overlooked if inadequate views are obtained.

The Judkins left guiding catheter is the initial choice for LAD angioplasty. Counterclockwise rotation, and advancing or withdrawing the catheter, will help to direct the guidewire optimally. The initial manipulations should always be carried out in a RAO view, since this gives a good idea about the position of the guiding catheter (which is seen in full profile), its relation to the left coronary ostium, and the anatomy of the left main stem and the proximal part of the LAD. Further manipulations may be carried out in other views. The balloon may be advanced in any view, although a RAO projection is preferable. However, if resistance is experienced to balloon advancement and force or deep intubation of the guiding catheter is required, such manipulations are best performed in an RAO view. Details of such maneuvers are described in Section 1.3.

1.8 LEFT CIRCUMFLEX CORONARY ARTERY ANGIOPLASTY

The proximal and mid LCx and the origins of the obtuse marginal branches are best defined in the RAO view with caudal angulation, which is the best projection for angioplasty in most cases. The ostium of the LCx and intermediate branch (IB) are well delineated in the LAO caudal ("spider") view (Fig. 30). The spider view is an excellent view for the delineation of the left main coronary artery and the origins of the LAD and LCx arteries, and should form part of every routine angiographic examination. A 61-year-old male presented with unstable angina. No coronary stenosis was visible except on the LAO caudal view, where a tight stenosis of the origin of the LCx was seen with some difficulty (Fig. 34a). The lesion was crossed with a 0.014-in. guidewire (Fig. 34b), and angioplasty performed with a 3.5-mm balloon (Fig. 34c), with an adequate result (Fig. 34d). The patient had recurrence of symptoms 3 months later. Angiographic evaluation revealed restenosis, with progression of the left

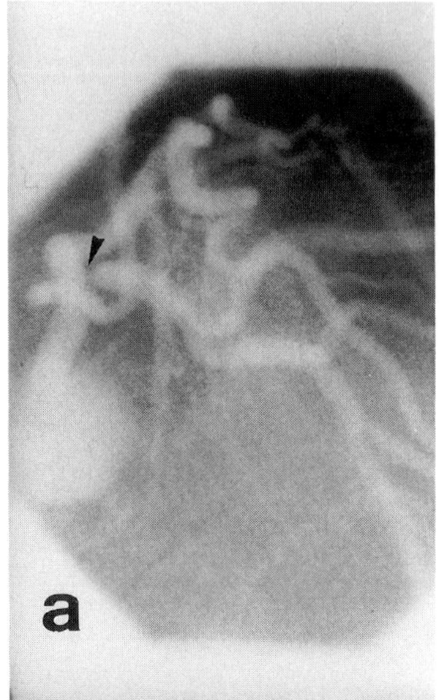

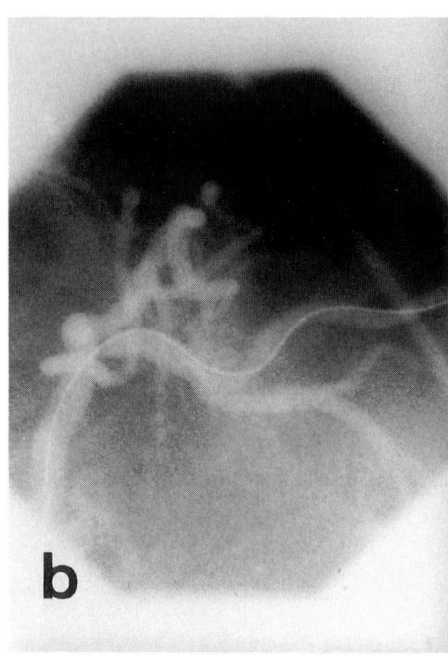

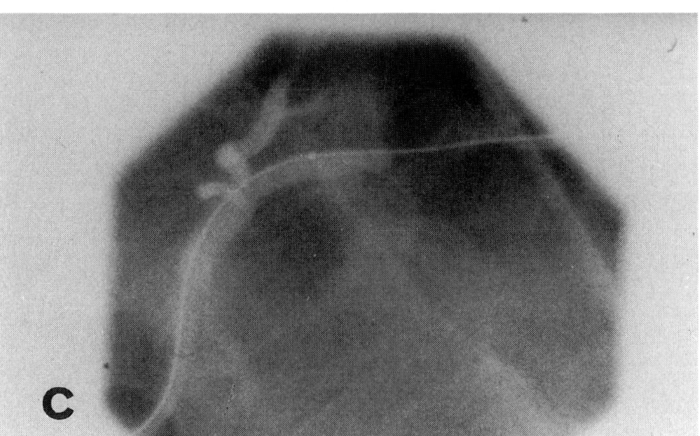

Figure 34

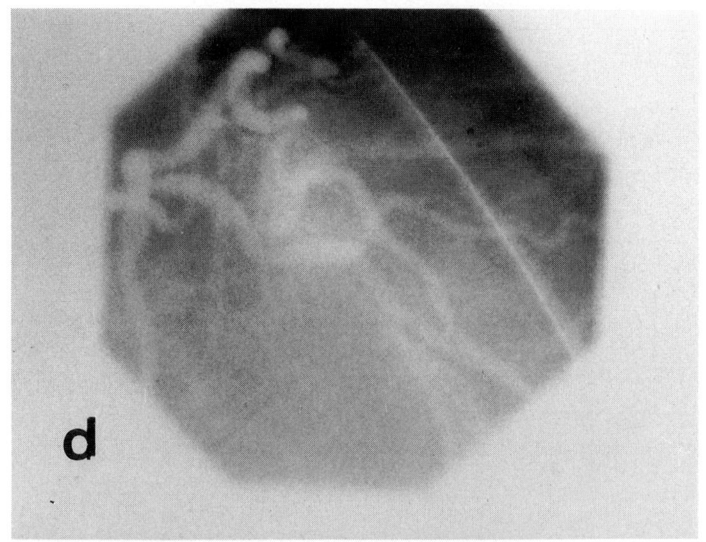

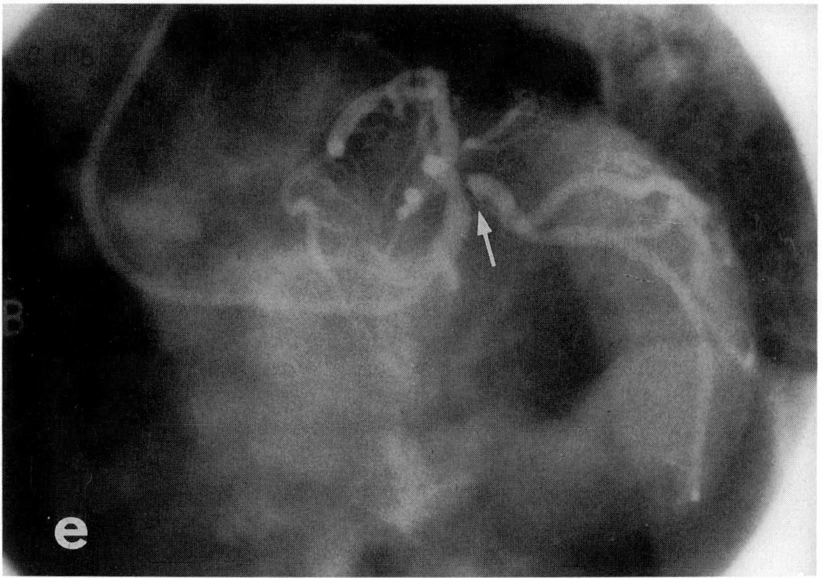

main stenosis (Fig. 34e). Elective CABG was performed.

The mid LCx is well seen in the LAO and lateral views (Fig. 31, arrows). For a left dominant coronary circulation, the posterior descending artery and the posterolateral branches can be separated by a LAO view with cranial angulation.

An Amplatz guiding catheter (type 2 curve for most aortas) is best suited for LCx lesions (Fig. 9). The tip may be made to point more favorably toward the LCx by pulling slightly on the catheter once it is engaged. However, pushing on the catheter may sometimes be better than pulling for directing the tip optimally toward the LCx. The Amplatz catheter affords good backup support, although it may be more traumatic than the Judkins shape (see Section 1.3). It is good practice to withdraw these catheters from the left coronary ostium by a pushing and rotating motion rather than pulling on it, since the catheter has a tendency to advance deeper on being pulled. This may result in dissection. The softer 6F catheters are less prone to such problems. Ideally, the withdrawal of an Amplatz catheter at the end of the procedure should be performed under fluoroscopy.

2
Special Indications

2.1
MULTIVESSEL ANGIOPLASTY

Although single-vessel angioplasty forms the great majority of PTCA procedures, multivessel angioplasty is also commonly attempted. Multivessel angioplasty can be performed in a single sitting or as a staged procedure. The decision should be based on the projected risk of both lesions closing simultaneously, and the amount of myocardium in jeopardy in such an event. The presence or absence of collaterals plays an important role in decision making.

Double-Vessel

A 40-year-old man with angina pectoris was detected to have an occluded RCA (Fig. 35a), collateralized from the LAD, which itself had a significant stenosis.

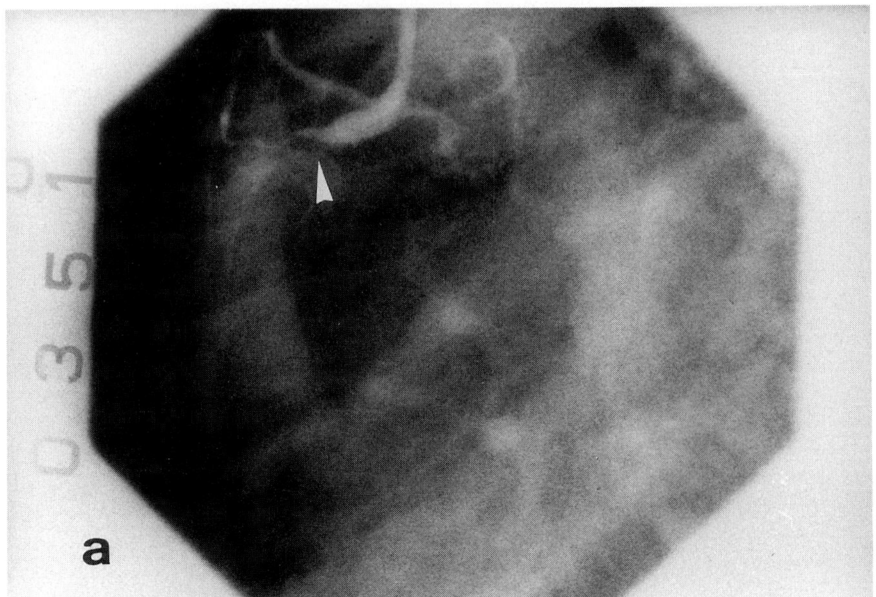

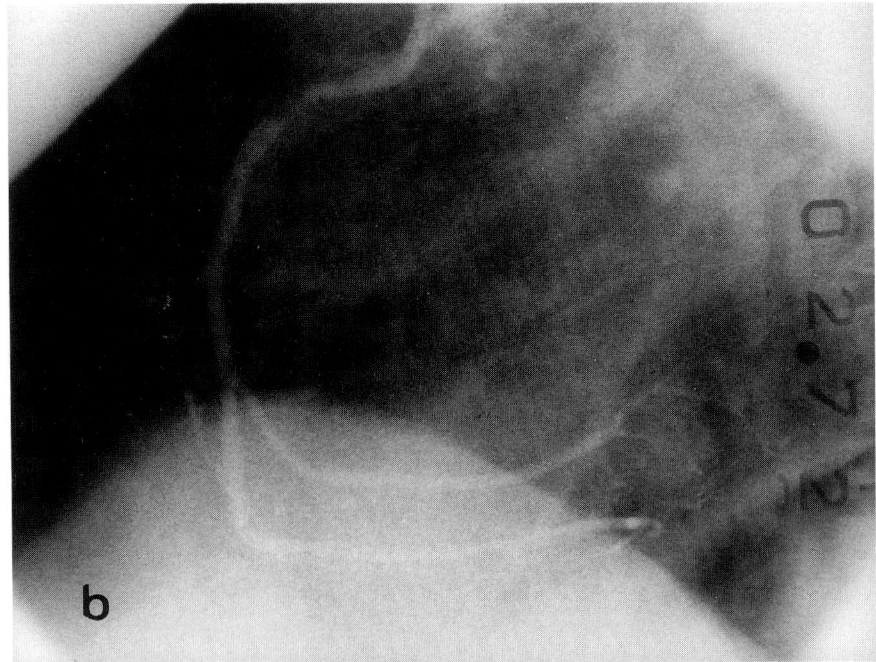

Figure 35

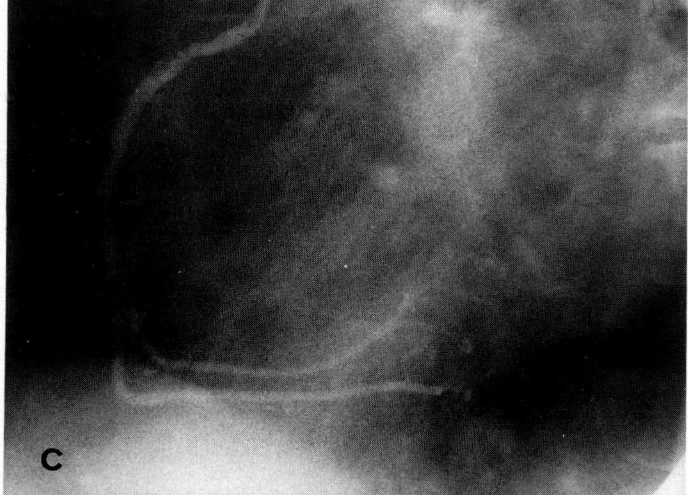

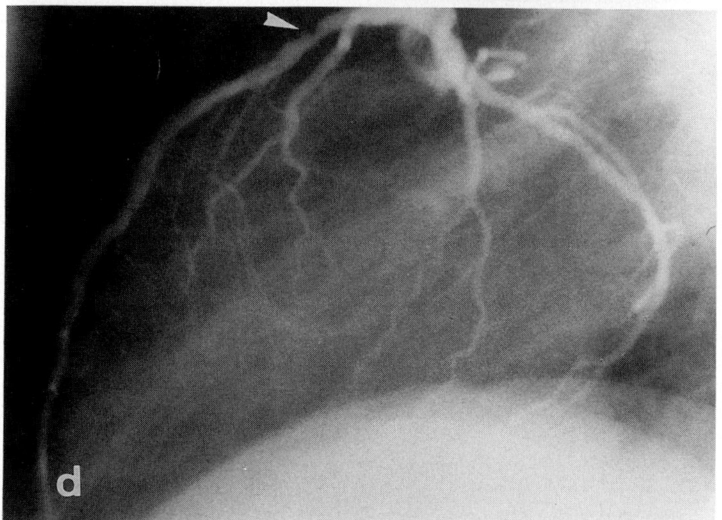

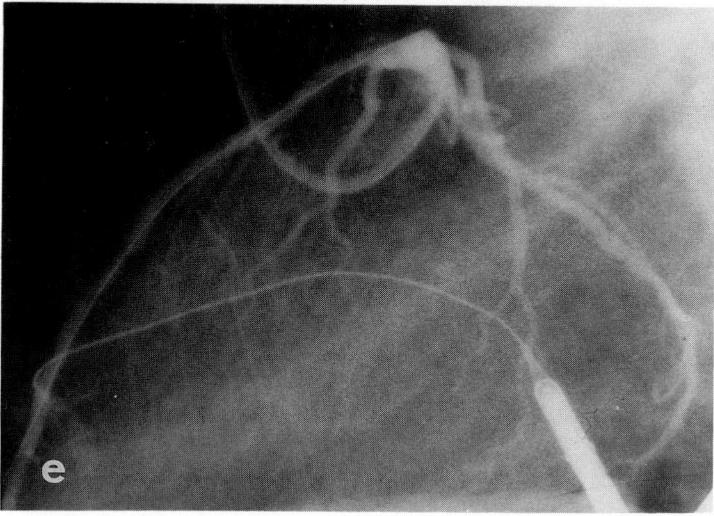

Staged angioplasty was planned for this patient, first tackling the RCA and subsequently, the LAD. The RCA was recanalized the first day, with an acceptable result (Fig. 35b). The next day, a control angiogram revealed a stable RCA angioplasty result (Fig. 35c), and the LAD lesion (Fig. 35d) was dilated with a good result (Fig. 35e). Such an approach is logical, especially in a situation where the collaterals between the LAD and the RCA can be used to support the vessel being dilated. The collaterals from the LAD were supporting the RCA in the first place, so that an acute reocclusion of that vessel would be inconsequential. Following successful recanalization of the RCA, these collaterals could have supported the LAD if it had closed following angioplasty. In such situations the presence of collaterals can be used advantageously.

Sometimes it may be relatively safe to dilate two vessels at the same sitting. Again, the projected risk of vessel closure, amount of myocardium at risk, and degree of collateralization should constitute the basis of decision making. The worse lesion, or the one supplying the greater amount of myocardium, should be dilated first and only if the result is good should the second vessel be attempted. A 62-year-old man with double-vessel disease had stenoses of the LAD (Fig. 36a) and RCA (Fig. 36b). The LAD received collaterals from the RCA via a branch that originated proximal to the stenosis (arrow). Following an adequate result of the LAD angioplasty (Fig. 36c), the RCA was dilated at the same sitting, with a good result (Fig.

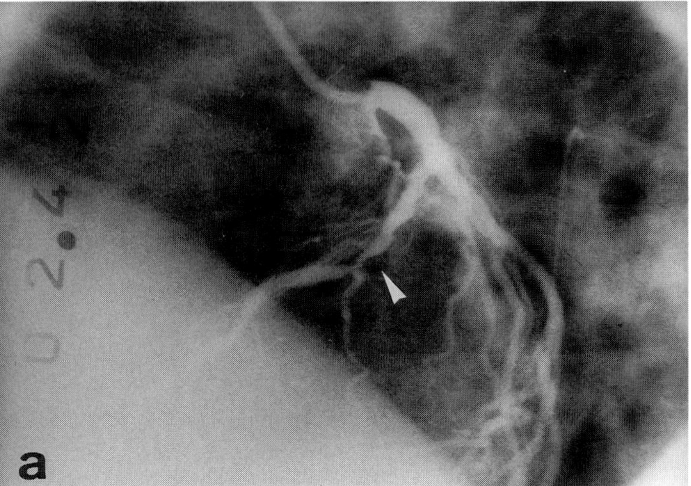

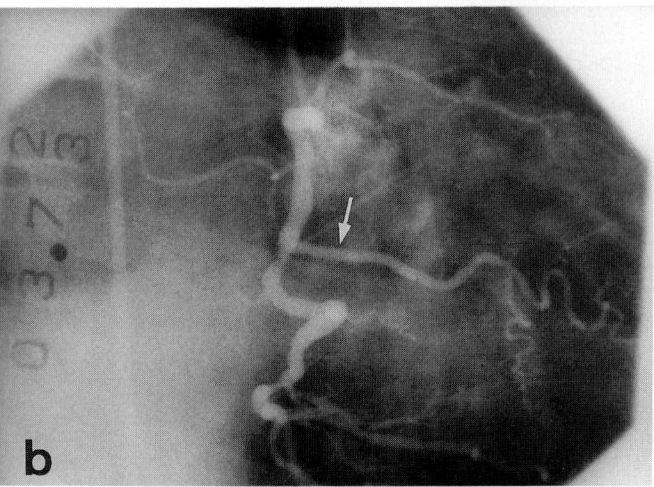

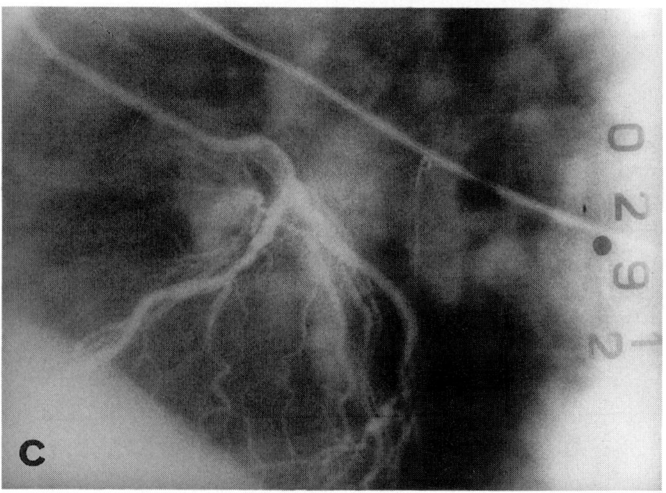

Figure 36

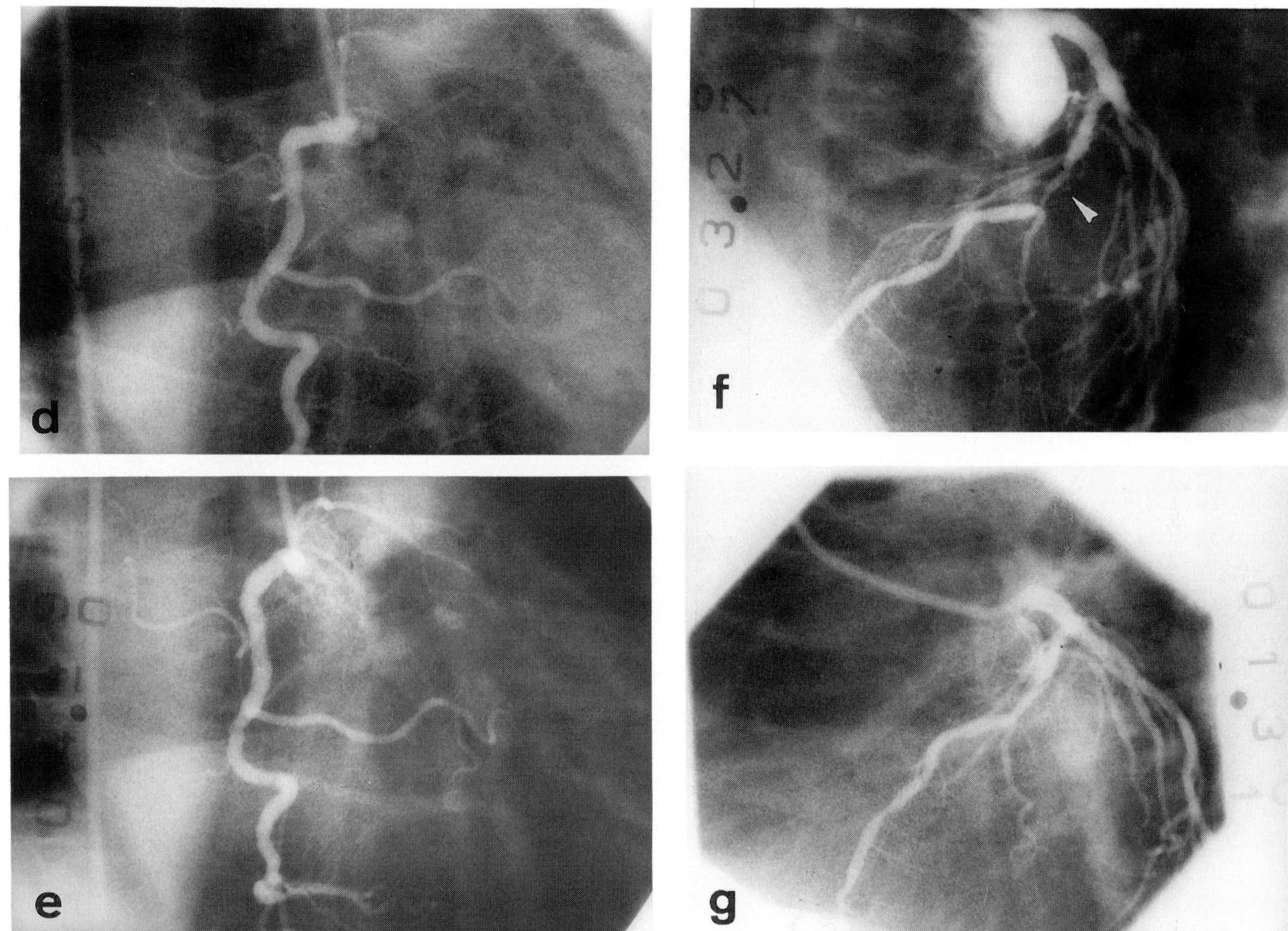

36d). Such an approach is safe, although the myocardium at risk is considerable, since the LAD was collateralized by the RCA branch, which originated proximal to the stenosis. In such a situation, even if acute closure of both dilated lesions occurred, the LAD would be protected by the collaterals. A 4-month follow-up for angina revealed a good long-term result of the RCA (Fig. 36e). An LAD restenosis was detected (Fig. 36f) and dilated (Fig. 36g). After 10 months, symptoms recurred. The RCA site was still widely patent (Fig. 36h), but a re-restenosis of the LAD (Fig. 36i) was seen and a third successful LAD PTCA performed (Fig. 36j). The patient remained asymptomatic following this intervention. This case also demonstrates another aspect of multivessel PTCA (i.e., the compounded incidence of restenosis and need for re-interventions).

Left Main Stem

Although technically easy, left main stem angioplasty is a high-risk procedure even with percutaneous cardiopulmonary support (CPS) systems. It should be left to the surgeons. However, it may be performed in a few selected cases where the distal circulation is protected by a bypass graft or abundant collaterals from the RCA. A 10-year-old boy with familial homozygous hypercholesterolemia had a tight left main stenosis (Fig. 37a) with an excellent collateral supply from the RCA (Fig. 37b). Angioplasty was performed using a 3.0-mm balloon. The patient tolerated balloon inflations of up to 10 minutes without pain or hemodynamic compromise, demonstrating the adequacy of the collateral supply.

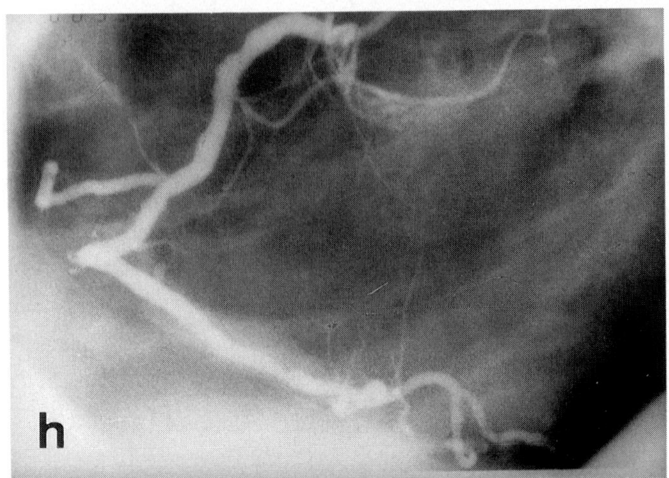

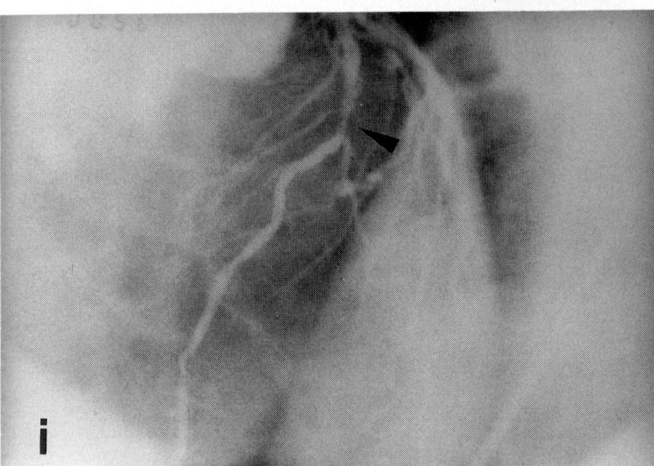

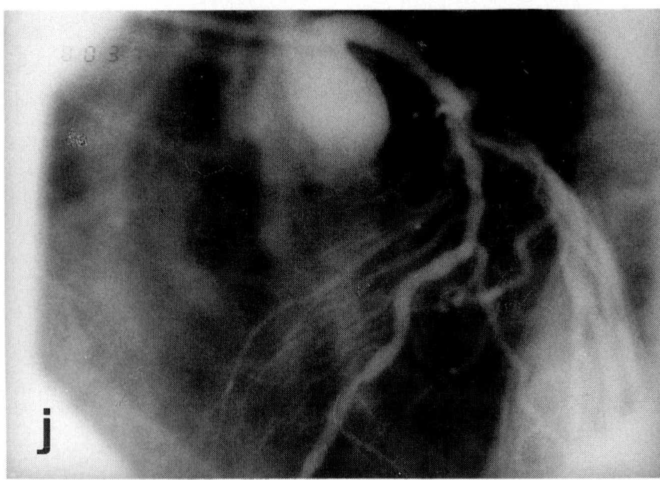

Figure 36 (Continued)

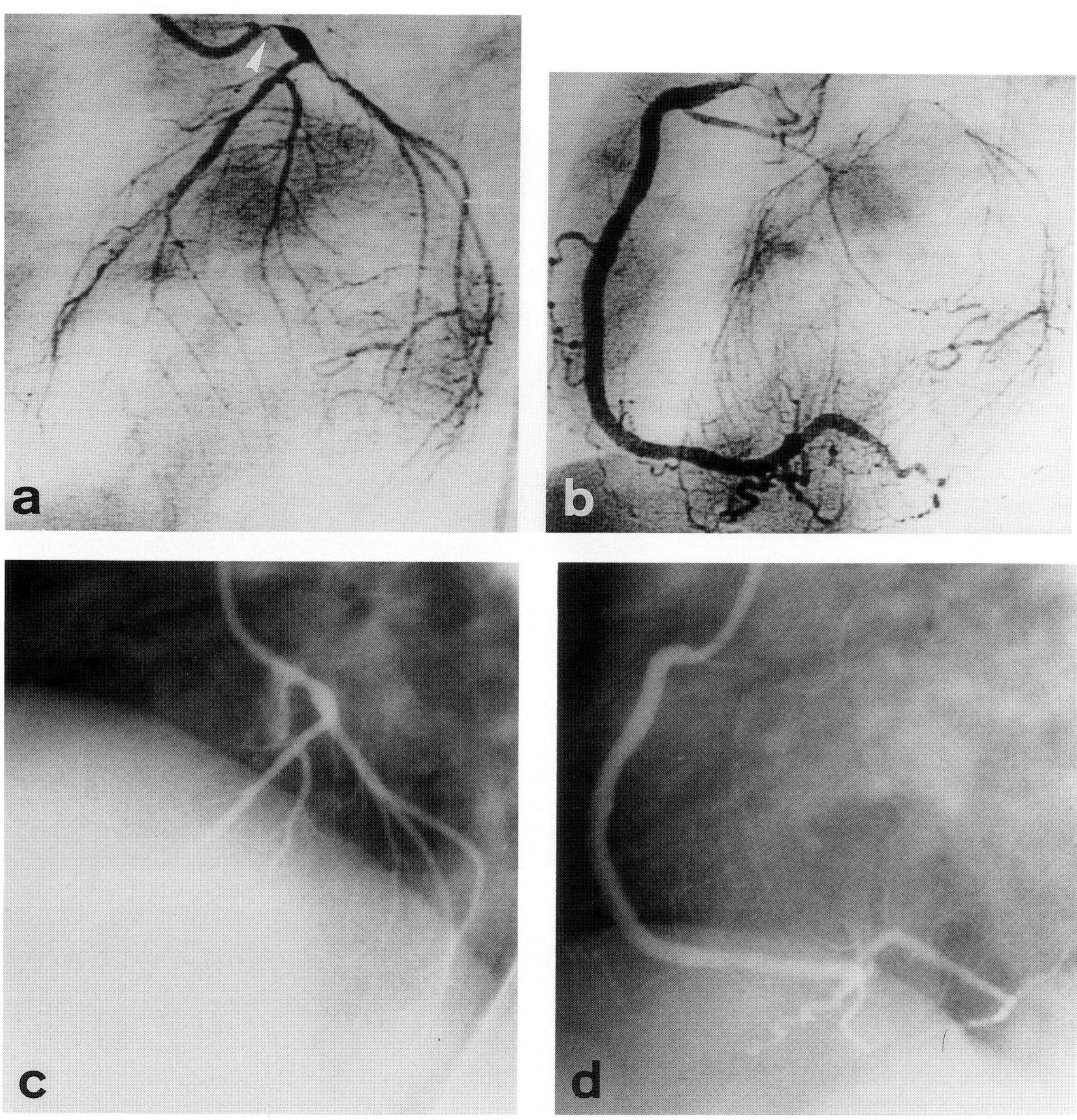

Figure 37

The final result was good (Fig. 37c), and was associated with a disappearance of collaterals from the RCA (Fig. 37d). The patient had no ischemia on stress testing and MIBI scintigraphy at a 5-month follow-up, and was still asymptomatic 2 years later. Another situation where angioplasty for a left main stem stenosis can be attempted is demonstrated in a 56-year-old man with an acute myocardial infarction with cardiogenic shock. Angiography revealed an occluded left main stem (Fig. 38a) which was dilated successfully (Fig. 38b). However, a thrombus from the left main stem was displaced down the LCx (Fig. 38c) and was pushed down farther by the force of the injection (Fig. 38d). The patient recovered subsequently.

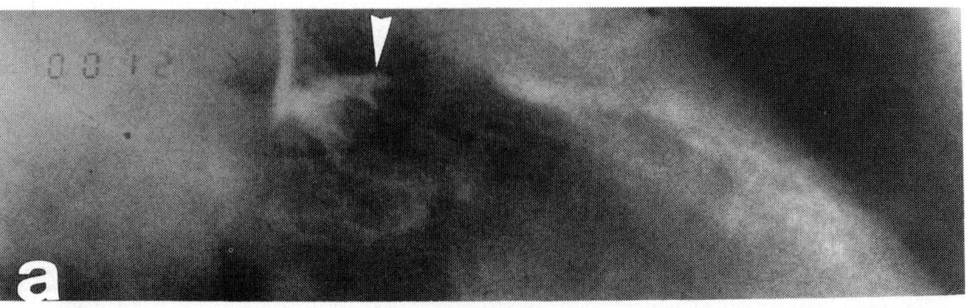

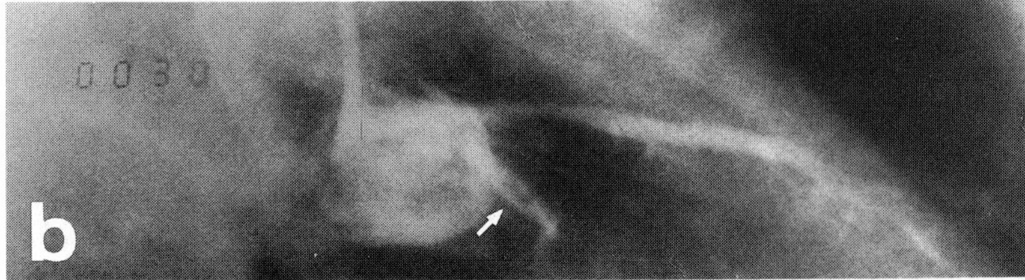

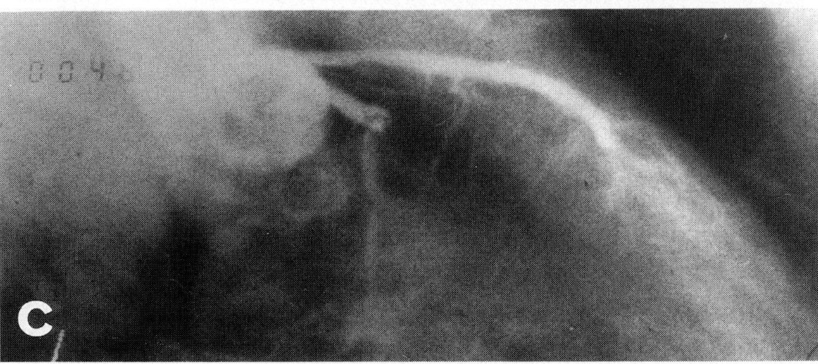

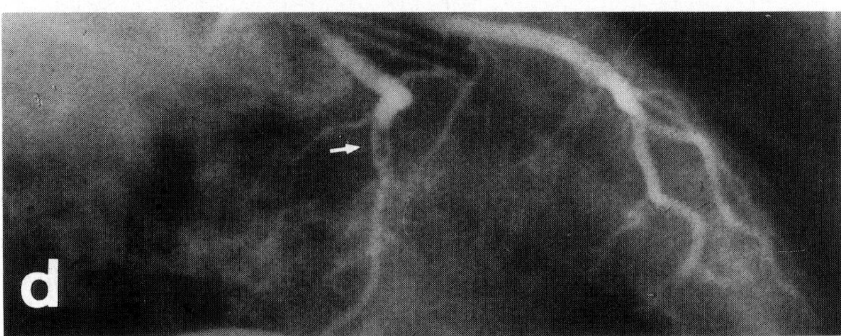

Figure 38

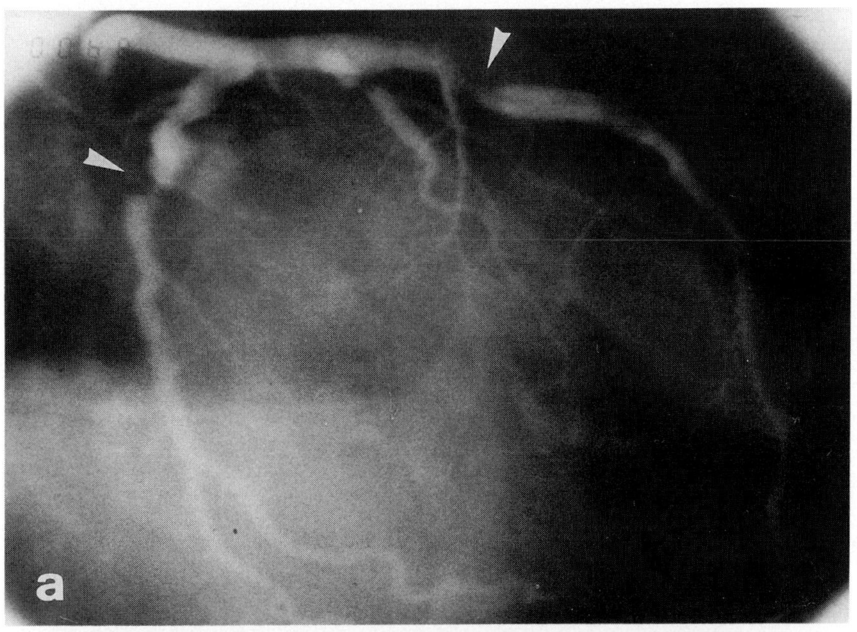

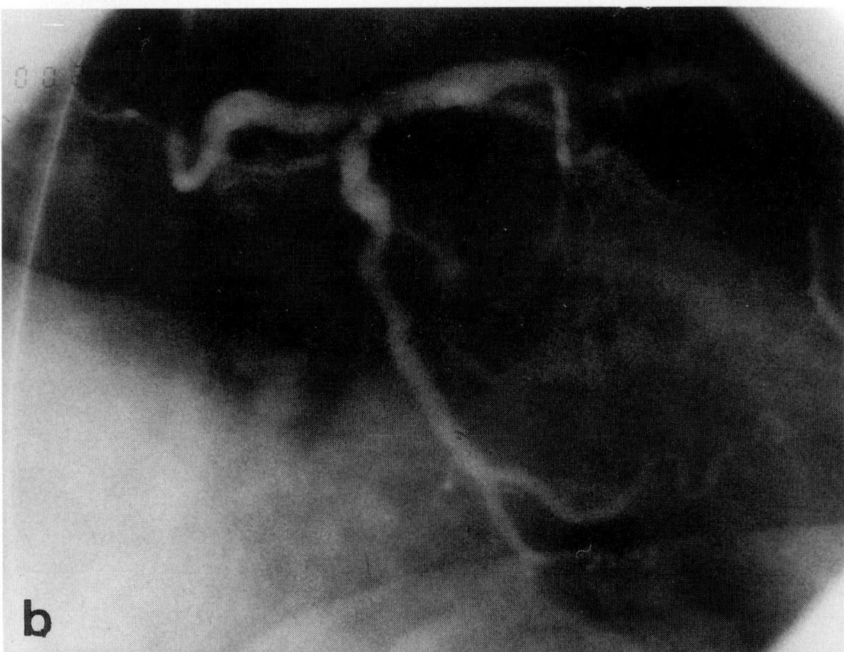

Figure 39

Left Main Equivalent

This refers to stenoses in the proximal LAD and LCx arteries such that simultaneous occlusion of both would equal an occlusion of the left main stem. However, the spontaneous risk of both lesions occluding simultaneously is low; hence clinically this situation is not truly equivalent to a left main stenosis. However, simultaneous angioplasty of both lesions converts this into a true left main equivalent, where the risk of simultaneous closure is real. It may be smaller than that of a left main stenosis, but occlusion of the first vessel may entrain closure of the second by causing hypotension. It is preferable to address the two lesions as a staged procedure. A 58-year-old man was detected to have a left main equivalent disease, with 80 to 90% stenoses of the proximal LCx and LAD (Fig. 39a). Successful angioplasty of the LCx was performed (Fig. 39b). Two weeks later, a repeat angiogram revealed a stable LCx lesion (Fig. 39c), and the LAD lesion was dilated (Fig. 39d). A 6-month follow-up study revealed no restenosis (Fig. 39e).

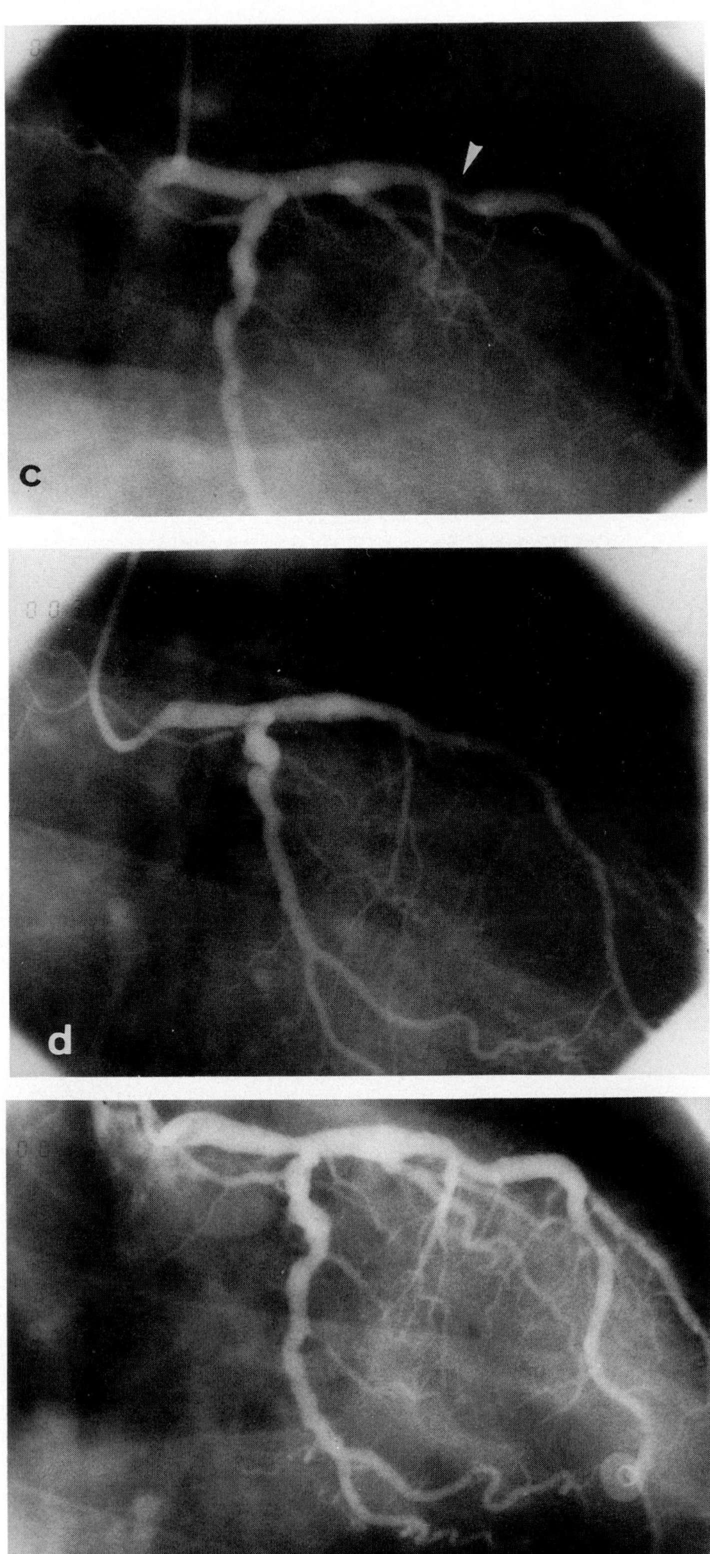

Figure 39 (Continued)

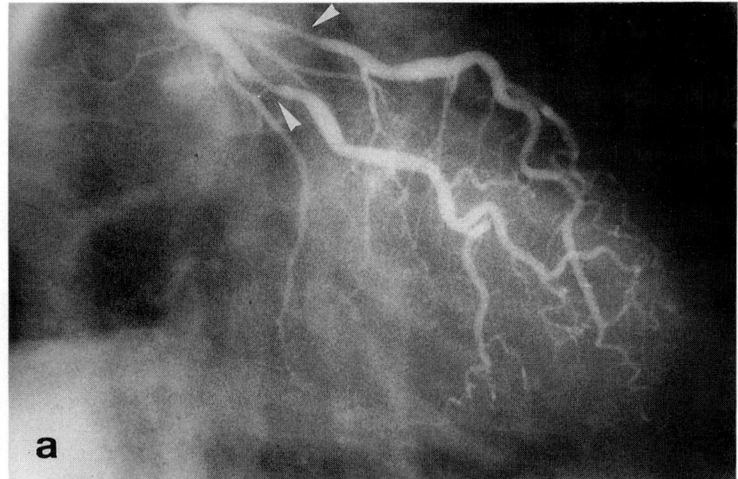

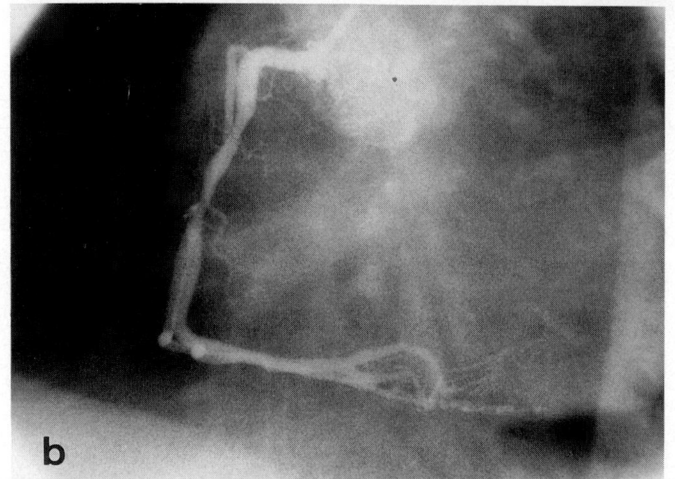

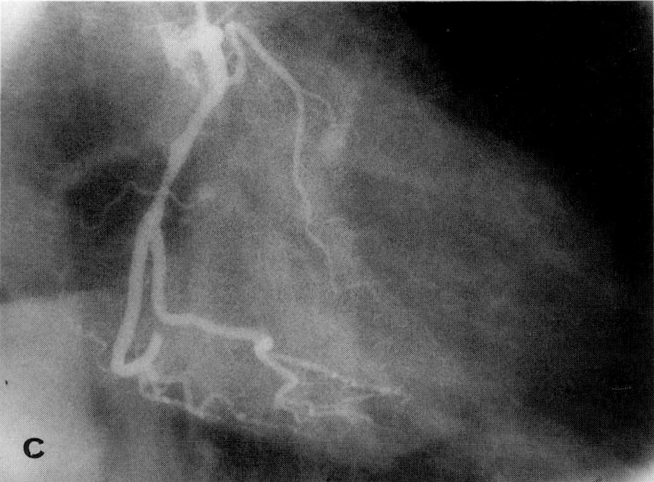

Figure 40

A 63-year-old man presented to another hospital with angina and significant stenoses of the LAD and LCx (Fig. 40a). In addition, the RCA had a nonsignificant stenosis (Fig. 40b,c).

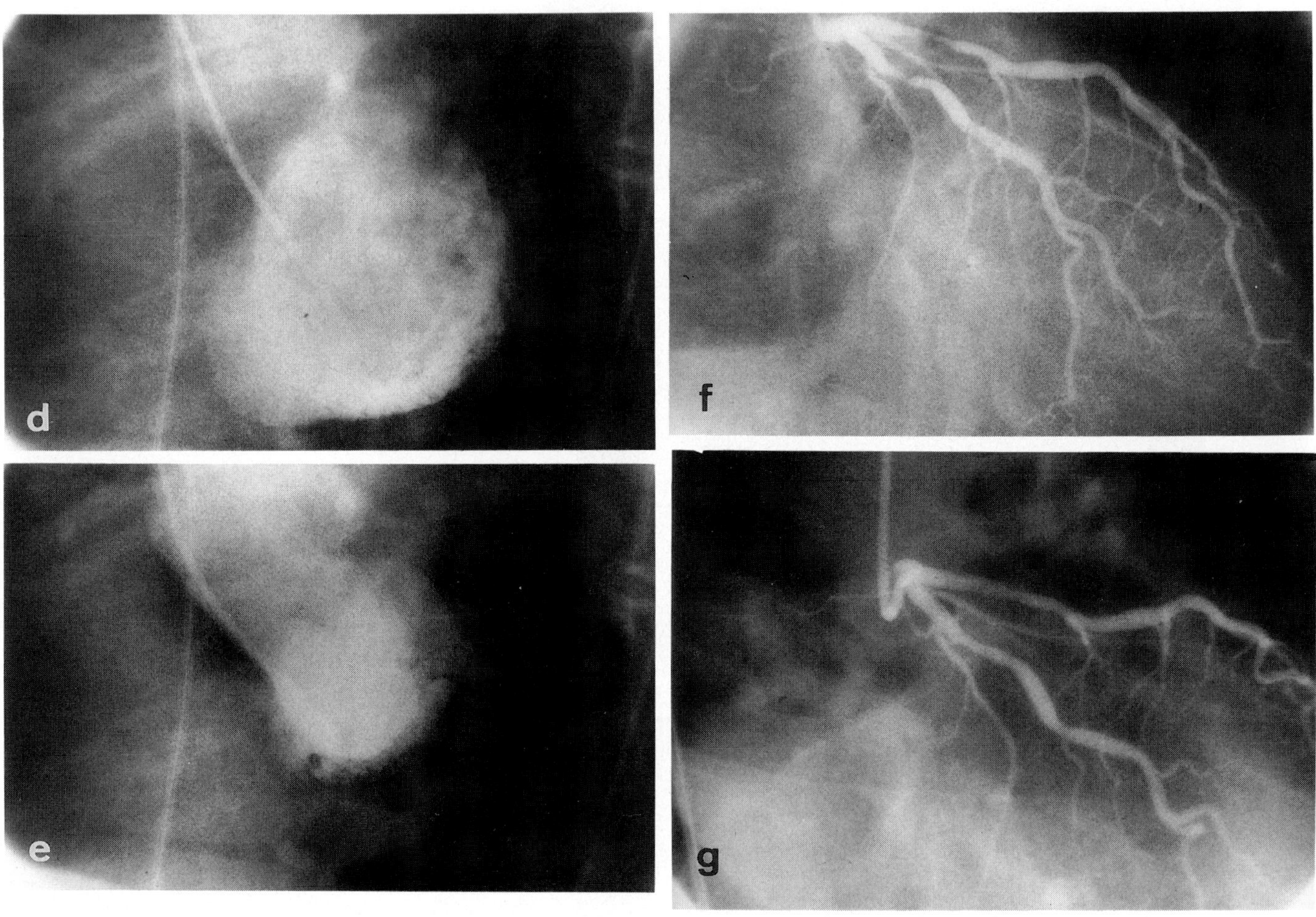

Figure 40 (Continued)

The left ventricular function was normal (Fig. 28d: diastole, Fig. 28e: systole). Five weeks later, angioplasty of the LAD and LCx was performed at the same sitting (Fig. 40f before, Fig. 40g after PTCA). The patient received heparin overnight. The next morning, 2 hours after discontinuation of heparin, the patient had acute chest pain,

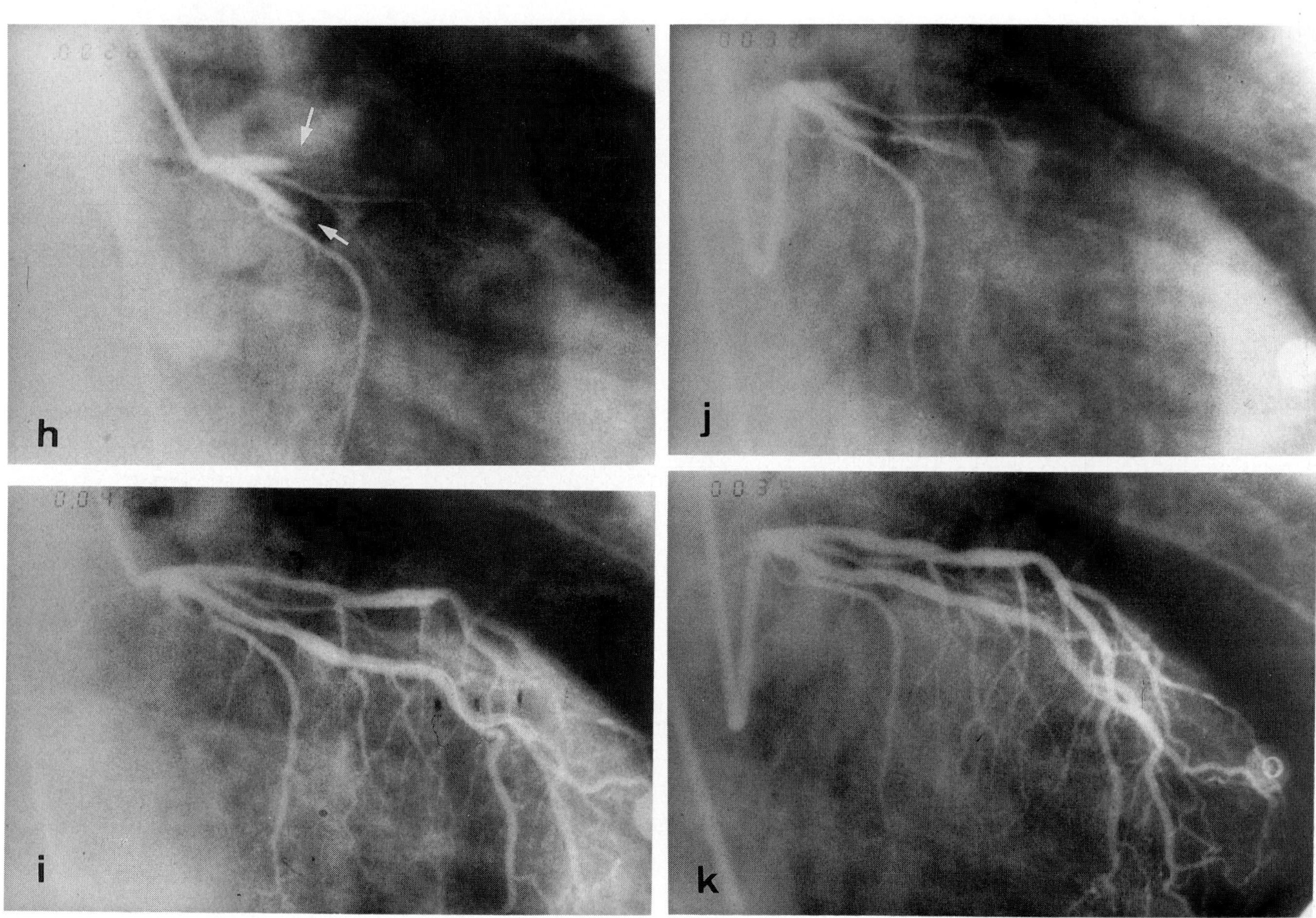

with ECG changes and hypotension with a systolic blood pressure of 60 mmHg. Angiography revealed occlusion of both vessels (Fig. 40h), which were redilated (Fig. 40i). However, both reoccluded immediately (Fig. 40j). The two vessels were then stented, with good immediate angiographic results (Fig. 40k). A control angiogram the next day revealed a good result (Fig. 40l). However, the left ventricular angiogram disclosed some hypokinesia of the territory supplied by the LCx (Fig. 40m: systole in RAO, Fig 40n: systole in LAO). On that occasion, the RCA lesion was seen to have progressed during the 5 weeks between the diagnostic study and the angioplasty (Fig. 40o,p) [to be compared with the earlier angiogram (Fig. 40b,c)]. It was planned to address this stenosis at a later session. A 6-month follow-up examination revealed restenosis at both dilated sites (Fig. 40q), the RCA stenosis had not progressed (Fig. 40r). The left ventriculogram still showed inferior hypokinesia (Fig. 40s: diastole, Fig 40t: systole), Elective CABG was performed. This patient demonstrates the possibility of simultaneous occlusion of two left main equivalent lesions and also the hazards of multivessel angioplasty, with increased procedural complications, future reinterventions, and often the need for CABG ultimately.

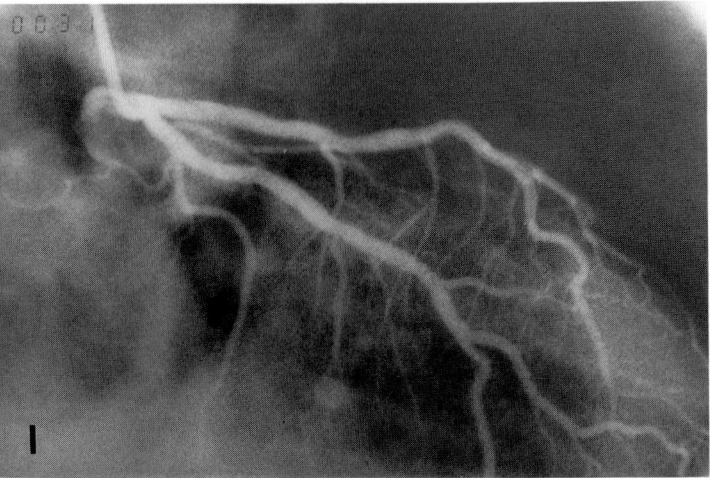

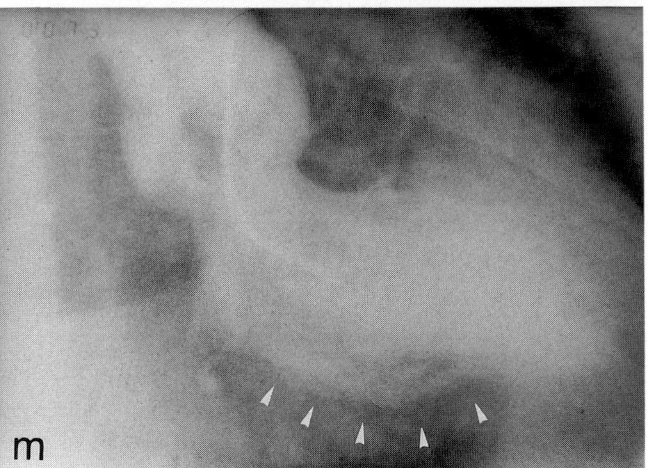

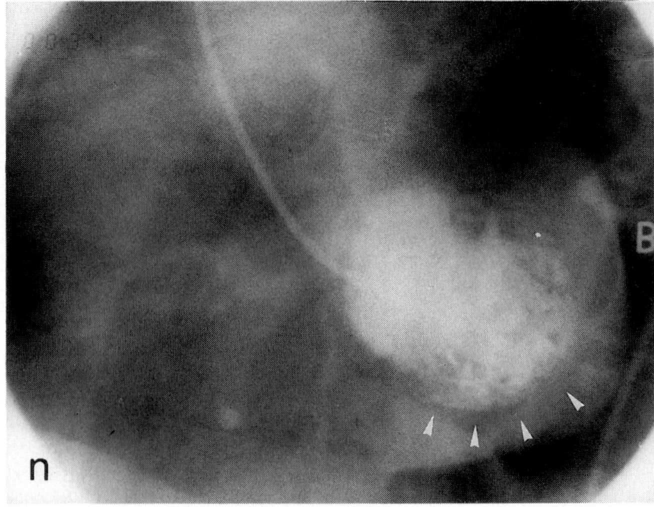

Figure 40 (Continued)

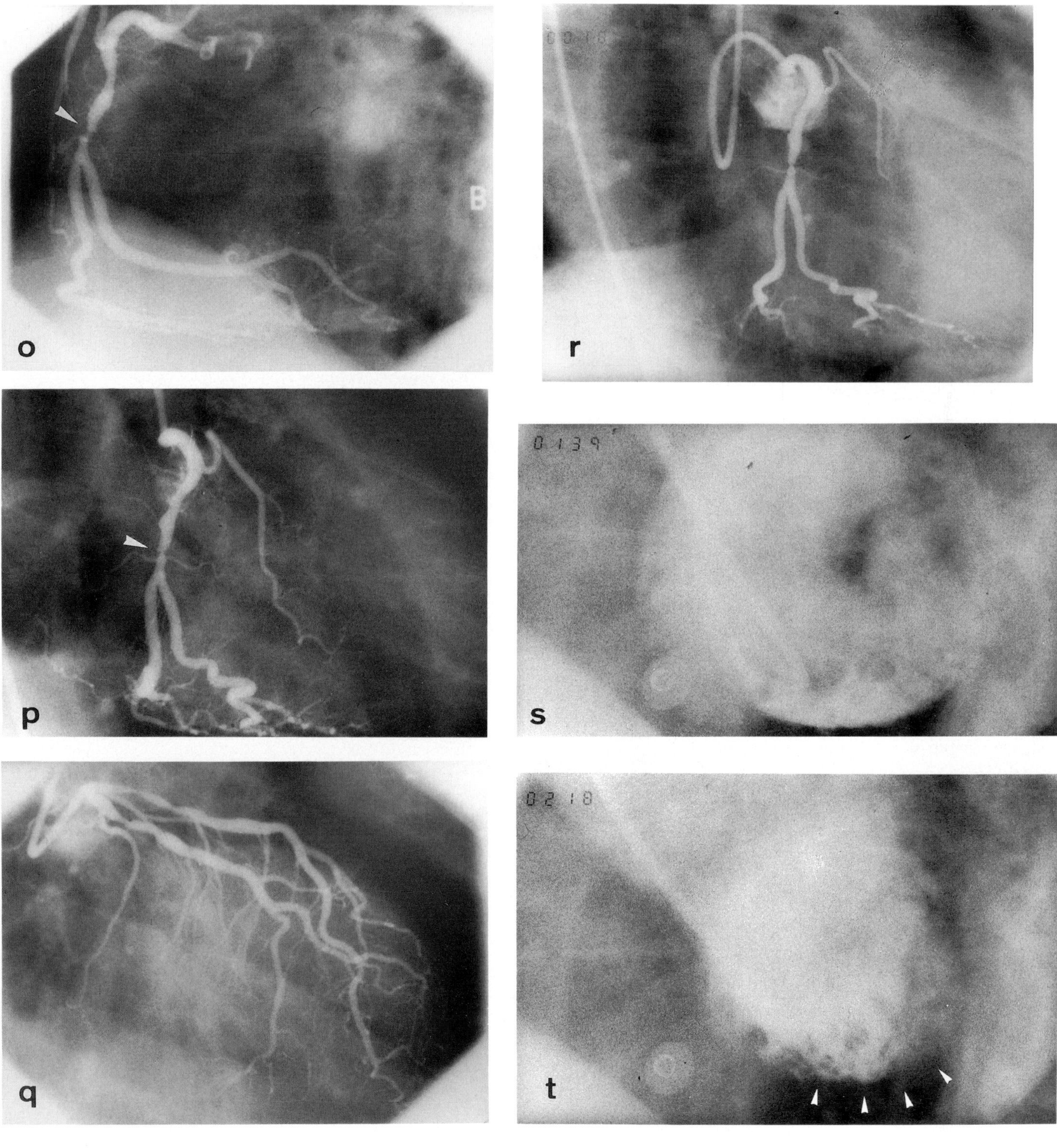
o
r
p
0 1 3 9
s
q
0 2 1 8
t

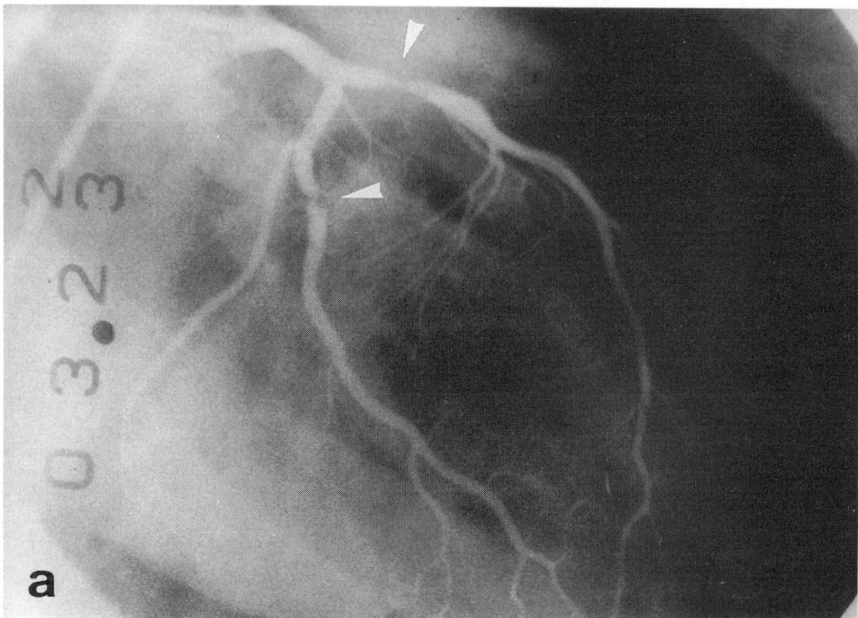
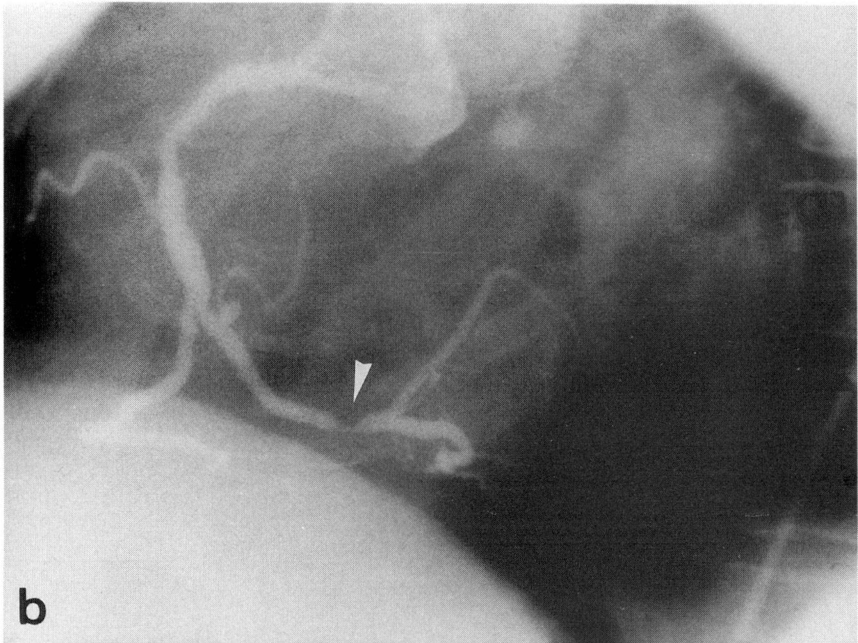

Figure 41

Triple-Vessel

Reports from several comparative and randomized studies suggest that bypass surgery is preferable to angioplasty in this setting. However, there are situations where angioplasty may be chosen over CABG. This includes patients with stenoses of distal vessels, following prior bypass surgery with graft attrition where the risk of repeat surgery is higher, or in patients in whom surgery is contraindicated due to old age or concurrent noncardiac disease. Triple-vessel angioplasty may be performed as a staged procedure. A 57-year-old man had stenoses of the proximal LAD, LCx (Fig. 41a), and distal RCA (Fig. 41b). The LAD stenosis was dilated first (since it supplied the major myocardial mass). Since the immediate result was good (Fig. 41c) the RCA lesion was dilated at the same sitting (Fig. 41d). The sheath was left

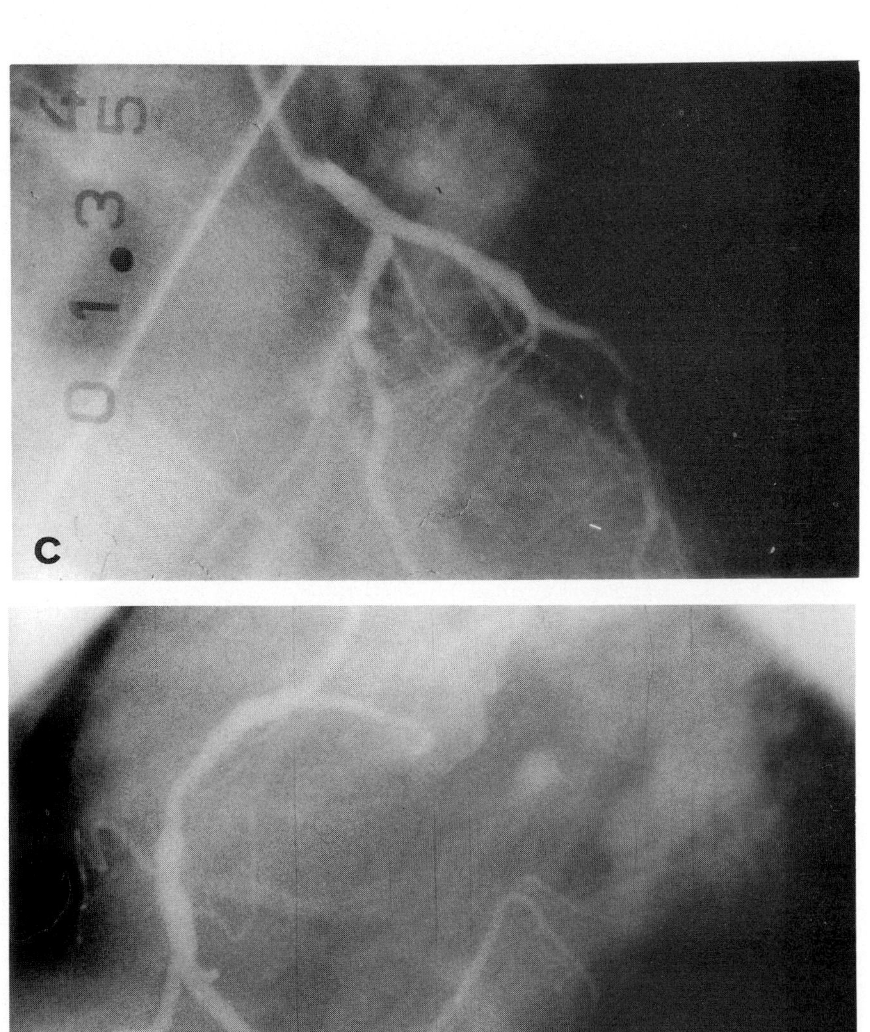
c
d

in place. The lesions were reassessed the next day, deemed stable, and LCx angioplasty performed (arrow) (Fig. 41e,f). The patient had an uneventful recovery. A routine angiogram performed 2 years later revealed an excellent long-term result with a normal left ventricular function (Fig. 41g,h).

The criteria to decide about which lesion should be approached first in a staged procedure are:

- The functional significance of the lesion, and the myocardial area subtended by the target vessel
- The complexity of the lesions
- The estimated probability of success (especially important with total occlusions)

The importance of each of these parameters will depend on the clinical setting. If multivessel angioplasty is chosen in a patient in whom bypass surgery is an option, the most difficult/

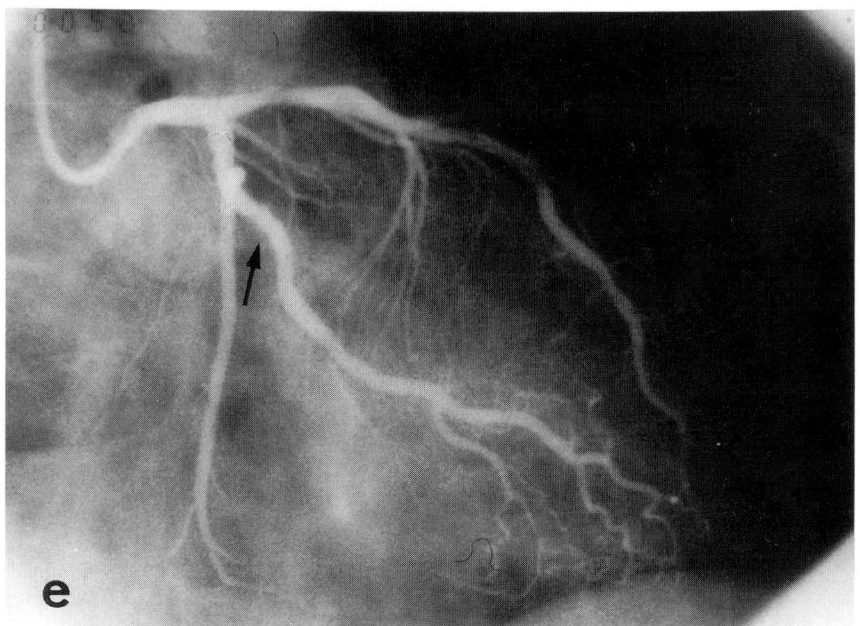

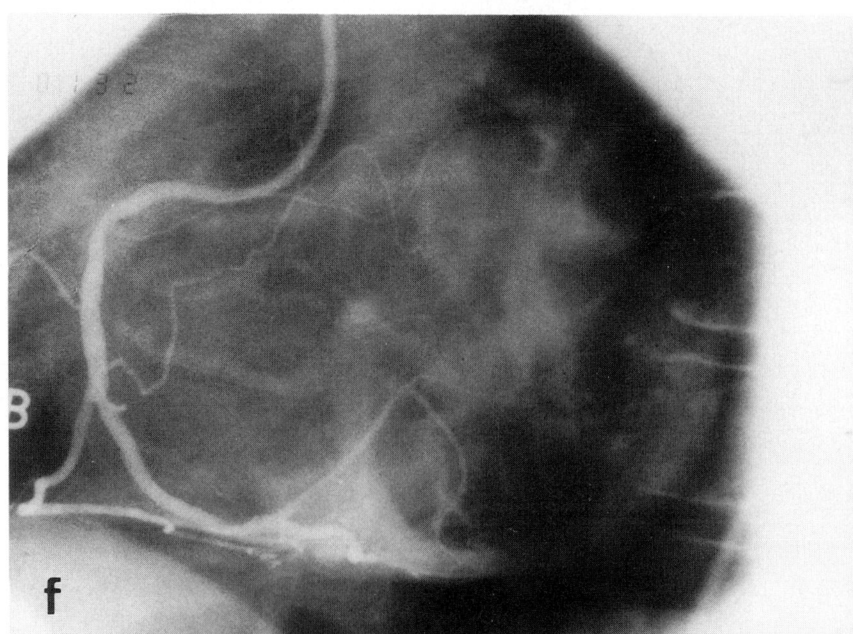

Figure 41 (Continued)

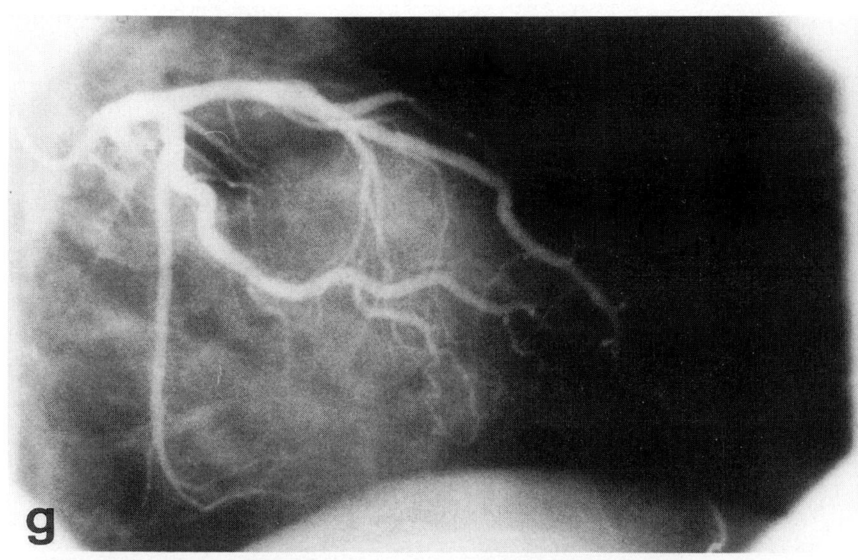

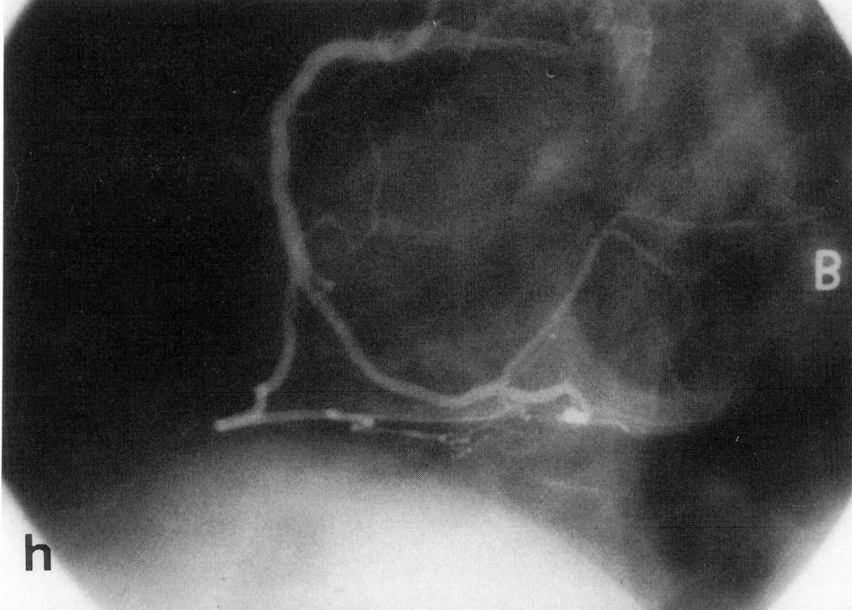

complex lesion should be attempted first ("worst first"), so that a failure or unacceptable result would qualify the patient for surgery. However, in a patient in whom surgery is not an option, or where one lesion is clearly more significant clinically than the others ("culprit lesion"), the stenosis that is hemodynamically most significant should be attempted first. If for some reason the other vessels cannot be addressed at the same sitting (dye load, borderline angioplasty result, excessively long procedure, etc.), the patient can still profit sufficiently from the intervention. Another benefit of a strategy to dilate the more important vessel first derives from the fact that this vessel can be closely surveyed for an extended period of time while the second vessel is treated. This affords the possibility to reintervene on it quickly should the result deteriorate or an acute occlusion occur.

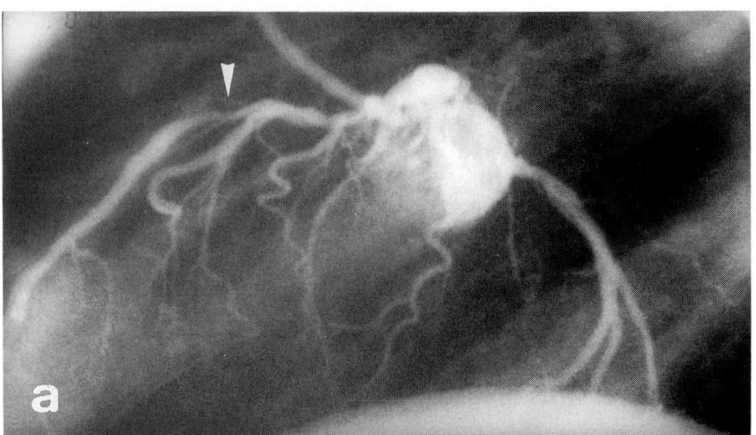

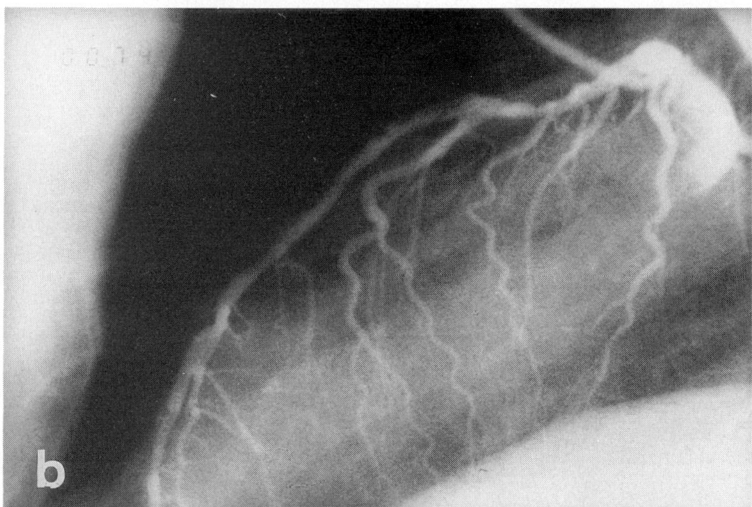

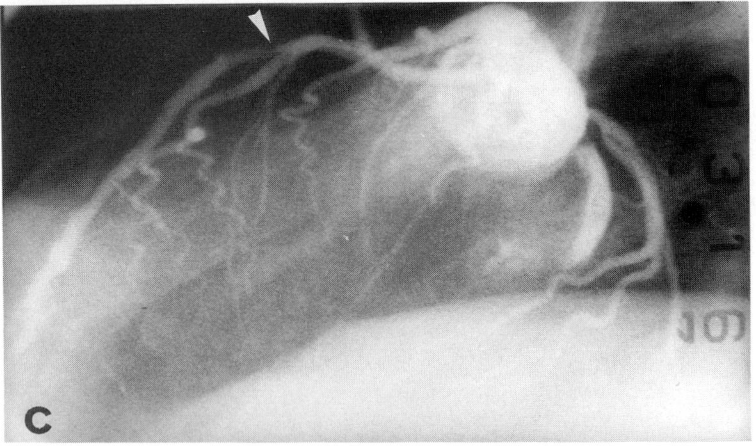

Figure 42

Multivessel angioplasty of a different kind may be performed over several years for progressive disease. A 60-year-old man with angina and an LAD lesion (Fig. 42a) underwent angioplasty with a resultant dissection (Fig. 42b), which was managed conservatively (no stent). A control angiogram 3 months later revealed restenosis (Fig. 42c), and repeat PTCA was performed with a good result (Fig. 42d). The patient presented 2 years later with angina. The LAD had remained patent (Fig. 42e). The LCx was found to be occluded (Fig. 42f), with good collaterization. It was recanalized successfully (Fig. 42g). Another 2 years later, while the long-term results in the other vessels looked good, angioplasty became necessary for a tandem lesion of

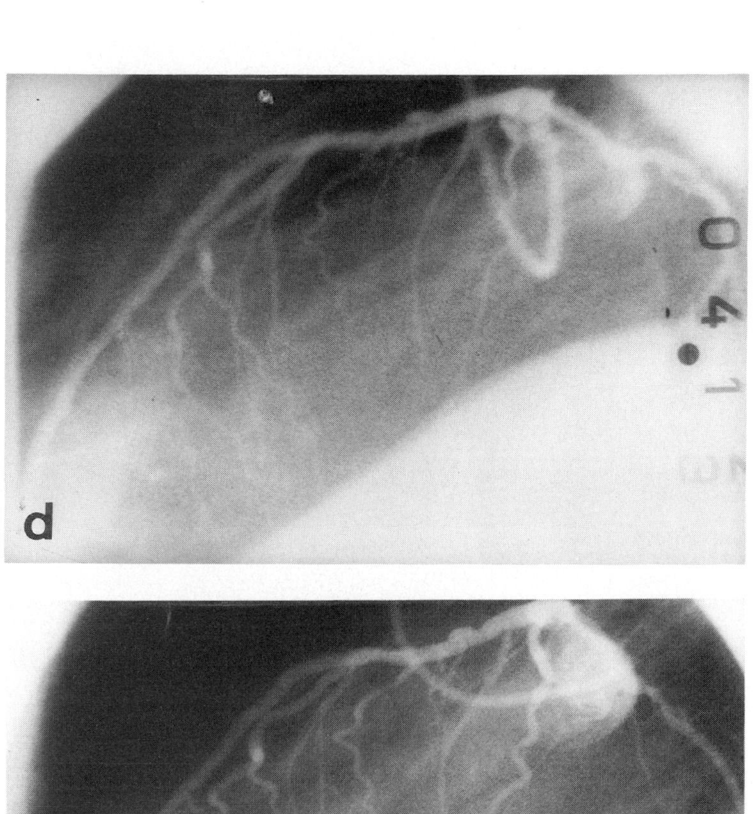
d

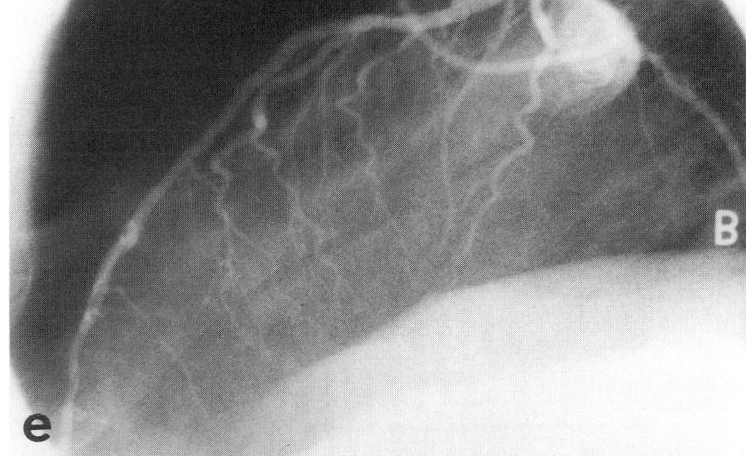
B
e

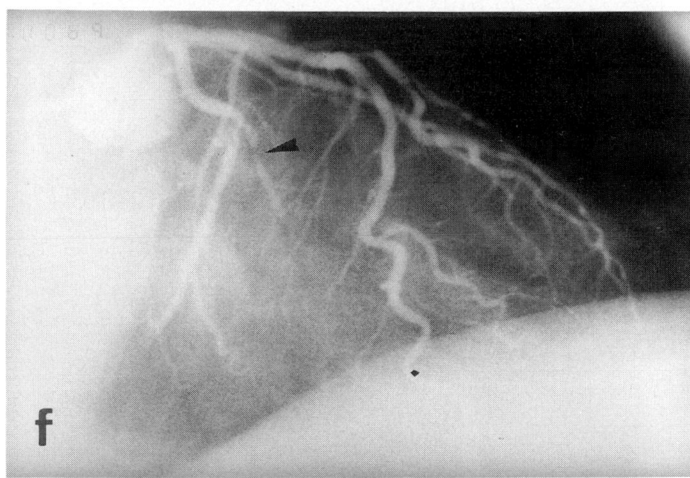
f

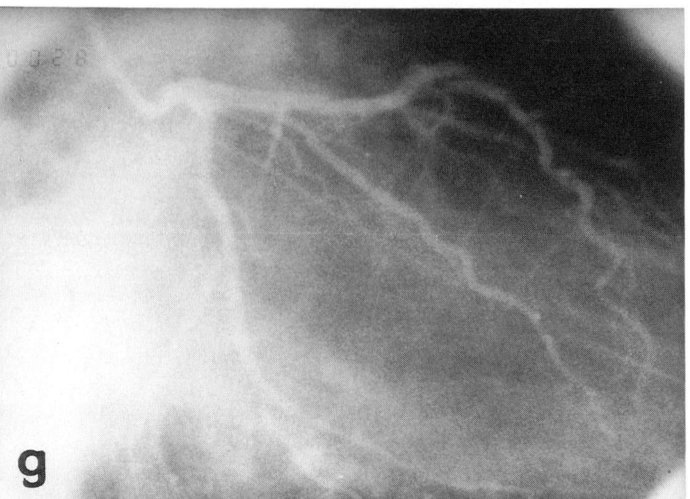

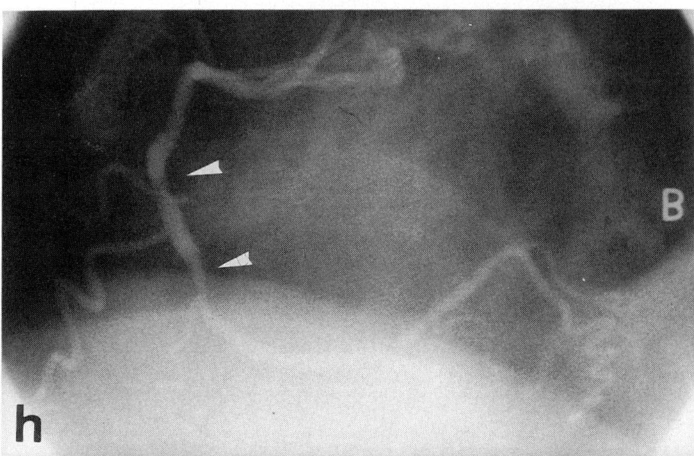

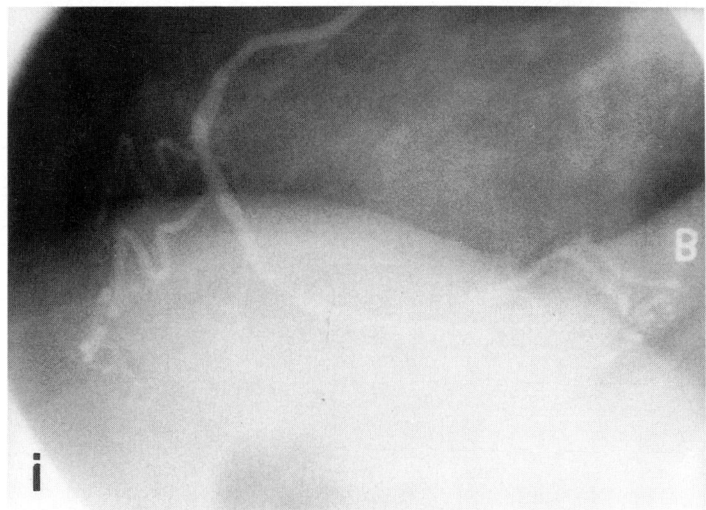

Figure 42 (Continued)

the RCA (Fig. 42h). This was performed with a good result (Fig. 42i). This example demonstrates another advantage of angioplasty over surgery. If the patient (or his referring physician) had selected surgery in the first place, the patient would have required another CABG (with its increased procedural risks) 2 years, or at least 4 years, later for disease progression. Although restenosis following angioplasty made the patient return for an additional intervention on the LAD, putting the total PTCA count up to 4, this was clearly the better option in the long run.

2.2 TOTAL OCCLUSION ANGIOPLASTY

When dealing with total occlusion angioplasty, success depends on several factors, primarily the duration of occlusion (which can be determined by the history and presence of bridging collaterals), the presence of a visible stump, and the length of the occlusion. Recent occlusions include occlusions less than 2 weeks old. These lesions are relatively soft and easy to cross.

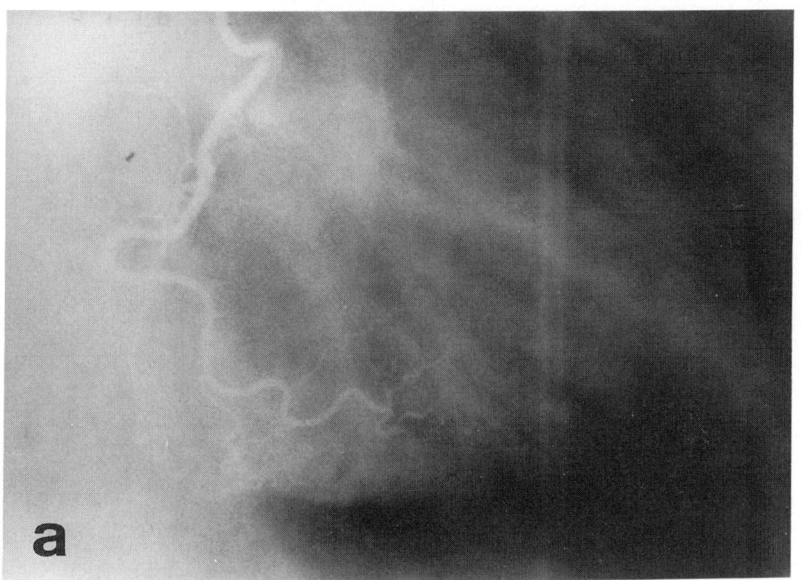

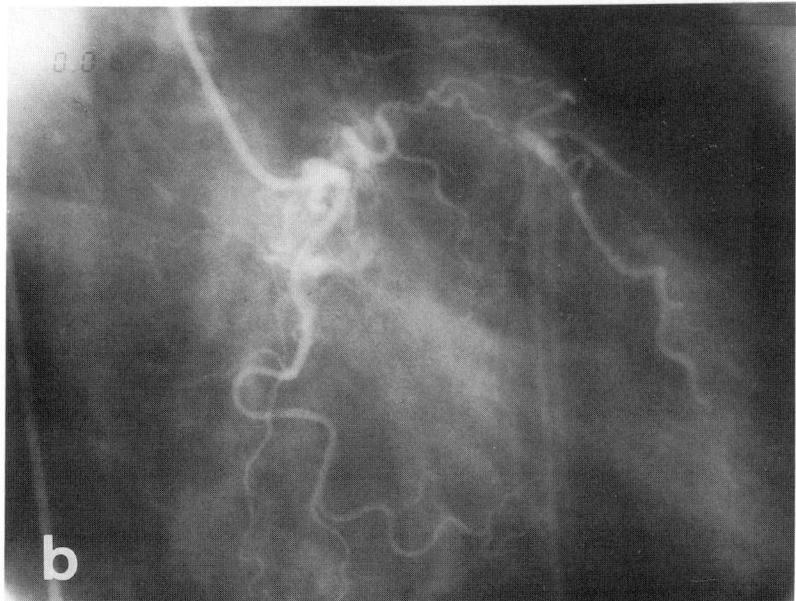

Figure 43

Nevertheless, a balloon can be used to brace the wire if it does not cross by itself. A success rate of greater than 90% can be expected for these lesions.

PTCA of chronic occlusions, defined as occlusions more than 2 weeks and less than several months old, is associated with success rates of about 70 to 80%. For old chronic occlusions (older than 3 months), the chances of success are lower, ranging between 30 and 70%, depending on lesion morphology and duration of occlusion.

For angioplasty of occlusions it is essential to have a viable region of myocardium, hence an akinetic or dyskinetic segment, and absence of visible collaterals to the occluded vessel should be considered contraindications to angioplasty. In this setting, the procedure would have no benefit even if technically successful. However, it is essential to look diligently for collaterals, especially when dealing with LAD occlusions, which may receive collaterals from the circle of Vieusens. If the conal branch of the RCA has a separate ostium, or the RCA is deeply intubated during injection, collaterals to the LAD may be overlooked (Fig. 43a). Injecting with the catheter less deeply intubated in the RCA showed

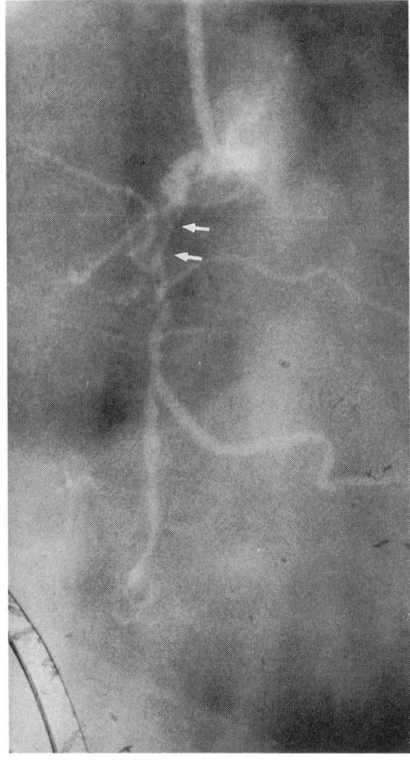

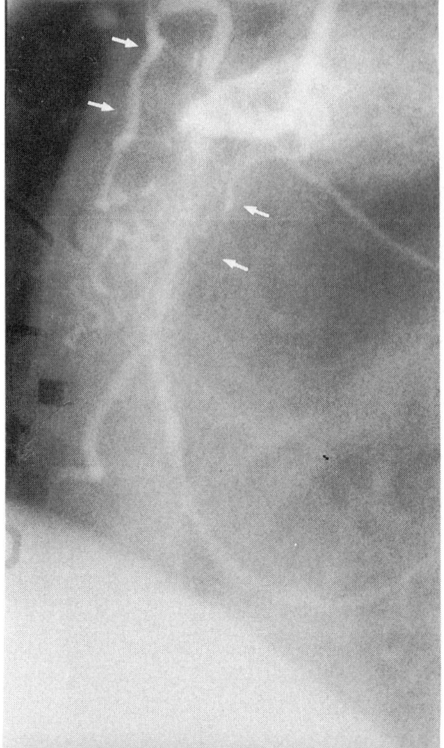

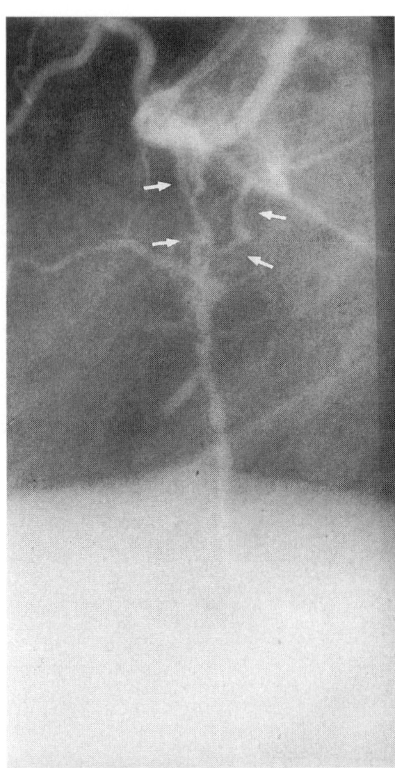

Figure 44

adequate collaterals to the LAD in this patient (Fig. 43b). Failure to have looked for the conal branch may have resulted in angioplasty not being offered to a suitable candidate. Similarly, the risk of LAD angioplasty in a patient with a nontotal LAD lesion may be overestimated by such an oversight.

The presence of bridging collaterals (Fig. 44) indicates long-standing occlusions. Such collaterals are harbingers of a lesion that cannot be crossed, and should contraindicate an angioplasty attempt. Sometimes a single bridging collateral (Fig. 45) can supply the distal vessel well, as in this patient with situs inversus and an occluded RCA. If angioplasty is attempted in such circumstances, it may compromise the collateral channel, leading to infarction.

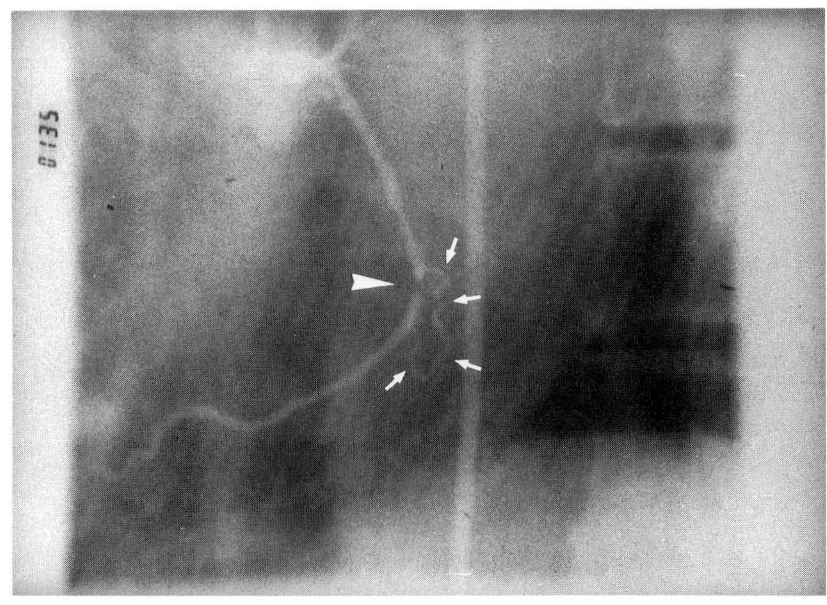

Figure 45

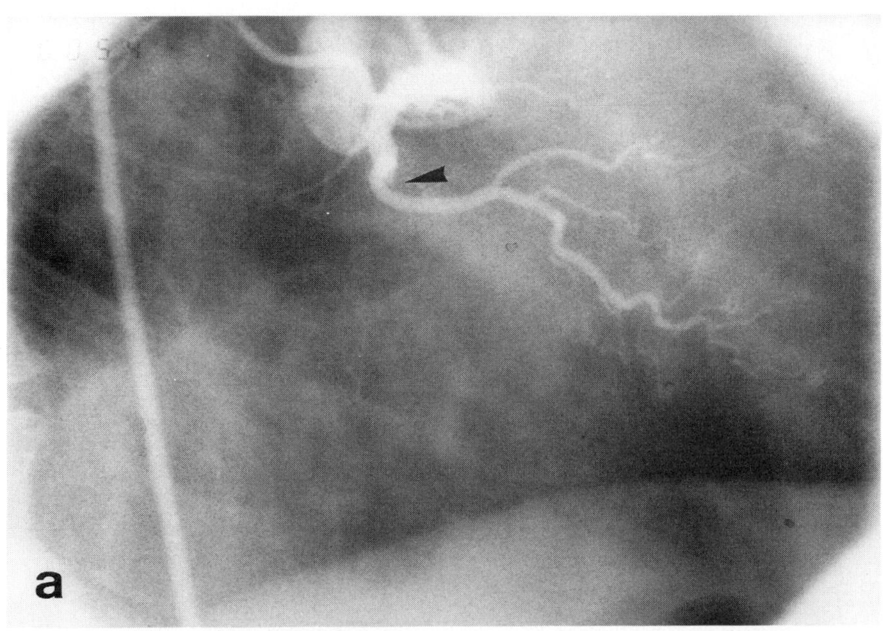

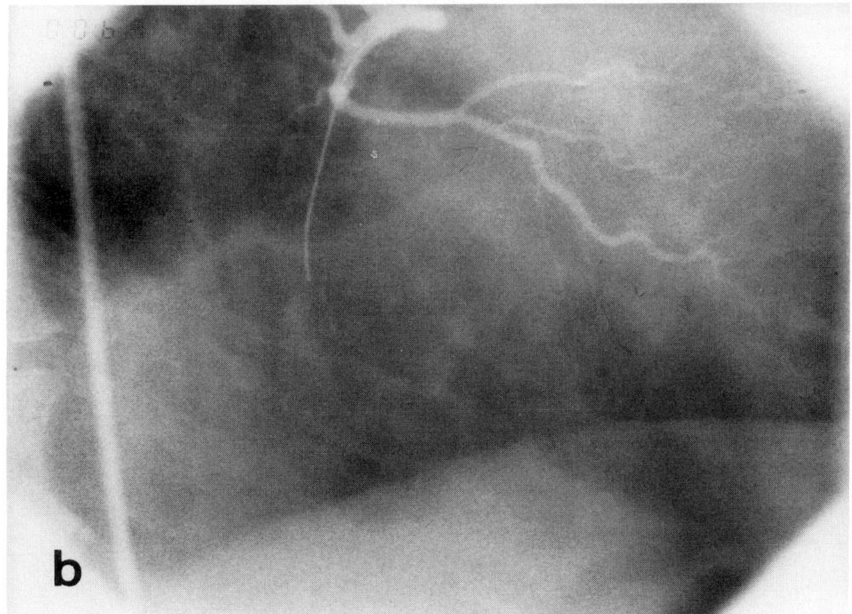

Figure 46

The chances of creating false (subintimal) channels during an angioplasty attempt are high while attempting chronic occlusions. Although fixed-wire balloons can be used for fresh occlusions, an over-the-wire or Monorail system is preferable for older lesions. A 66-year-old man with a freshly occluded RCA (Fig. 46a) underwent recanalization using a fixed-wire system (Omniflex-Medtronic). The wire was advanced across the obstruction, where it got stuck. A test injection was unable to define whether the true lumen had been found (Fig. 46b) until a "blind" balloon inflation had been carried out (Fig. 46c) with the risk of not being correctly placed. The result was good in this case (Fig. 46d). Disadvantages of using a fixed-wire system for recanalization of occlusions include the impossibility of stiffening the wire tip for crossing tough lesions. Additionally, a distal injection cannot be made, and the wire has to be advanced in a more-or-less blind fashion. A technique for avoiding wire passage in a false lumen is to inject dye after each advance of the guidewire. In a Monorail system the dye tracks along the balloon lumen into the distal artery as a faked distal injection, which reveals whether one is in the correct channel. This is demonstrated by a 45-year-old man who presented with a

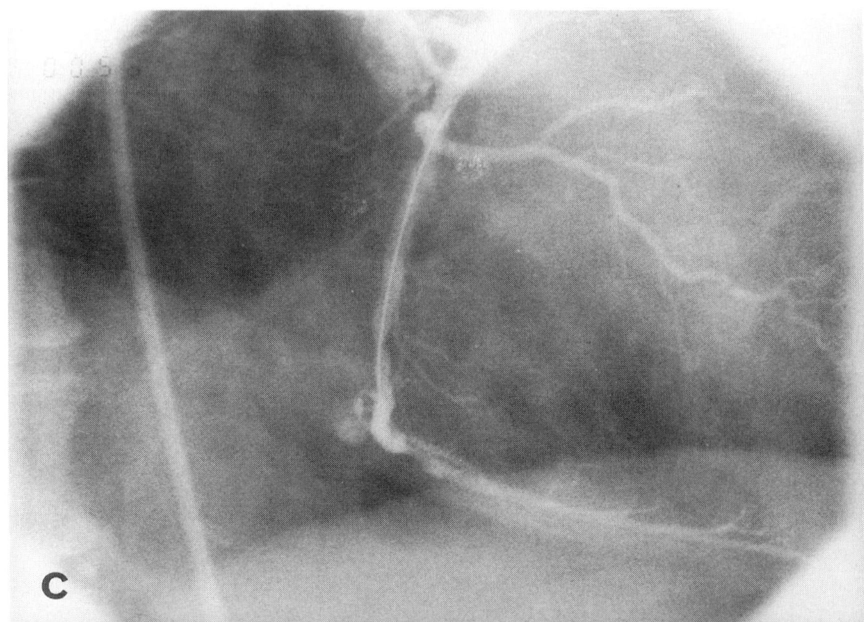

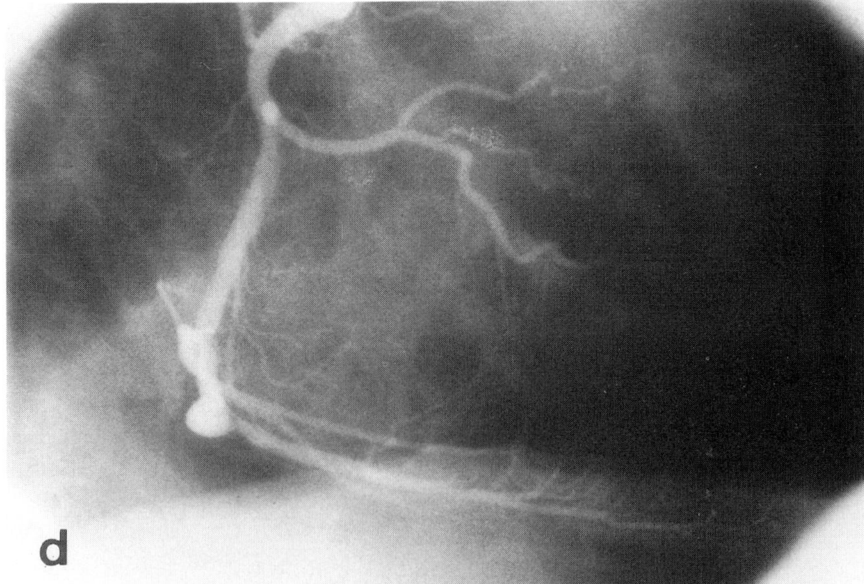

Figure 46 (Continued)

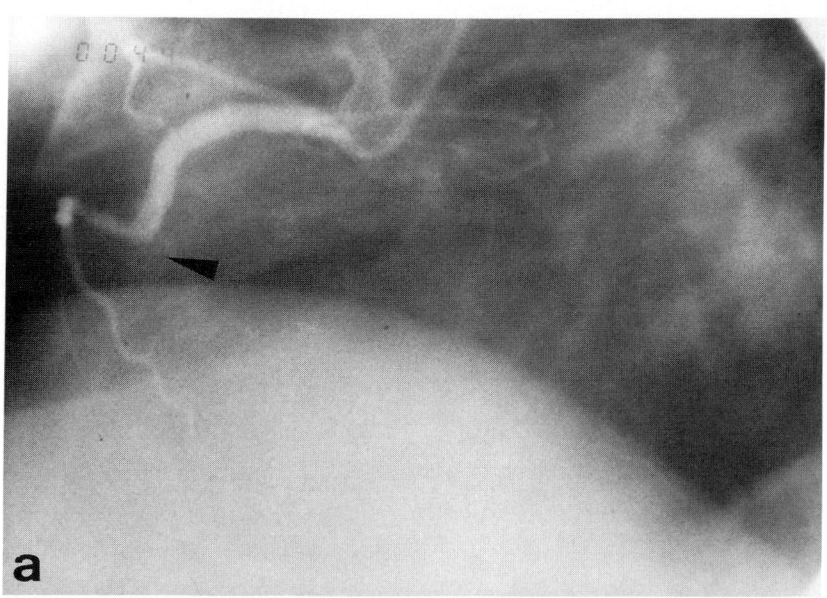

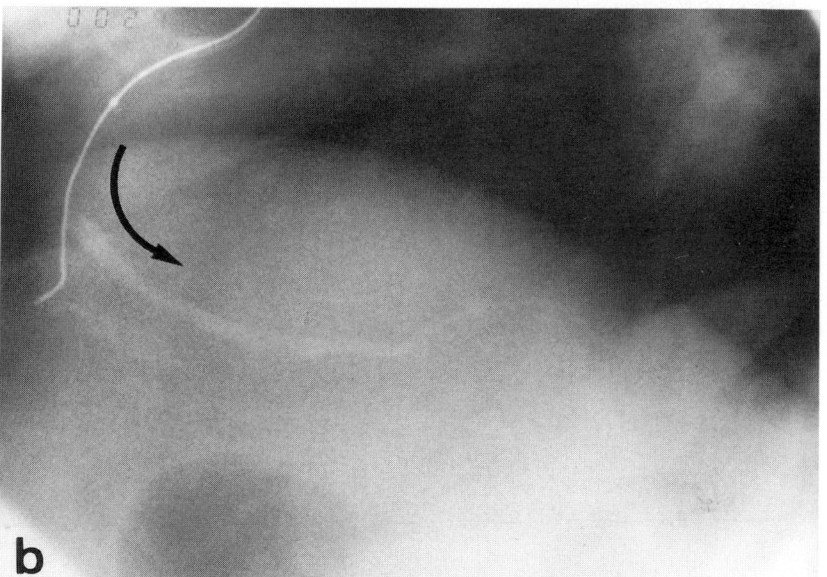

Figure 47

2-week-old occlusion of the RCA (Fig. 47a). The lesion was approached with a Magnum wire with a nonopaque ball tip. The Magnarail balloon was advanced over the wire up to the stenosis, for increased backup support to the wire. The wire was then advanced into the occlusion. At this stage, slight resistance was felt, and an injection was performed through the guiding catheter to obtain a faked distal injection. The reason for the difficulty in advancing the wire now became evident (Fig. 47b), it being in a side branch. The wire was repositioned, and angioplasty performed (Fig. 47c), with a good final result (Fig. 47d) (the arrow points to the branch in which the wire had entered previously). The technique of faked distal injection is also useful to distinguish between wire passage in the true lumen (where the faked distal injection distinctly shows the distal vessel) to that in a false lumen (where the faked distal injection results in staining of the vessel wall, with dye holdup). In such an event the true lumen can sometimes be reentered by acutely curving the guidewire and attempting another angle of entry.

Sometimes, pushing along a dissected plane may result in reentry into the true lumen distally. This can safely be attempted when dealing with occlusions since no worse can happen than a failure in an already occluded vessel. Subsequent balloon dilatation may re-

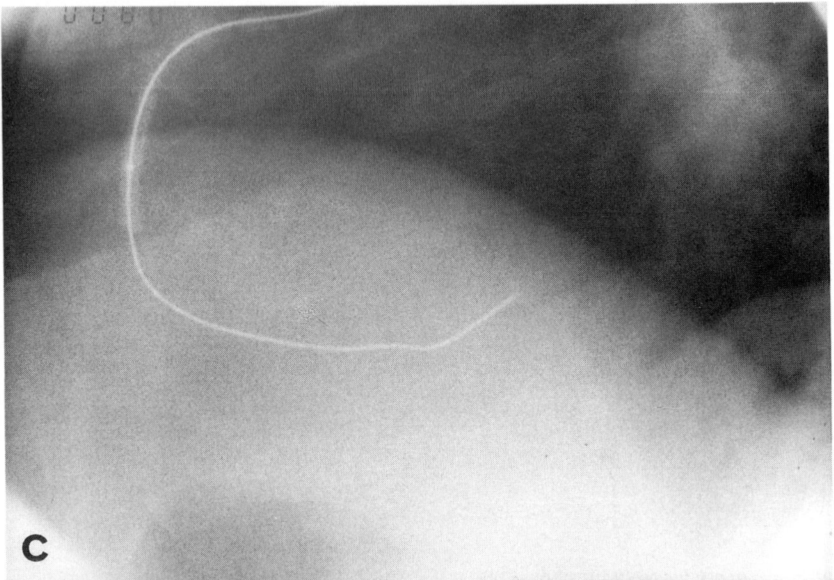

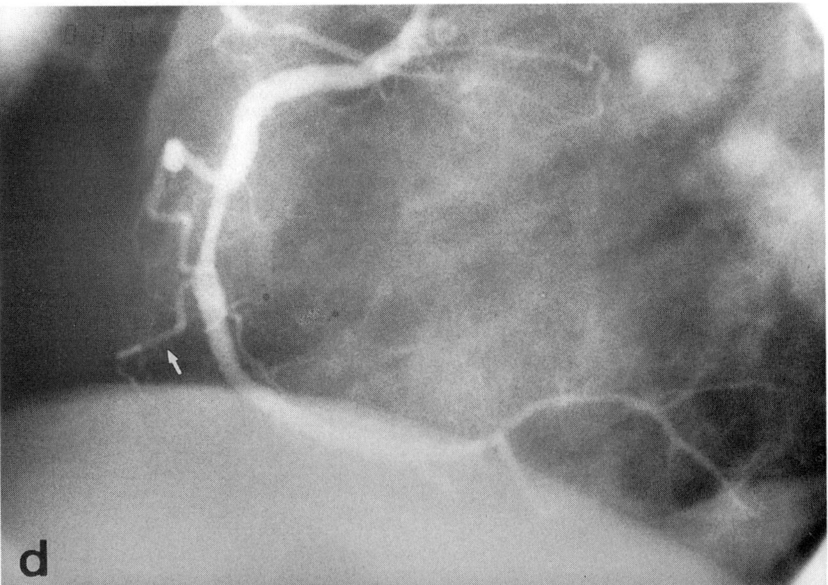

Figure 47 (Continued)

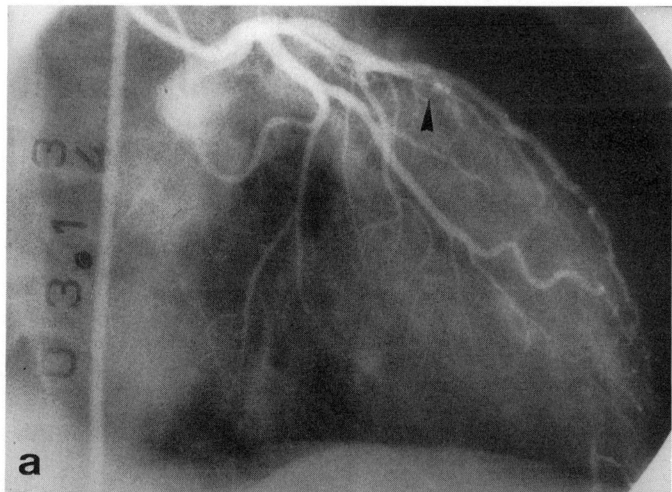

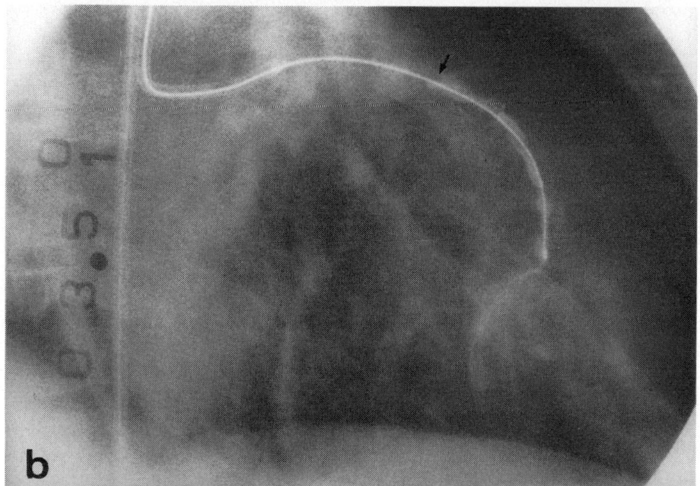

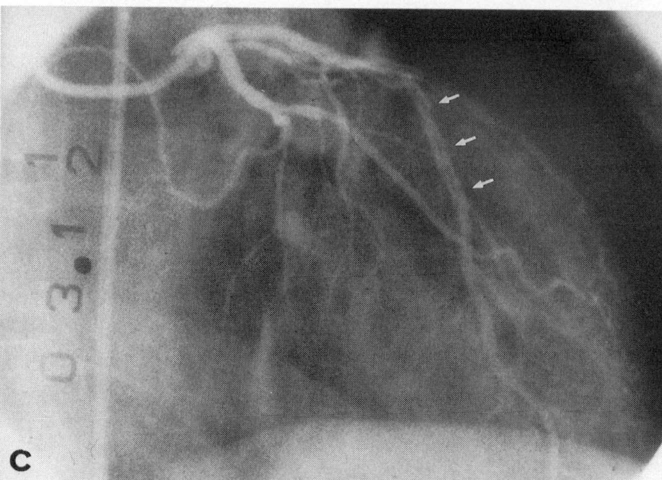

Figure 48

sult in a large dissection and a patent vessel. Such dissections may ultimately heal, with surprisingly good results. A 64-year-old man underwent angioplasty for an occluded LAD (Fig. 48a). However, the Magnum wire entered into a false lumen (Fig. 48b), evident by intimal staining and holdup of dye. By pushing the wire further, it suddenly reentered the true lumen, and angioplasty was performed, with a resultant long dissection (Fig. 48c). The distal flow was good. Such a result is acceptable in a vessel that was occluded in the first place and may heal spontaneously. Other cases may not turn out so favorably, as in a patient with an occluded RCA (Fig. 49a). An-

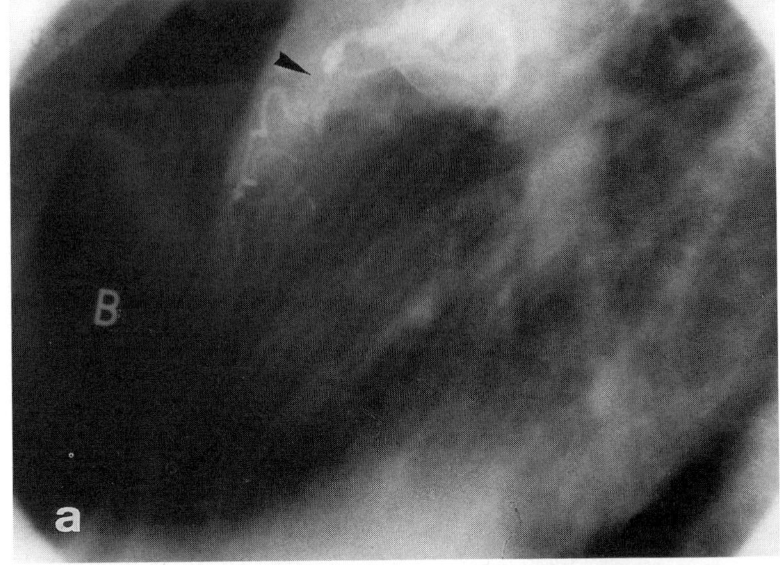

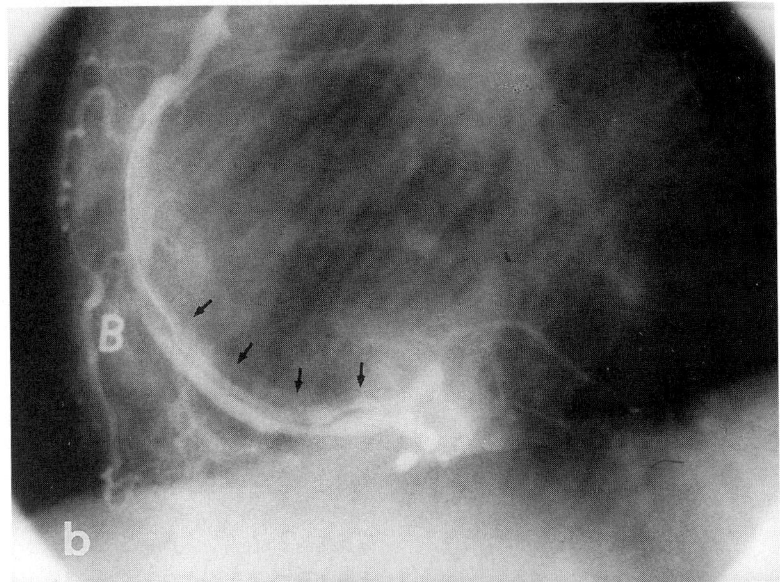

Figure 49

gioplasty resulted in a long dissection (Fig. 49b), with a high probability of acute closure. However, this is not dangerous, since the vessel had been closed and vessel reocclusion is innocuous in such cases.

A Magnum wire–Magnarail balloon system is well suited for occlusion angioplasty. Figure 50 describes the steps in using this system. The wire is initially steered into the stump of the occluded vessel (Fig. 50a,b). Crossing the lesion is briefly attempted with the wire alone. If this is not successful (typical to occlusions more than a few days old), a Magnarail balloon of adequate size is advanced onto the tip of the wire, and lesion crossing is reattempted with the added support offered by the balloon (Fig. 50c). Successful crossing of the lesion is evident

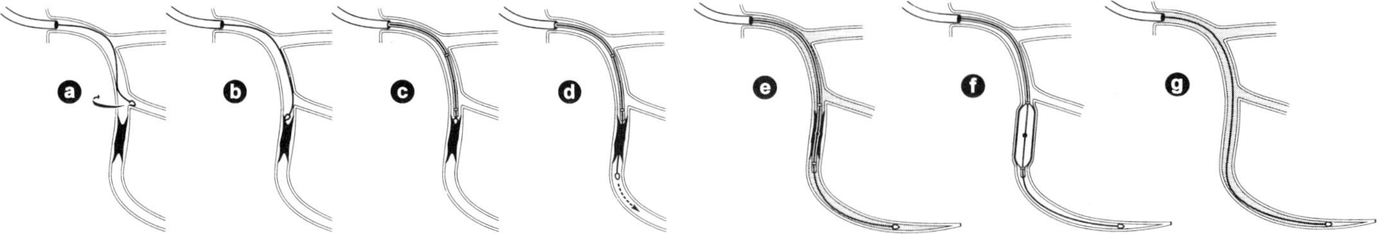

Figure 50

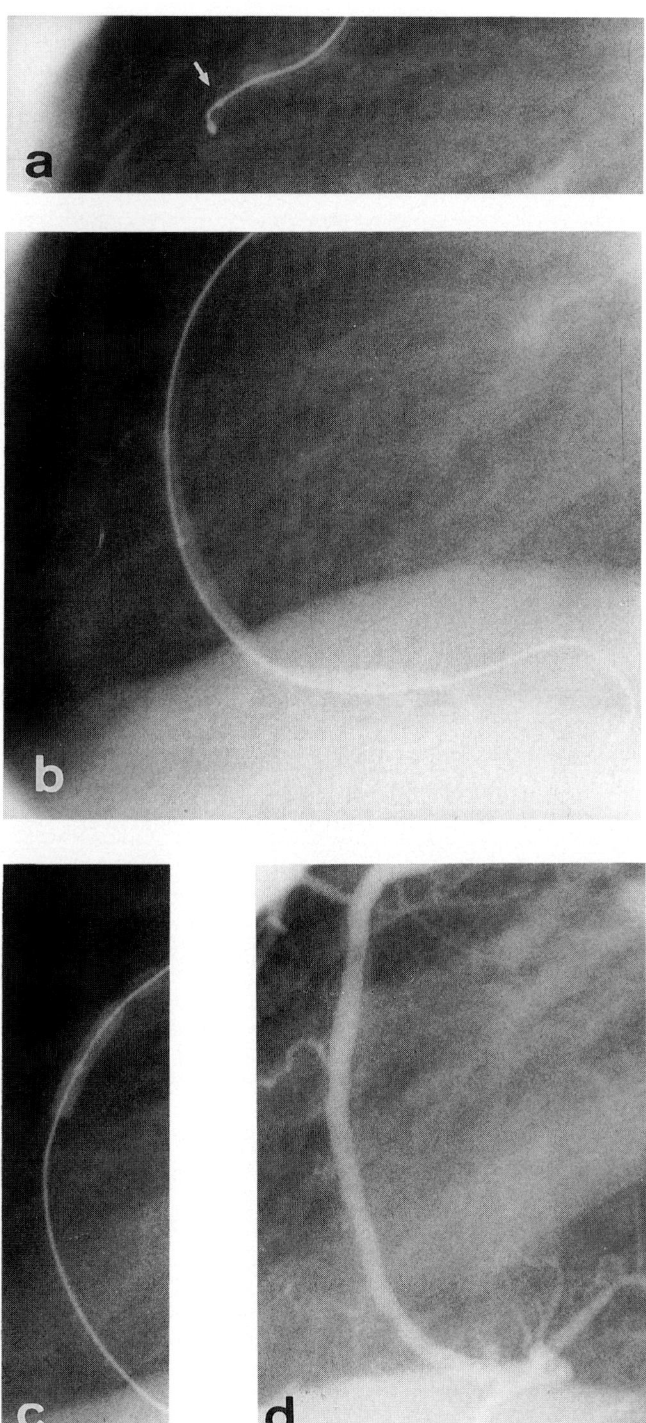

Figure 51

by a popping sensation in some cases and free distal passage of the wire (Fig. 50d). The location of the wire within the true vessel lumen can be further confirmed by advancing the balloon into the lesion and making a faked distal injection (Fig. 50e). Dilatation is then carried out (Fig. 50f) and the result assessed with a dye injection after removal of the balloon (Fig. 50g).

Another method of using the Magnum wire, especially in cases in which the projected chance of success is low, is demonstrated in a 35-year-old patient with an occluded RCA. A Magnum wire was advanced onto the occlusion but could not cross it alone. The wire was supported with a Magnarail probing catheter (which has a distal marker) (Fig. 51a). This helps in supporting the Magnum wire for additional pushing power, similar to a Magnarail balloon. Additionally, the catheter lumen can be used to make a distal dye injection (Fig. 51b) to confirm the position of the catheter in the true lumen. Successful angioplasty was performed with a 3.0-mm Magnarail balloon (Fig. 51c), with a good result (Fig. 51d). Such an approach using a Magnarail probing catheter instead of a Magnarail balloon is cost-effective in cases with a low probability of success, since it saves the cost of the balloon in case of failure. However, if recanalization does succeed, it will ultimately result in the added expenditure of the probing catheter in addition to a balloon.

2.3 COLLATERALS

Collaterals play a pivotal role in the approach to occlusion angioplasty. As described above, the total absence of a collateral supply to the occluded artery (indicating a nonviable myocardium), or the presence of local bridging collaterals (indicating a chronic occlusion with a low chance of success) constitute contraindications to angioplasty. Collaterals serve as markers of viable myocardium, and if adequate, supply the recipient artery with blood equal to a 90% stenosis. Additionally, knowledge of collaterals to the myocardium supplied by a nonoccluded vessel is of great importance in general pre- and post-PTCA risk stratification. Angioplasty to a vessel with a good collateral supply reduces the risk of a major infarction in the event of acute closure.

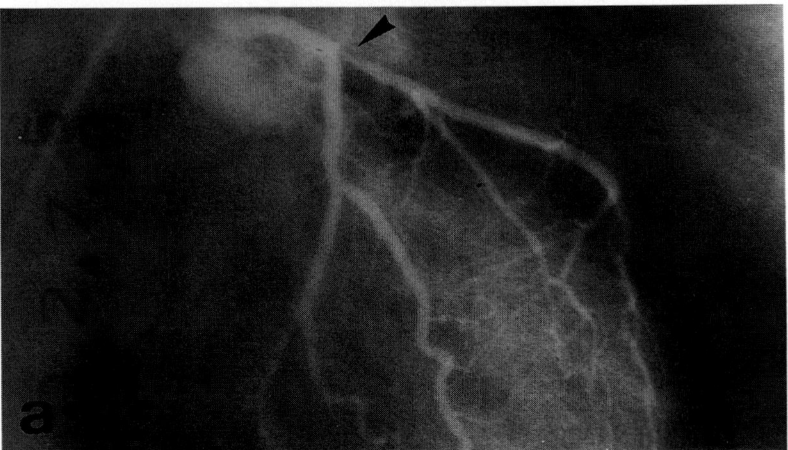

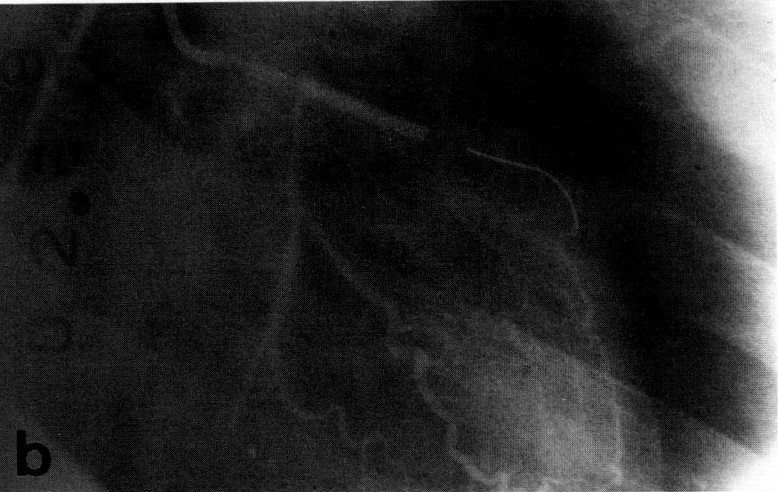

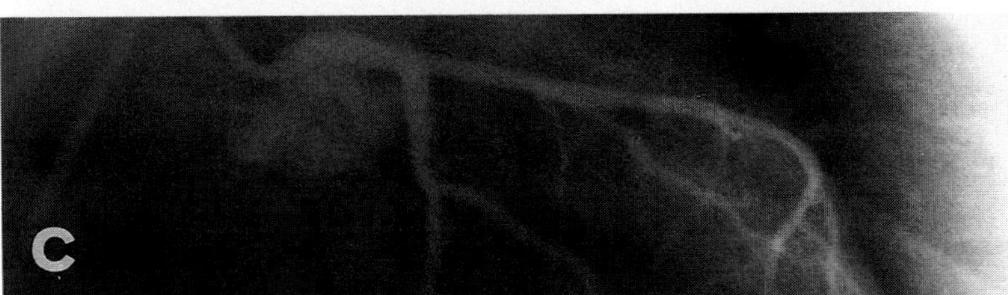

Figure 52

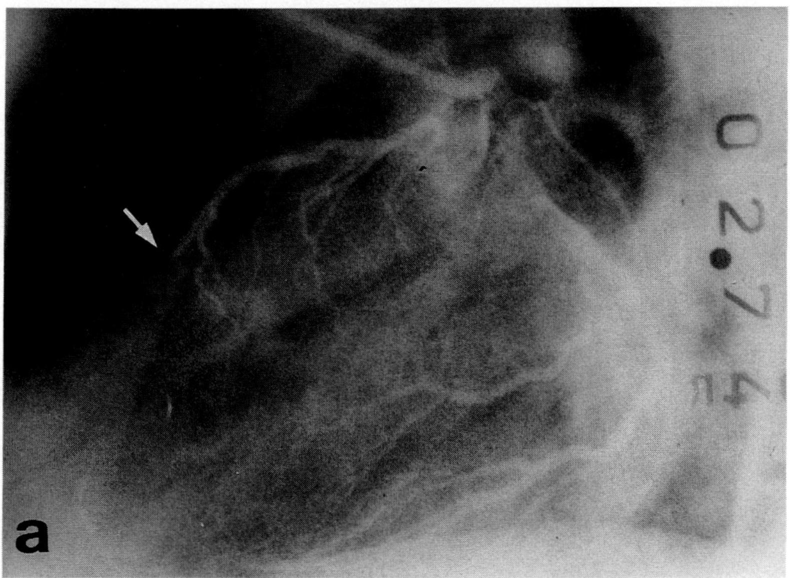

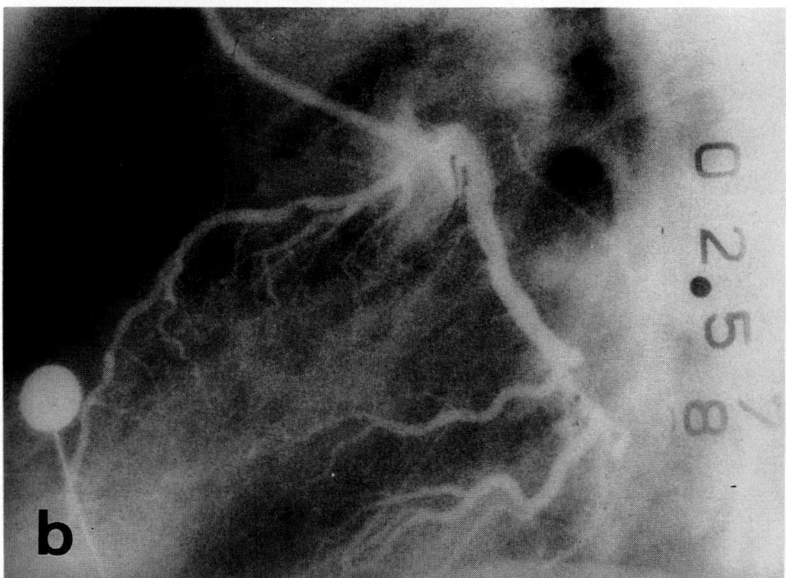

Figure 53

In such a situation one can rest assured that vessel closure will have little hemodynamic significance. If such collaterals are not seen on the diagnostic film, it is helpful to inject dye into the coronary artery while the balloon is inflated. If a Monorail system is used the dye trickles down the catheter into the distal vessel as a faked distal injection. If the dye gets washed out rapidly from the distal vessel, this indicates a good collateral supply, be it ipsilateral or contralateral. If the dye hangs up distally, with no clearing off, the collateral supply is poor. If using a fixed-wire system or a non-Monorail balloon, ipsilateral collaterals can be demonstrated by injecting into the vessel with the balloon inflated and looking for opacification of the vessel distal to the balloon, as in a patient with an LAD stenosis dilated through a diagnostic 5F catheter (Fig. 52a), with opacification of the distal vessel (Fig. 52b) revealing a good collateral supply. Similar information can be obtained from the patient's symptoms and ECG changes during the balloon inflation. A well-tolerated inflation without significant ECG changes indicates good collaterals unless the reperfused myocardium is already infarcted.

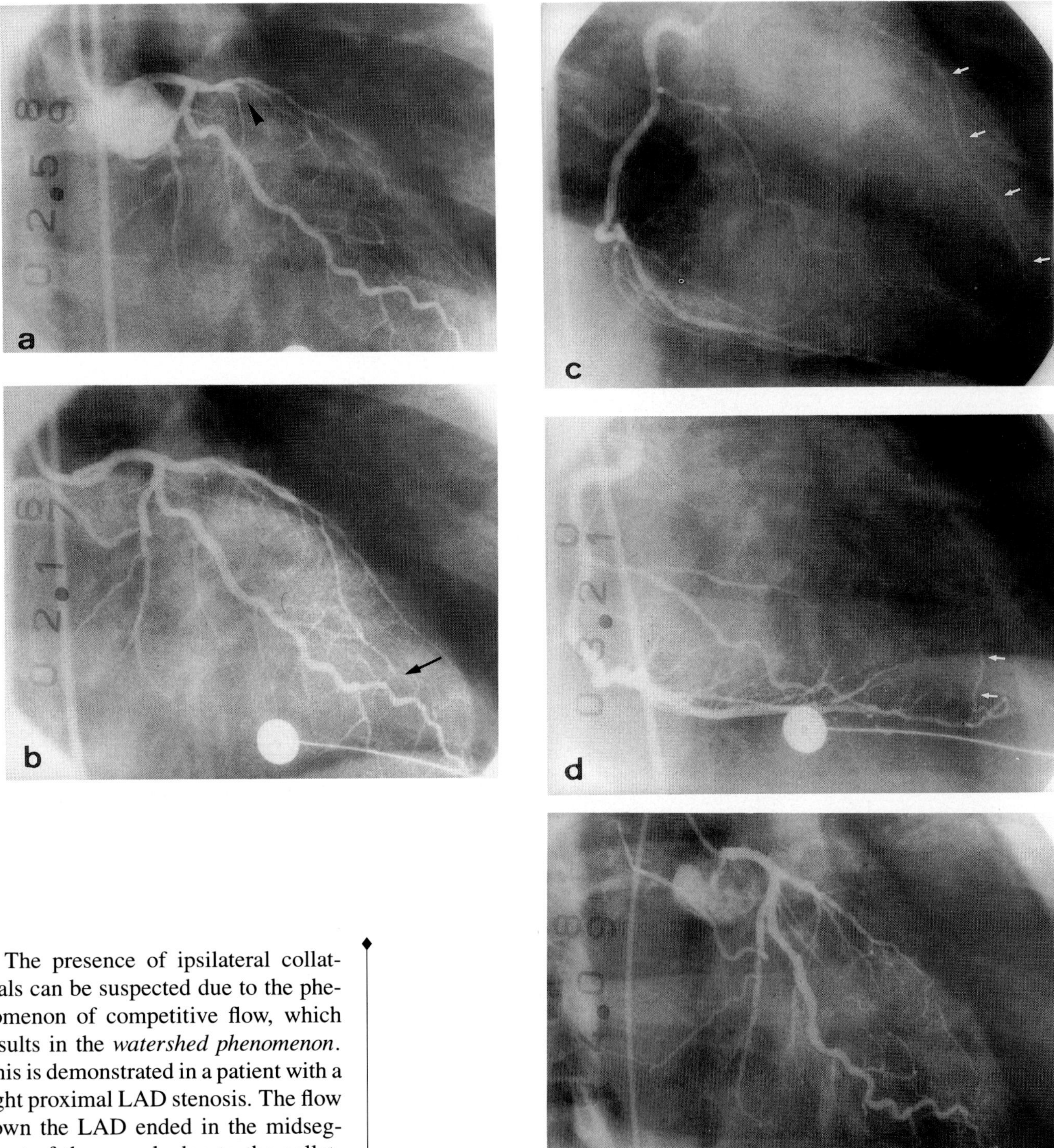

Figure 54

The presence of ipsilateral collaterals can be suspected due to the phenomenon of competitive flow, which results in the *watershed phenomenon*. This is demonstrated in a patient with a tight proximal LAD stenosis. The flow down the LAD ended in the midsegment of the vessel, due to the collateralization from the LCx (Fig. 53a). This marked the *watershed zone*. Following successful angioplasty of the LAD lesion, antegrade flow to the distal LAD was reestablished: the water-

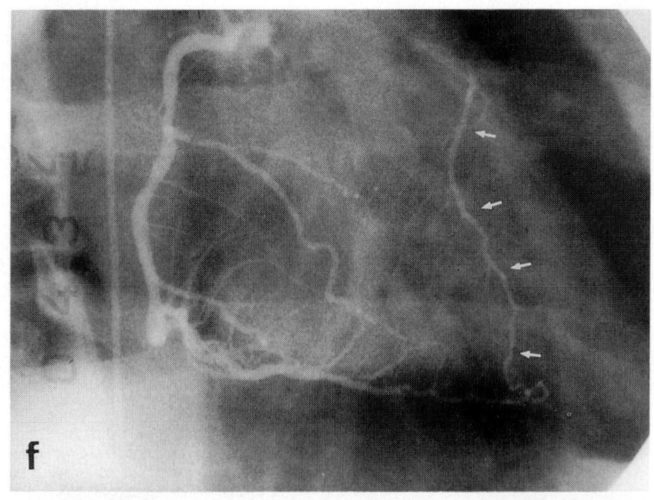

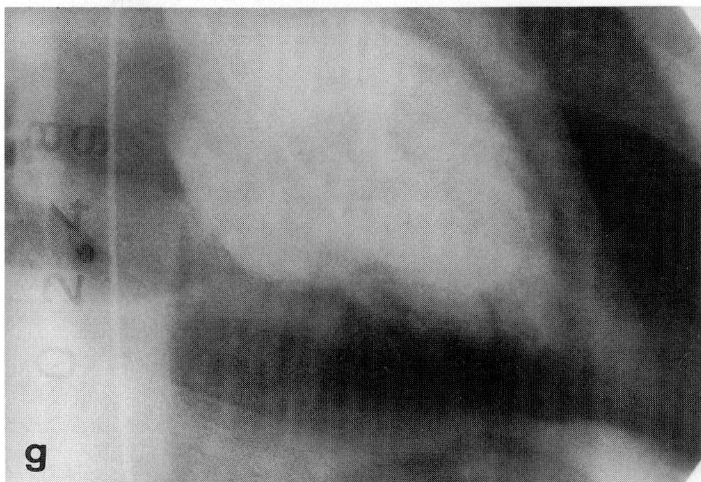

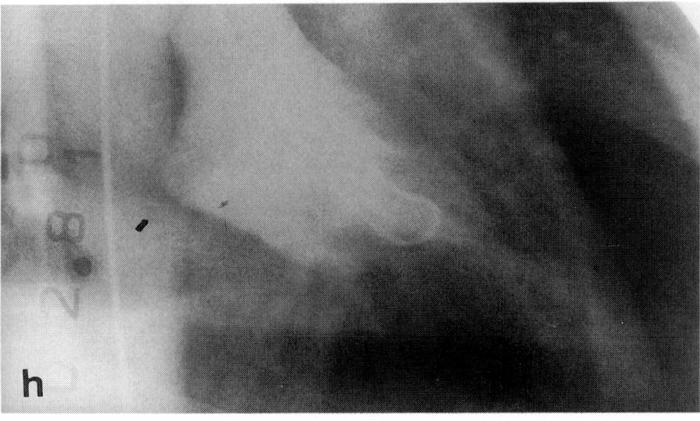

shed zone shifted back to its normal position at the apex.

Collaterals disappear following angioplasty of the native vessel. The disappearance of collaterals can be utilized as a marker of adequate angioplasty. Partial disappearance of collaterals is an indication of a suboptimal angioplasty result. The partial persistence of ipsilateral collaterals can also be detected by the watershed phenomenon. Recanalization of an occluded LAD (Fig. 54a) was carried out with an acceptable result (Fig. 54b). The LAD, however, was seen to stop short of the apex (arrow). The collaterals from the RCA prior to the angioplasty (Fig. 54c) were much reduced, but persisted, supplying the distal part of the LAD (Fig. 54d, arrows). The persistence of these collaterals could have been judged from the left coronary angiogram, since the distal LAD was not seen, being supplied by the collaterals. In other words the watershed zone remained in the distal LAD (Fig. 54a, arrow). It came as no surprise when the LAD was seen to be reoccluded at a 6-month follow-up evaluation (Fig. 54e). The collaterals from the RCA had been recruited again and supplied the entire LAD (Fig. 54f).

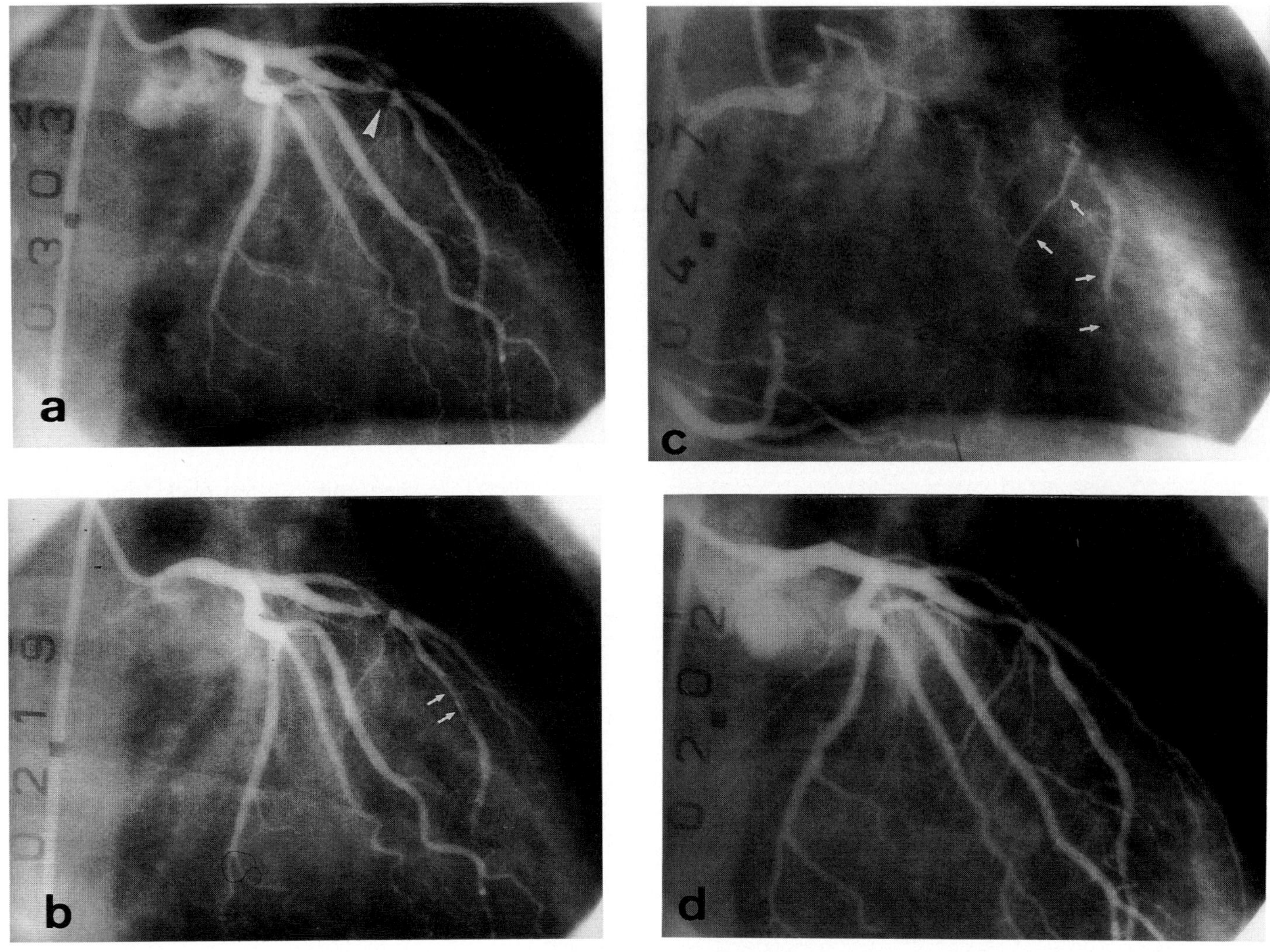

Figure 55

The left ventricular function was normal (Fig. 54g: diastole; Fig. 54h: systole) since the collaterals had prevented an infarction.

The presence of collaterals and streaming can sometimes lead to a peculiar flow pattern in the vessel, as seen in this patient with a tight LAD stenosis (Fig. 55a, systolic frame). In diastole, the collateral flow into the LAD created a competitive flow pattern simulating a dissection (Fig. 55b, arrows). The RCA angiogram revealed

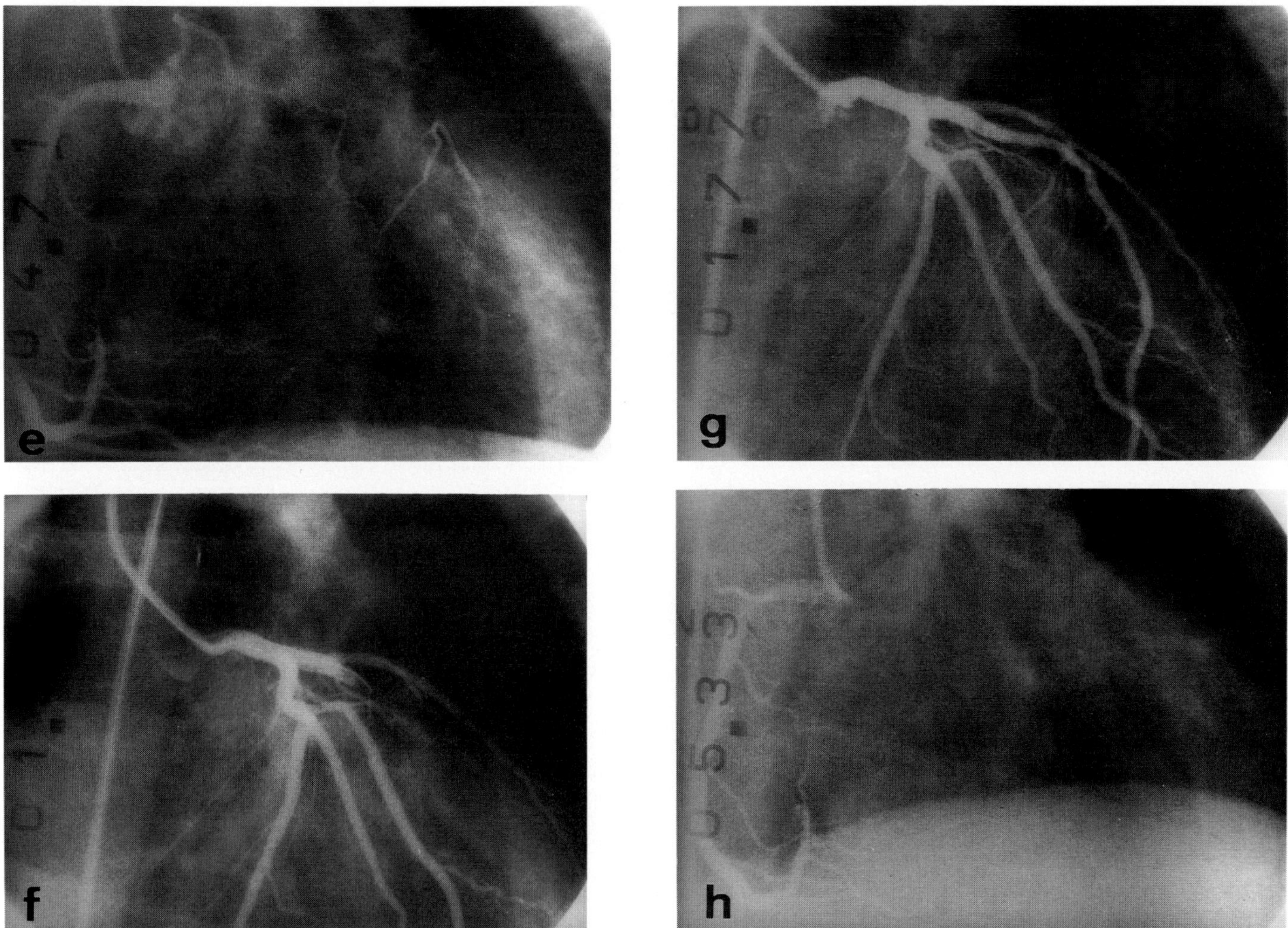

the collateral supply to the LAD (Fig. 55c). The result after one balloon inflation revealed an insufficient result, with persistence of the "pseudo-dissection" due to the competitive flow pattern (Fig. 55d). The persistence of collaterals was confirmed by the RCA injection (Fig. 55e). The vessel occluded shortly afterward (Fig. 55f), with no signs of ischemia, as predicted. It was redilated, with a good result (Fig. 55g) and disappearance of the collaterals (Fig. 55h).

The disappearance of collaterals as an index of successful angioplasty is also demonstrated by the following case. Angioplasty was performed for a functional occlusion of the LAD (Fig. 56a), with a good result (Fig. 56b). The occluded LAD had been adequately supplied by collaterals from the RCA (Fig. 56c), which disappeared following angioplasty (Fig. 56d), confirming a good angioplasty result. The importance of collaterals in this patient is evident from the normal left ventricular function (Fig. 56e: diastole, Fig. 56f: systole), despite the occluded LAD.

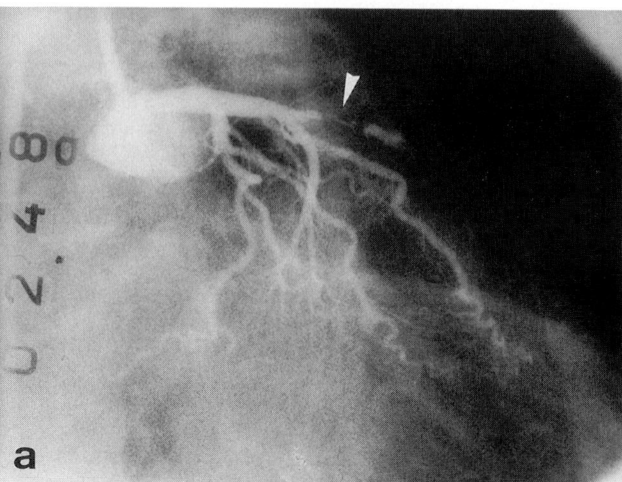

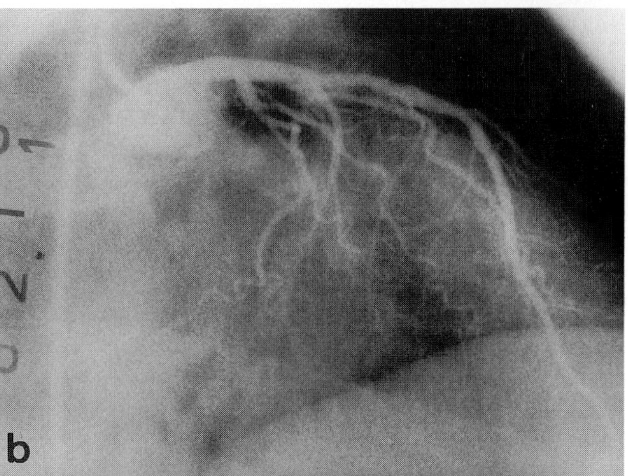

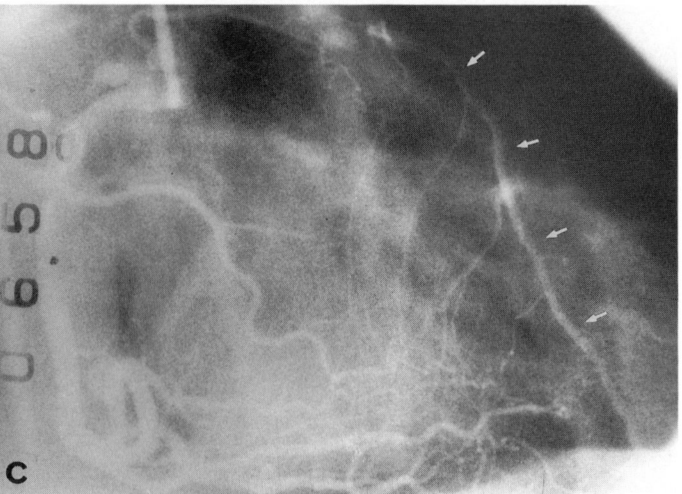

Figure 56

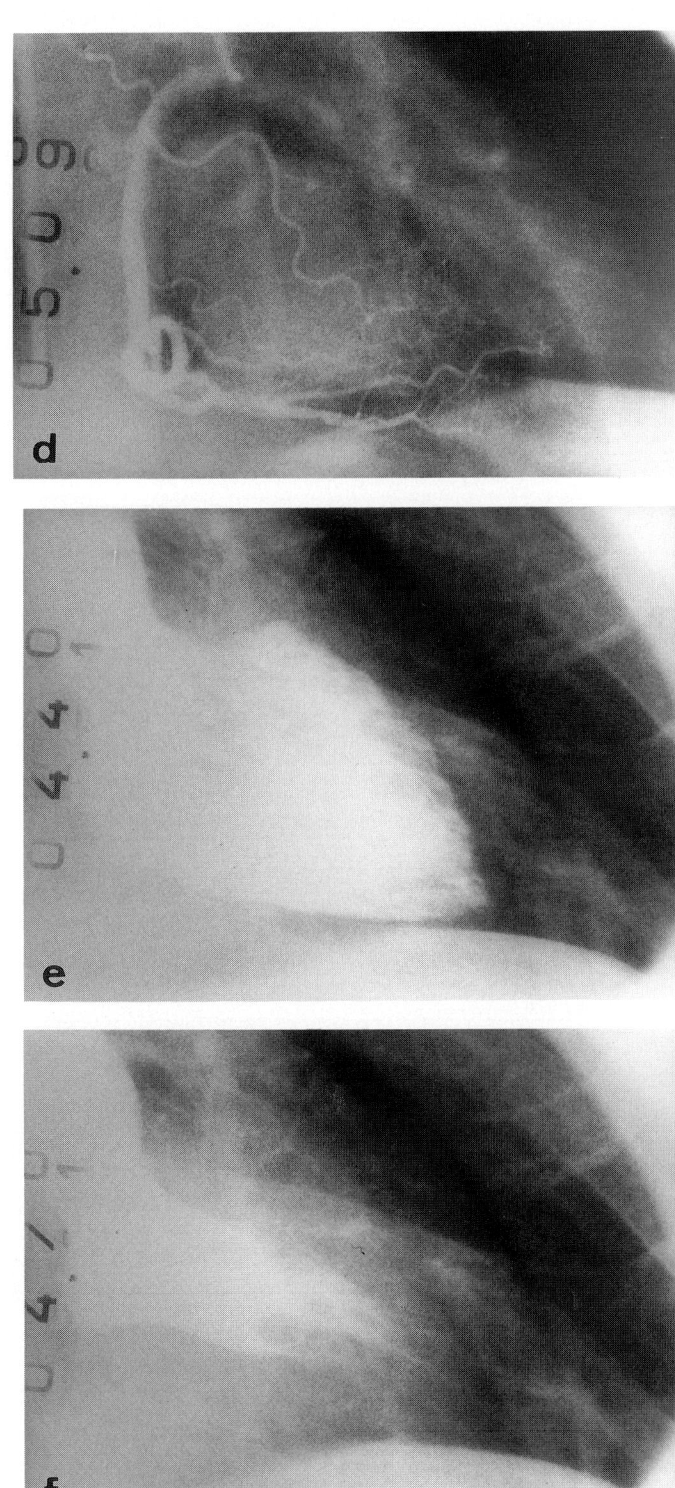

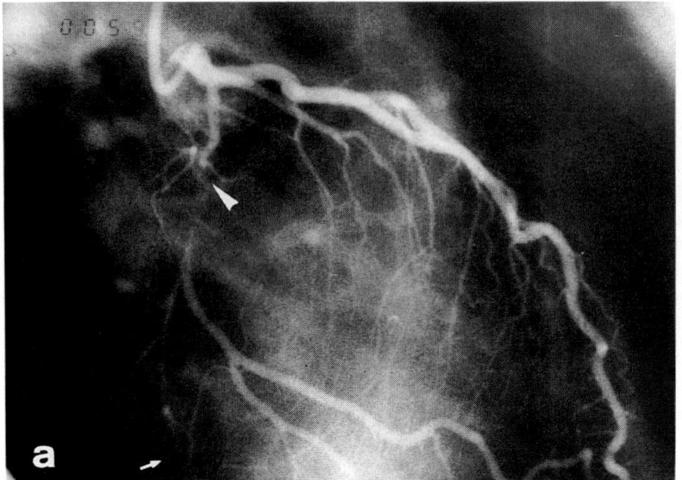

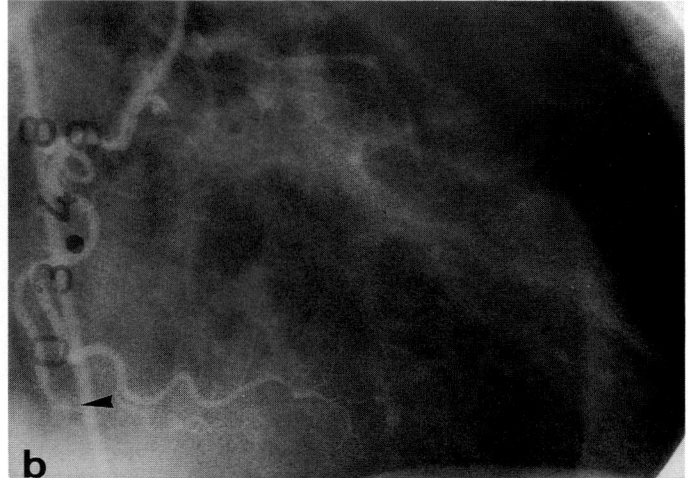

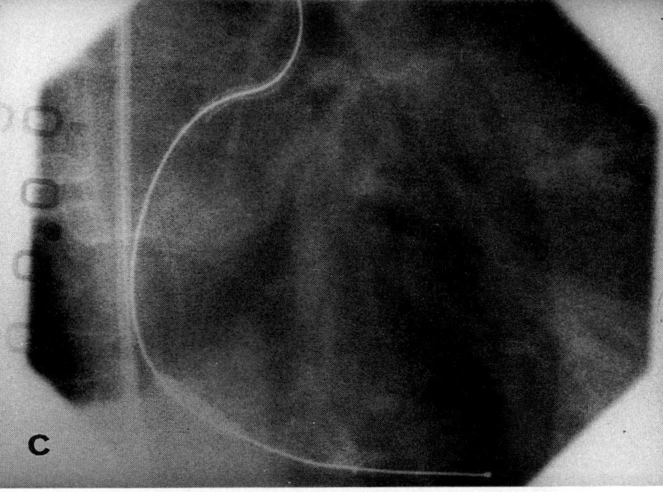

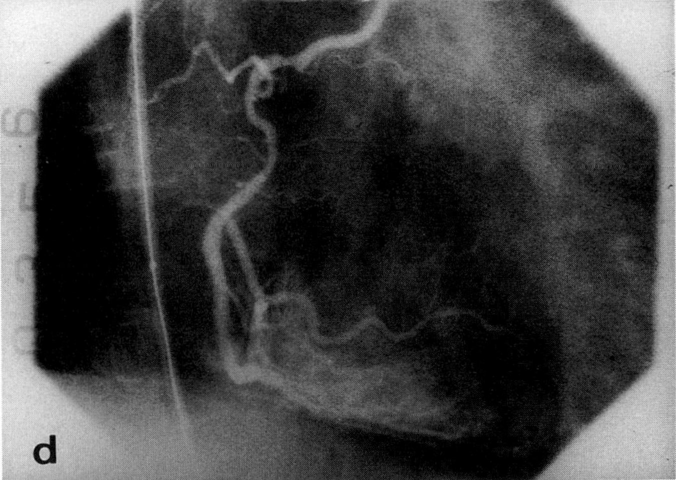

Figure 57

In case of an acute reocclusion, collaterals are instantly recruitable. This is well demonstrated in the example of a 46-year-old man with occlusions of the LCx (Fig. 57a) and the RCA (Fig. 57b), both receiving good collateral supply from the LAD (Fig. 57a). The RCA was recanalized using a Magnum–Magnarail system (Fig. 57c), with a good result (Fig. 57d). A repeat left coronary angiogram revealed disappearance of the collaterals to the RCA (Fig. 57e). The LCx was then recanalized, with the same system (Fig. 57f), with a good result (Fig. 57g). However, collaterals to the RCA were seen again (arrows), indicating reocclusion of the RCA. A control injection of the RCA revealed a distal occlusion (Fig. 57h). This was redilated successfully (Fig. 57i). A repeat left coronary angiogram confirmed the absence of collaterals (Fig. 57j). This case demonstrates how collaterals work and how they should be looked for carefully and monitored throughout the intervention.

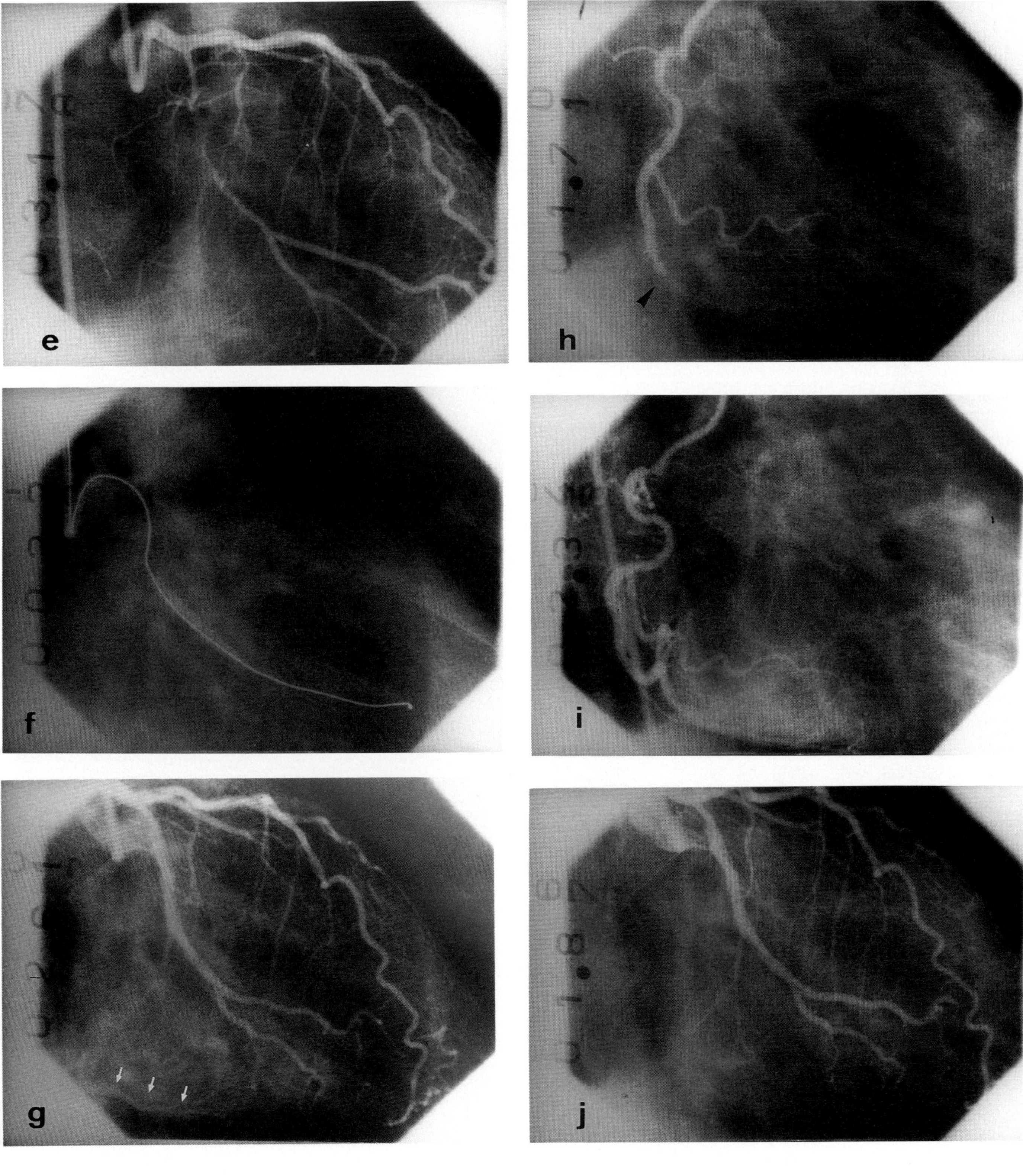
e
h
f
i
g
j

Collaterals become dormant once antegrade flow is established and remain dormant as long as antegrade flow is maintained. This is demonstrated in the case of this 48-year-old man with an occluded LAD (Fig. 58a) which was recanalized successfully (Fig. 58b). The LAD had received collaterals from the RCA (Fig. 58c), which disappeared following angioplasty (Fig. 58d). At a 1-year follow-up, the long-term result of the LAD angioplasty was good (Fig. 58e) and the collaterals remained undemonstrable (Fig. 58f). In case the vessel later reoccludes, these collaterals will again be re-

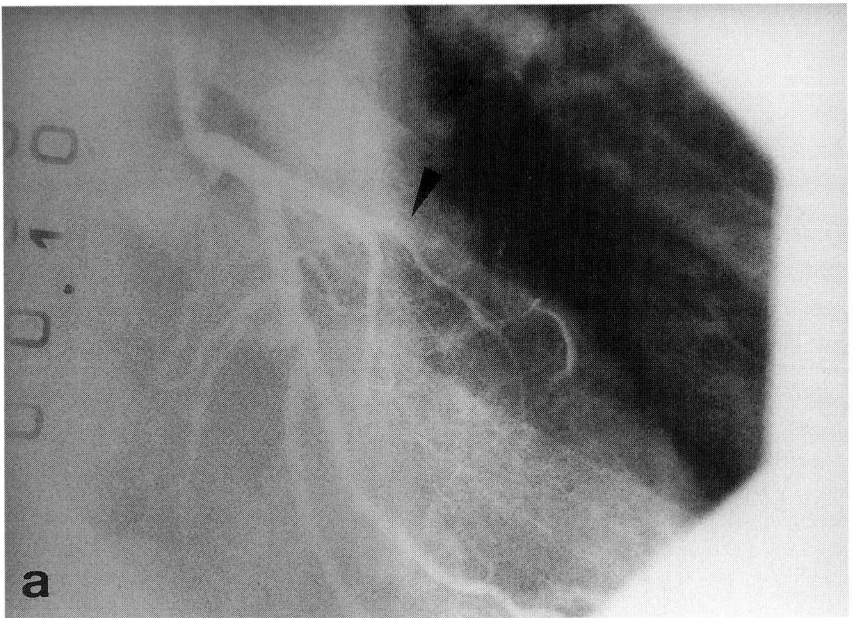

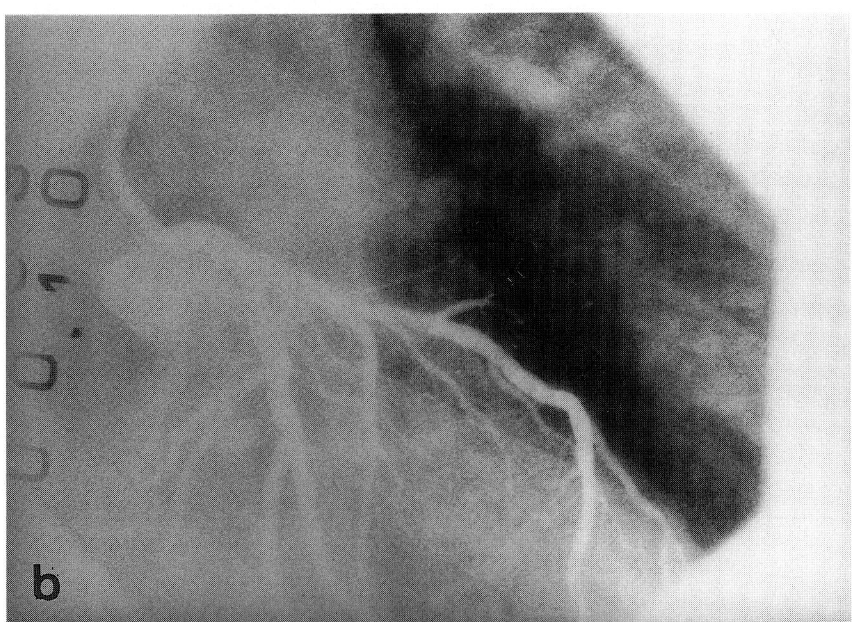

Figure 58

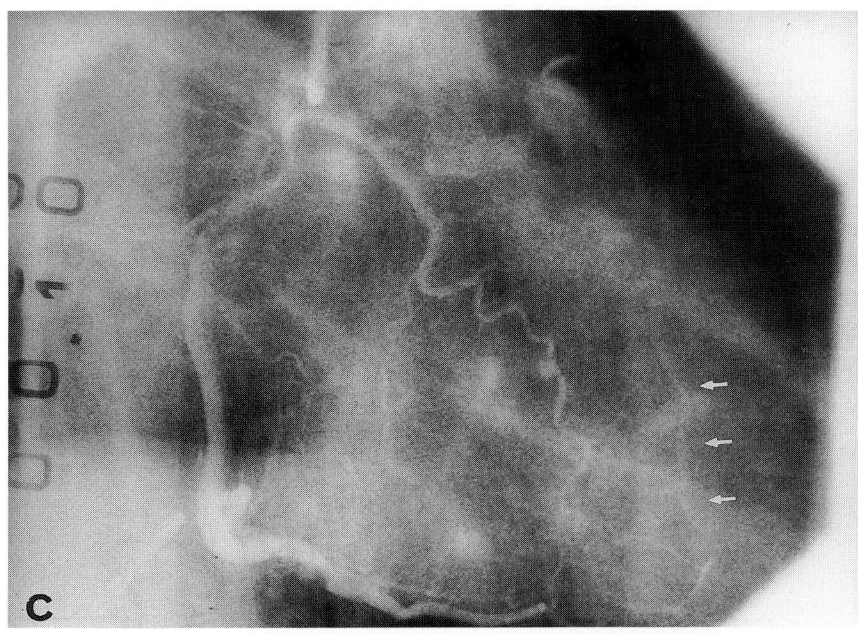
c

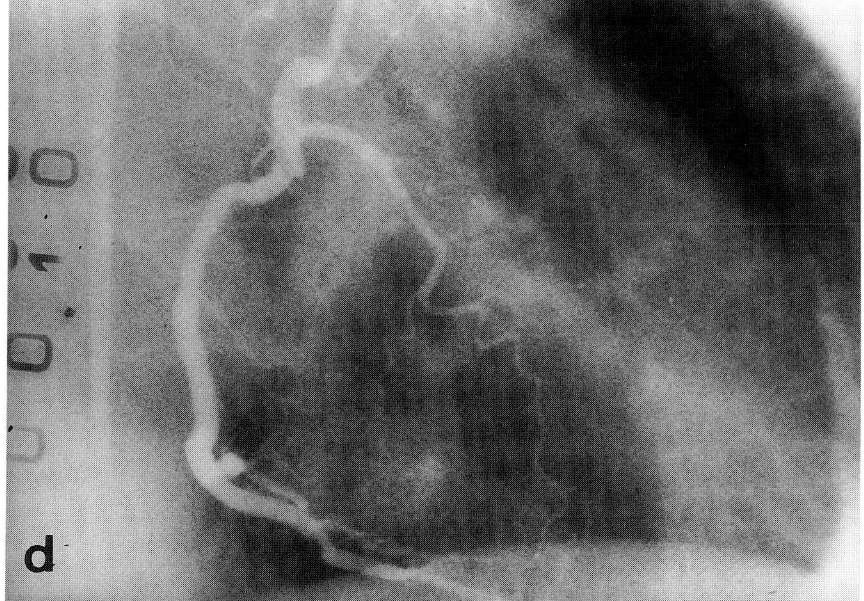
d

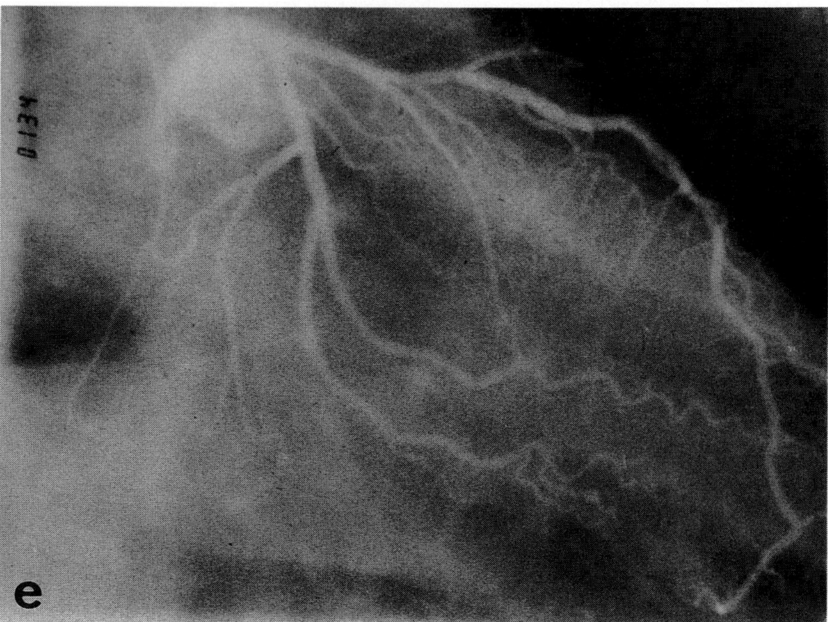

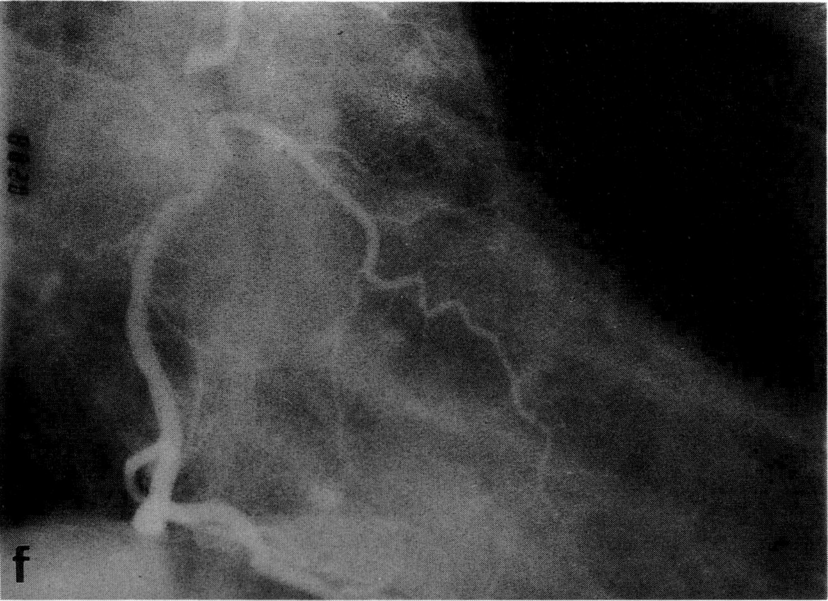

Figure 58 (Continued)

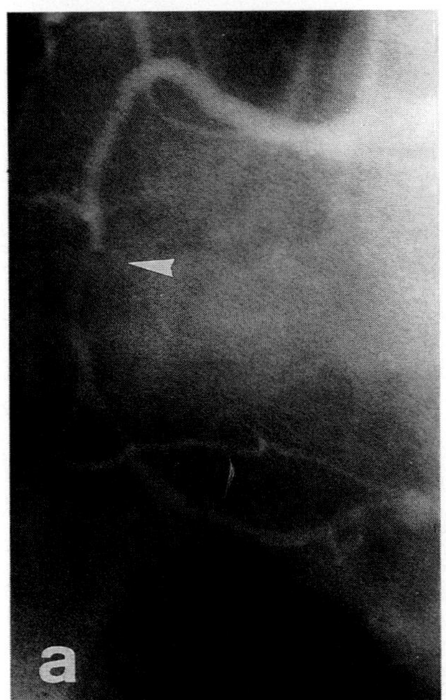

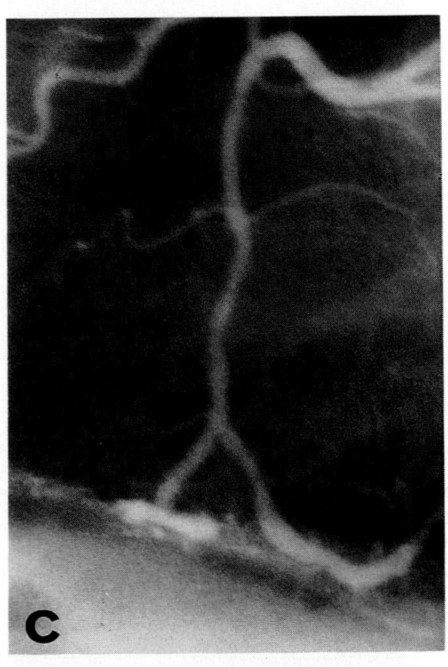

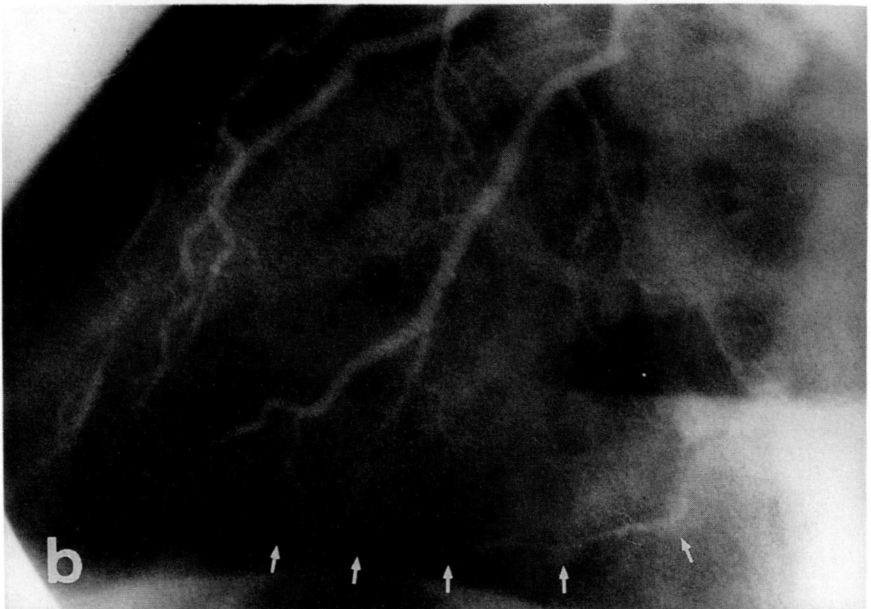

Figure 59

cruited. This is demonstrated by a 63-year-old man with a severe stenosis of the RCA (Fig. 59a) which received collaterals from the LAD (Fig. 59b). After successful angioplasty of the lesion (Fig. 59c) the collaterals from the LAD disappeared. Three months later symptoms recurred, the RCA was seen to be functionally reoccluded (Fig. 59d), and the collaterals were again present (Fig. 59e). The vessel was successfully redilated (Fig. 59f). Six months later the patient was recatheterized for angina. The RCA was again occluded (Fig. 59g), and the collaterals were again present (Fig. 59h). This case demonstrates the repeated reliable recruitment of dormant collaterals in case of need.

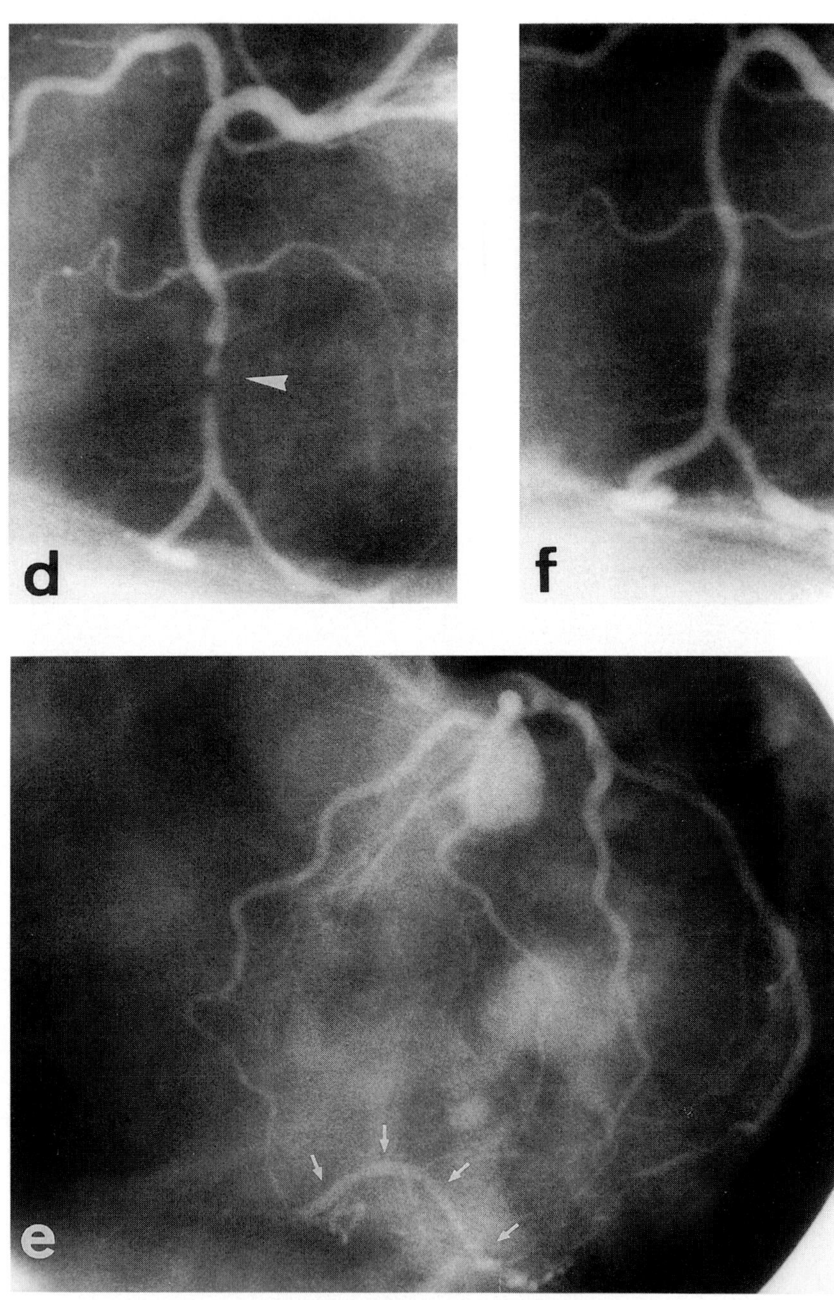

Figure 59 (Continued)

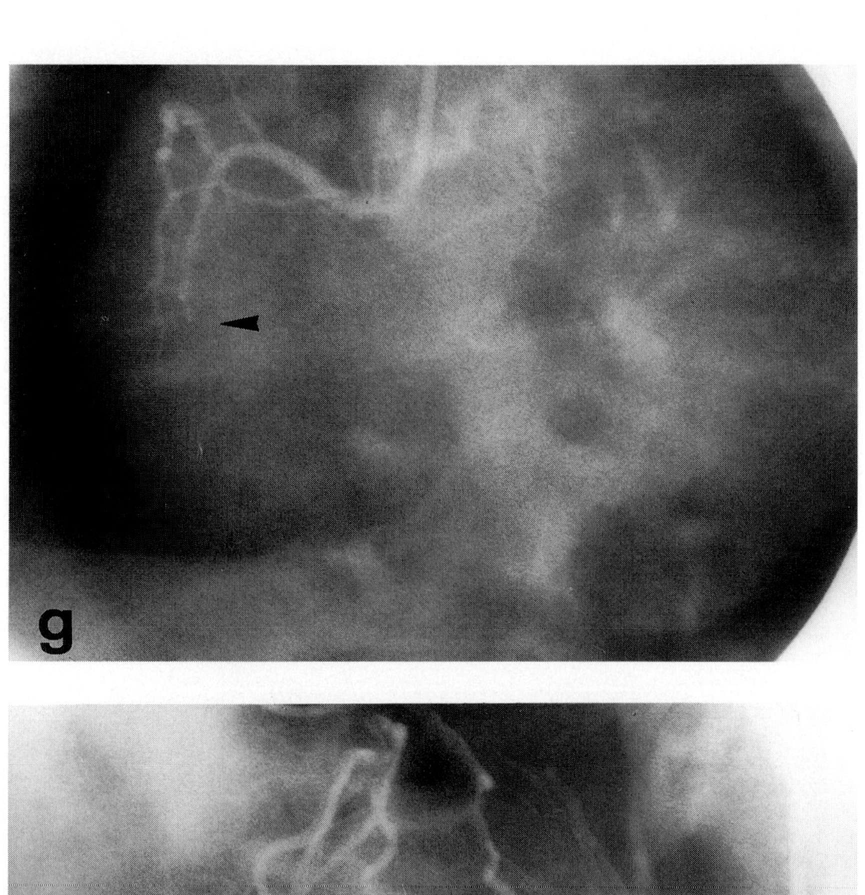
g

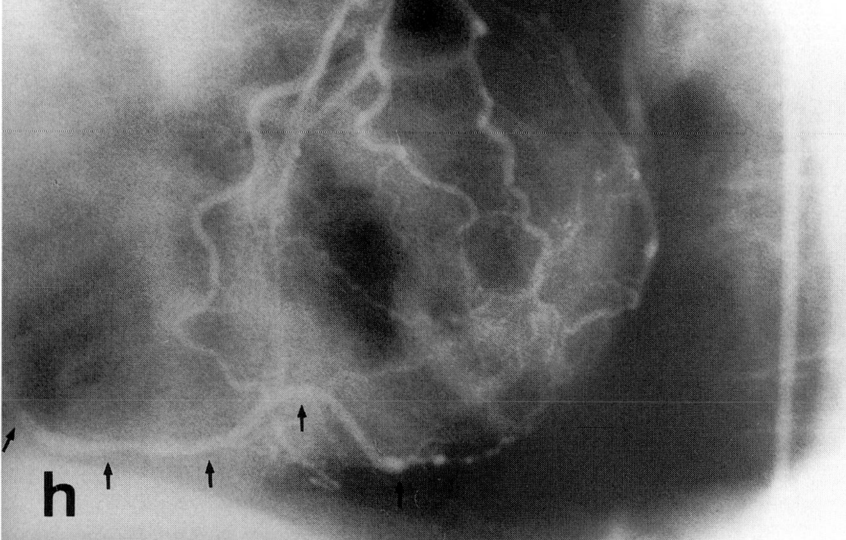
h

Collaterals are instantly reversible, as demonstrated by a 64-year-old patient with an occluded RCA supplied by collaterals from the LAD (Fig. 60a). Following successful angioplasty of the RCA (Fig. 60b), the collaterals were instantly reversed. The reversal is distinctly demonstrated in this patient due to a forceful RCA injection despite the fact that the stenosis of the proximal LAD was not critical.

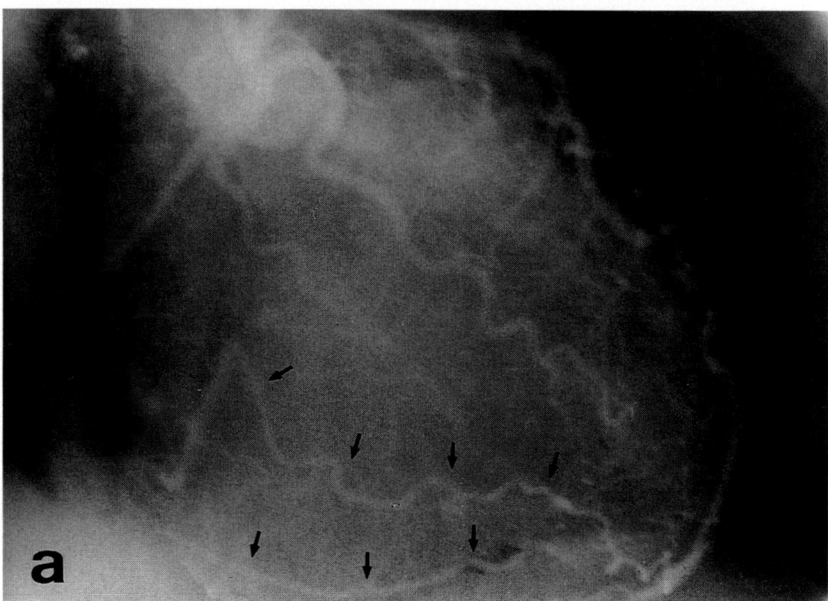

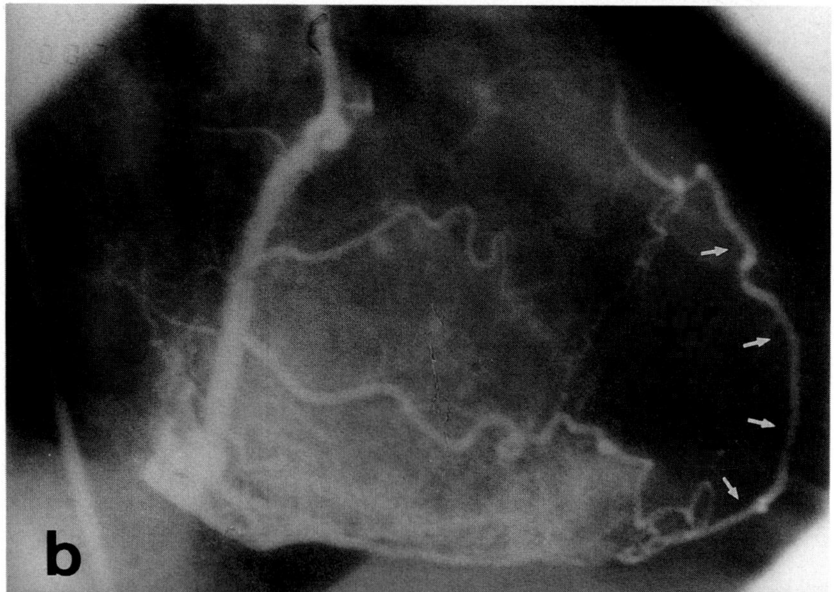

Figure 60

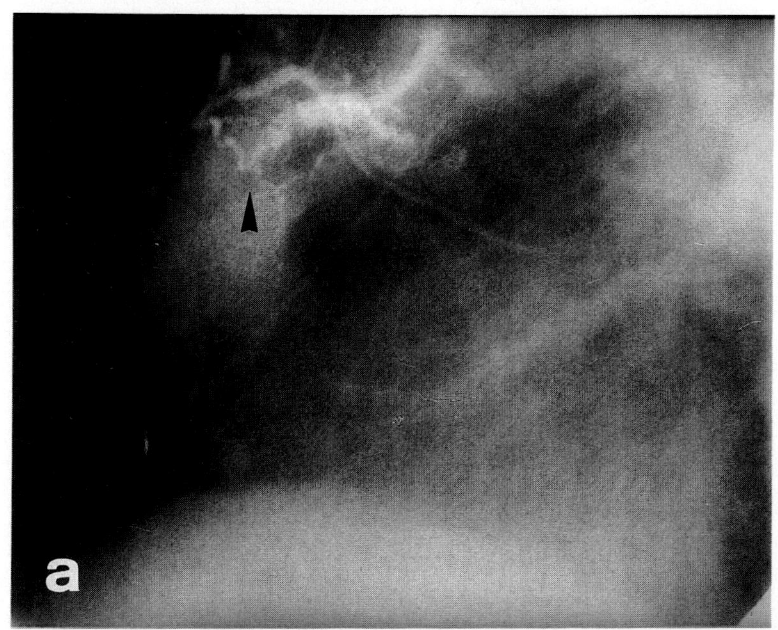

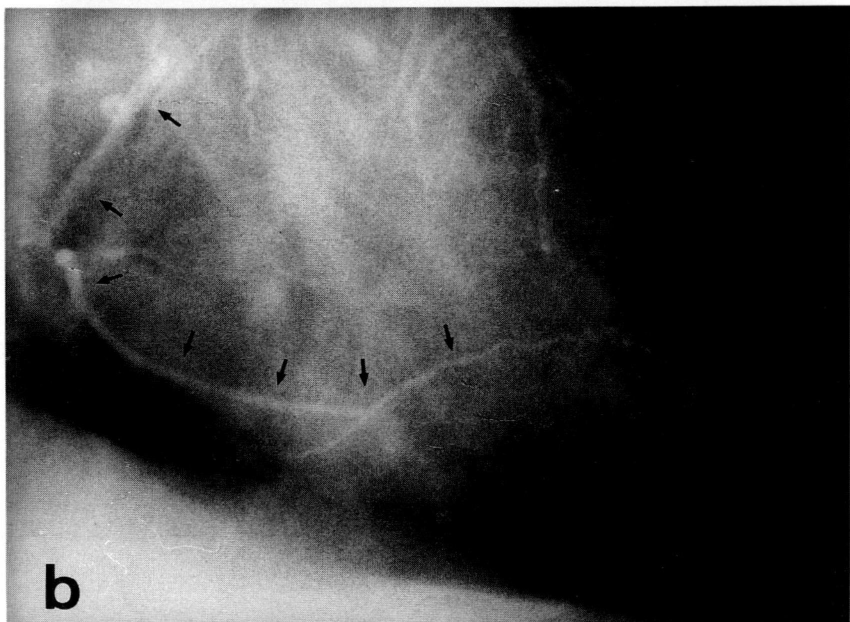

Figure 61

The presence of such reversed collaterals can be demonstrated even after longer periods of time. A 67-year-old man underwent angioplasty for an occluded RCA (Fig. 61a), which was supplied by collaterals from the LAD (Fig. 61b). The left ventricular angiogram revealed inferior hypokinesia (Fig. 61c: diastole, Fig. 61d: systole). Successful recanalization was performed (Fig. 61e), with a good result (Fig. 61f). This was associated with a disappearance of collaterals (Fig. 61g). The patient presented with angina 7 months later. The left ventricular function was improved, with a reduction of the inferior wall hypokinesia, suggesting a previously hibernating myocardium (Fig. 61h: diastole, Fig. 61i: systole).

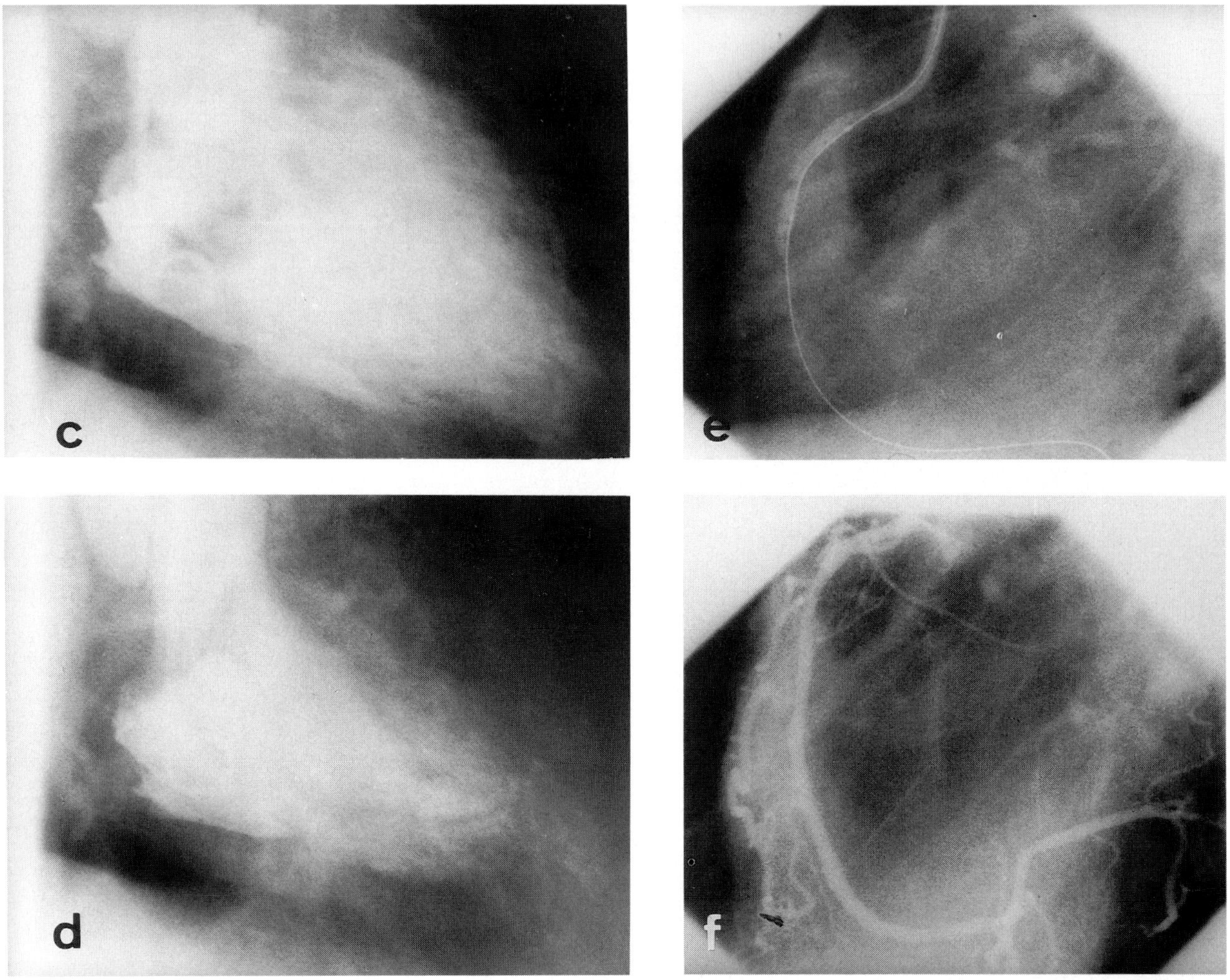

The collaterals had prevented a complete infarction of the territory. This also demonstrates the advantages of reopening occluded vessels, especially if they are well collateralized. However, there was a stenosis of the mid LAD (Fig. 61j). The RCA was patent, and there were no collaterals to the LAD (Fig. 61k). The presence of the dormant, and immediately recruitable collateral supply was demonstrable (arrows) by a RCA injection while the balloon was inflated in the LAD (Fig. 61l). The LAD angioplasty result was satisfactory (Fig. 61m). Reversed col-

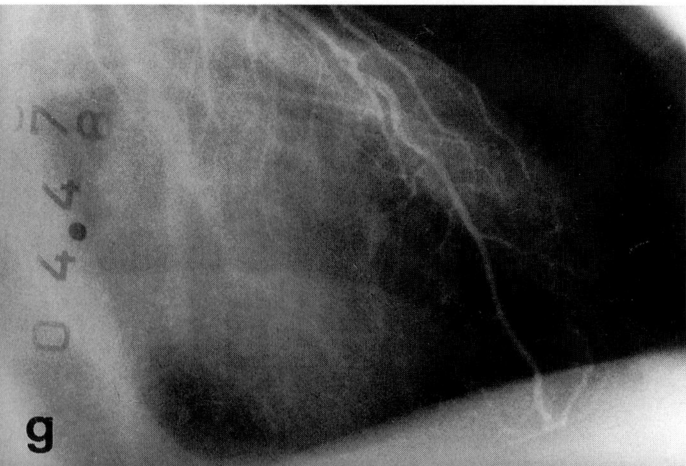

Figure 61 (Continued)

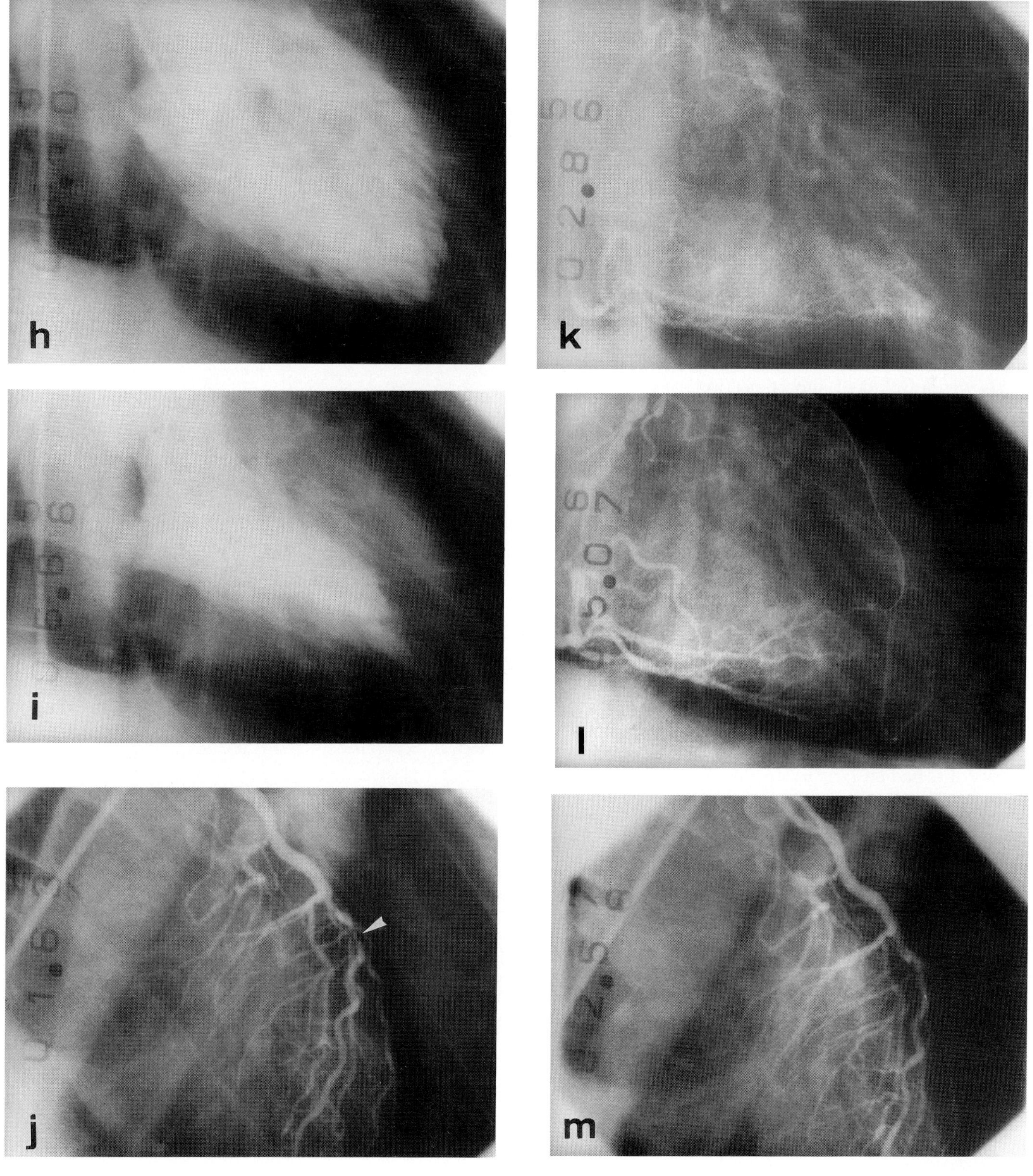
h
k
i
l
j
m

laterals were of clinical importance in a 61-year-old woman with an occluded RCA that was supplied by collaterals from the LAD (Fig. 62a). The occluded RCA (Fig. 62b) was reopened successfully (Fig. 62c). The patient presented 3 years later with angina. Angiography revealed an occluded LAD (Fig. 62d), which received a rich collateral supply from the RCA (which it had supplied earlier) (Fig. 62e). The ventriculogram revealed only mild anterior hypokinesia, the collateral supply having prevented an infarction in the LAD territory (and in the RCA territory if it had still been dependent on the LAD).

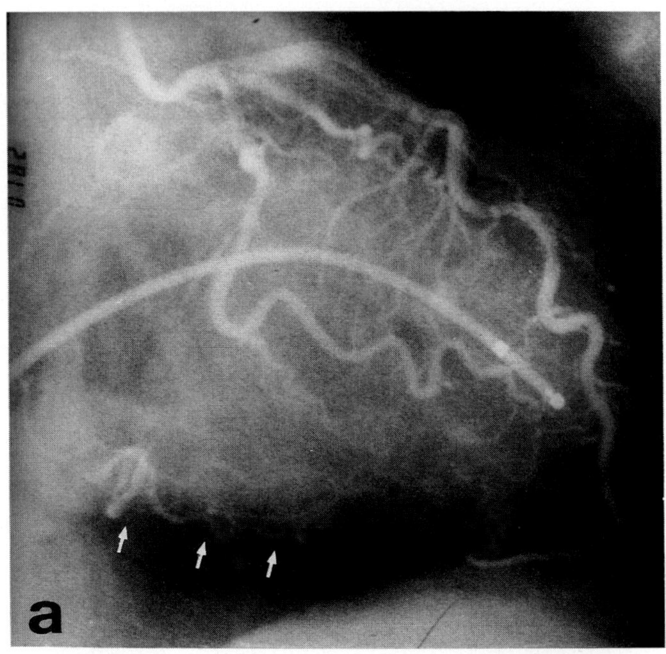

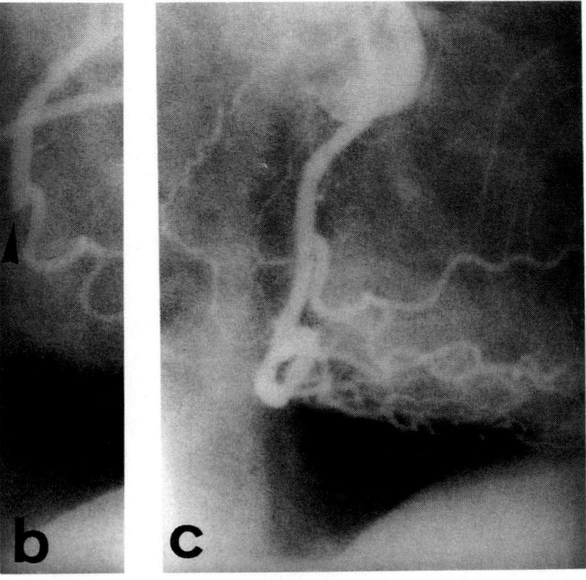

Figure 62

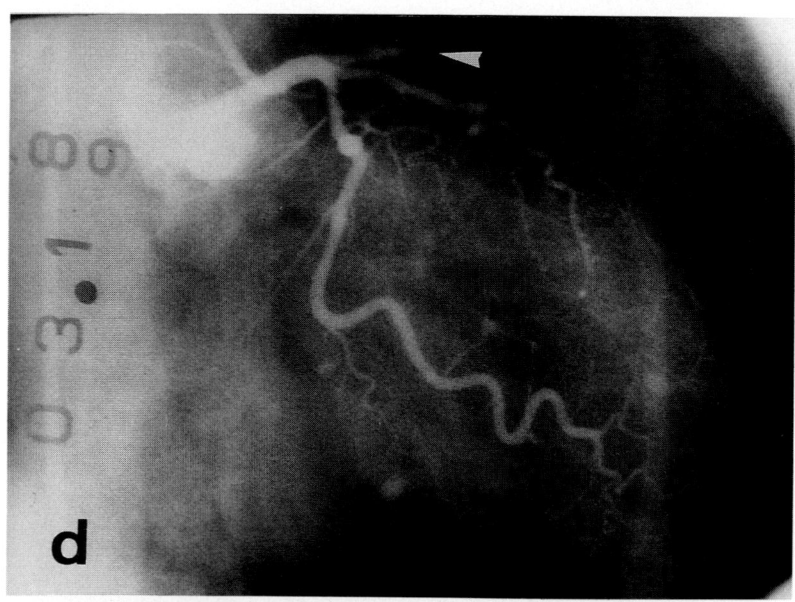
d

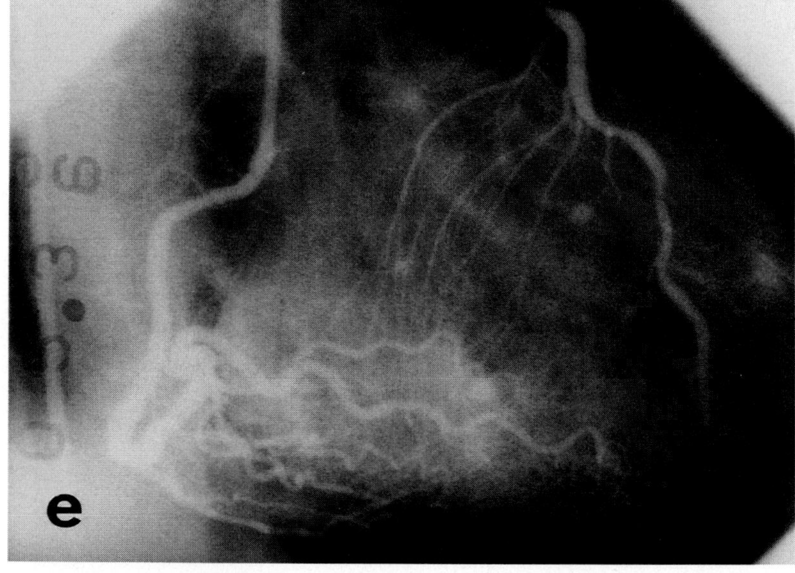
e

Collaterals may remain dormant for many years. A 58-year-old man underwent successful angioplasty for an occluded LAD (Fig. 63a) which received collaterals from the RCA (Fig. 63b). This was associated with the disappearance of collaterals from the RCA. The patient underwent a repeat examination 6 years later, which revealed a good long-term result of the LAD angioplasty (Fig. 63c). However, collaterals were seen supplying the RCA from the LAD (Fig. 63d). A selective LCx injection did not result in any collateral flow to the RCA (Fig. 63e), confirming that the collaterals originated from the LAD. The RCA was confirmed to be occluded and successful angioplasty performed (Fig. 63f, arrow marks the site of occlusion). This case demonstrates how collaterals can lie dormant for long periods of time, are reversible, and can be recruited when needed.

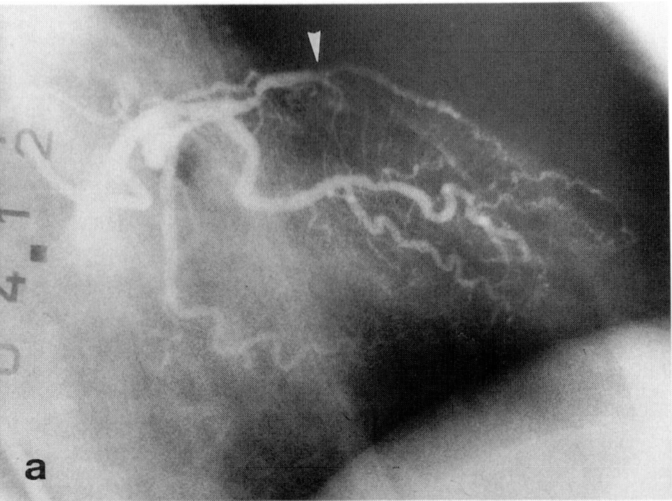

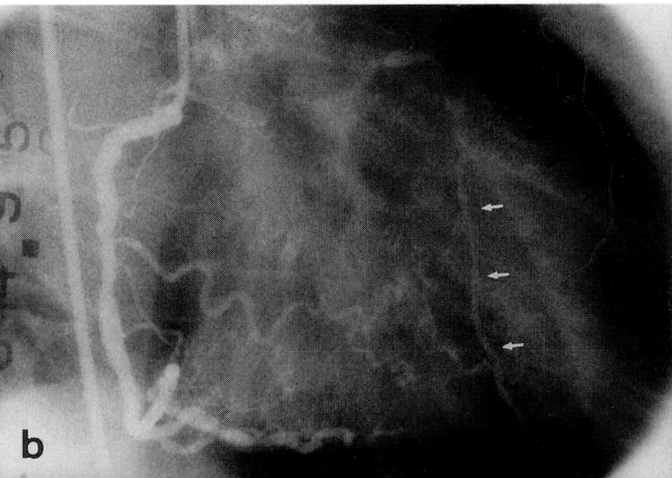

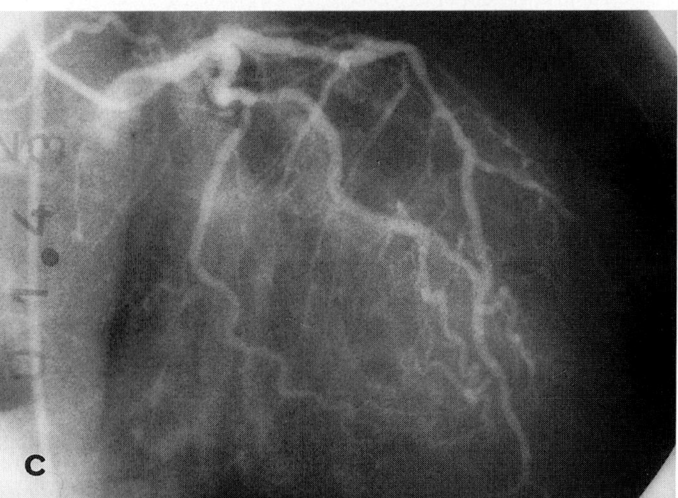

Figure 63

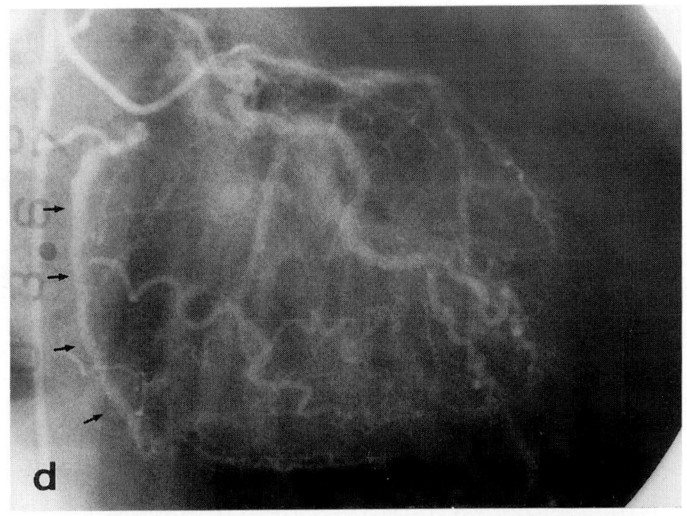
d

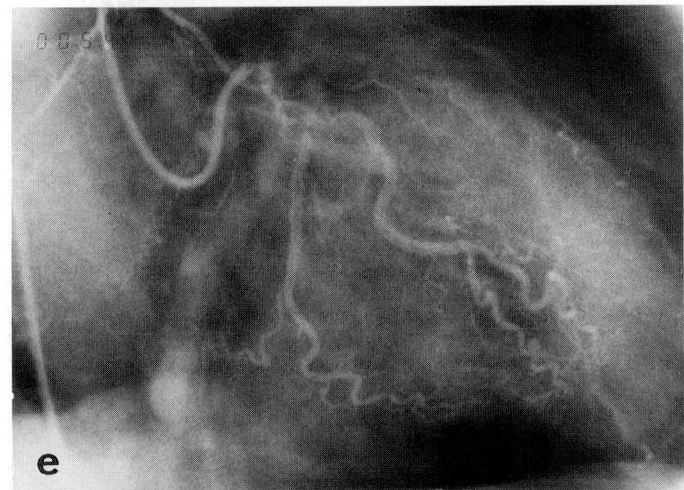
e

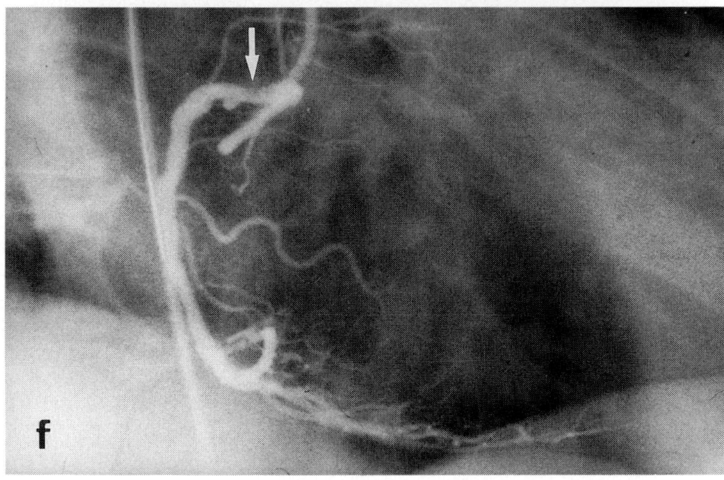
f

Collateral flow, even if interrupted due to dissection during an angioplasty attempt, has a tendency to recover, especially if the angioplasty result is poor. On the one hand, this results in an increased risk of restenosis of a lesion with an initially poor result, but on the other hand, it affords ongoing protection to the myocardium at risk. A 57-year-old man had an occluded marginal branch of the LCx, which received collaterals from the LAD (Fig. 64a). Following an unsuccessful attempt at recanalization of the vessel, which resulted in a long local dissection (Fig. 64b), the collaterals disappeared (Fig. 64c), probably due to a compromise of the distal vessel by the dissection, which obstructed the collateral inflow. A repeat angiogram 1 year later showed the collaterals to have reappeared, with a "healing" of the dissection and distal perfusion of the vessel (Fig. 64d). This demonstrates that collaterals tend to fill the true lumen and seal off the false lumen distal to an occlusion.

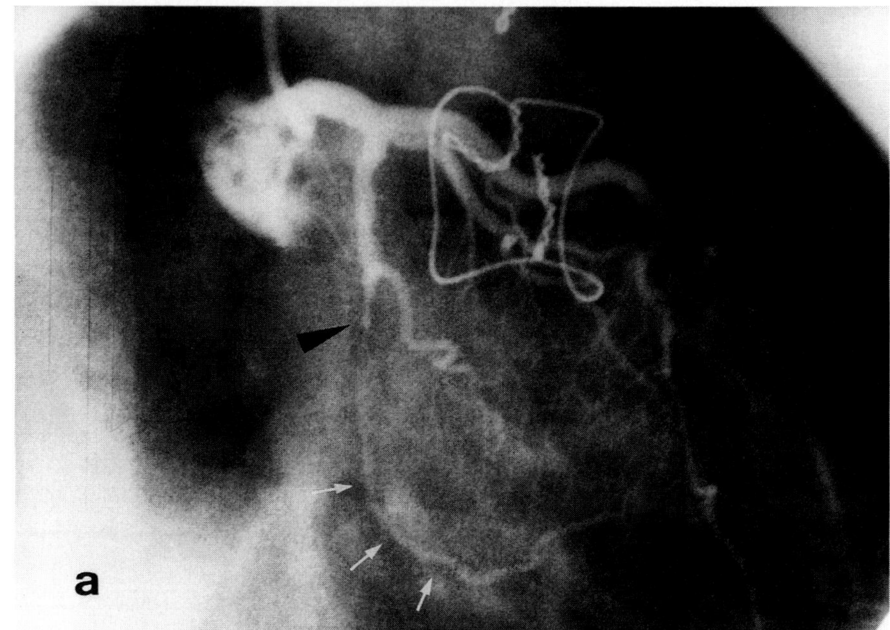

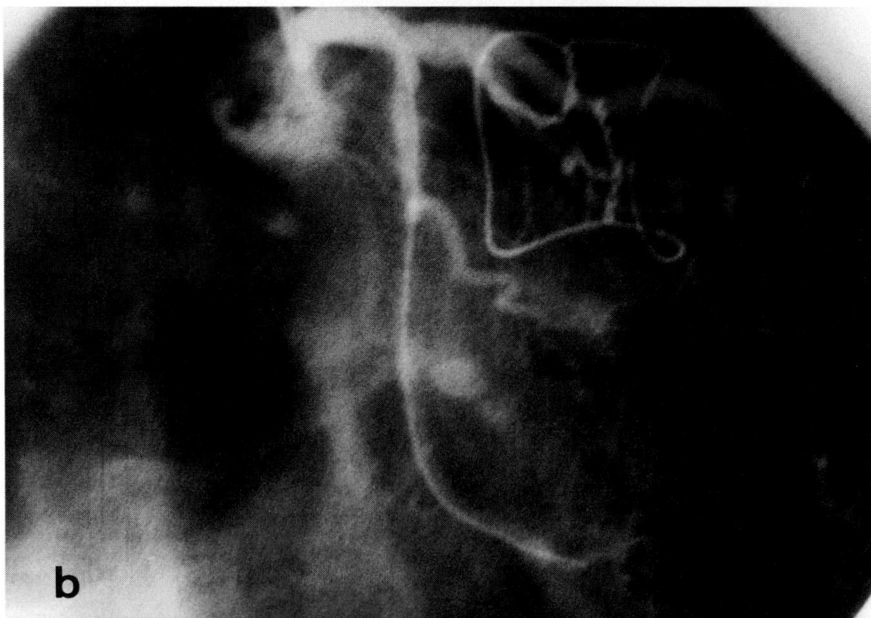

Figure 64

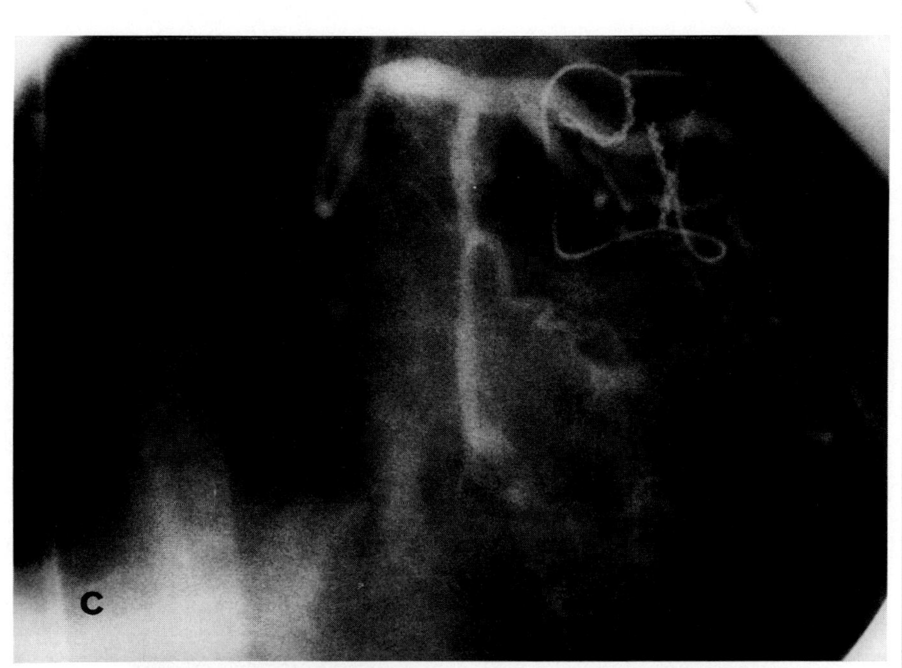
c

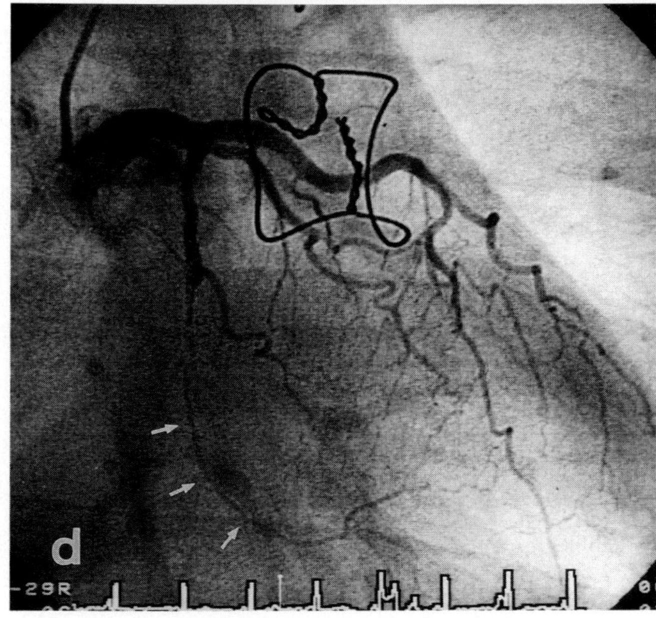
d
-29R

2.4 GRAFT ANGIOPLASTY

Vein Grafts

Stenoses of venous grafts are frequently addressed by angioplasty. For most bypass grafts, a multipurpose guiding catheter is best suited, but others, such as an Amplatz catheter, a venous bypass graft catheter, or a right Judkins catheter may be preferable for some cases.

The results of venous bypass graft angioplasty are best for discrete stenoses of the distal anastomotic site. Angioplasty was performed for stenosis of the distal anastomotic site of a 6-month-old venous graft to the RCA (Fig. 65a) with a 3.5-mm balloon (Fig. 65b). The result was good (Fig. 65c). A 6-month follow-up study revealed an excellent long-term result (Fig. 65d).

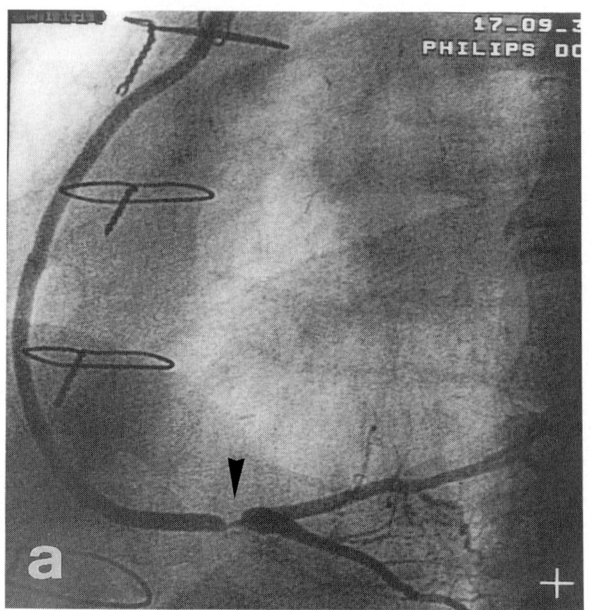

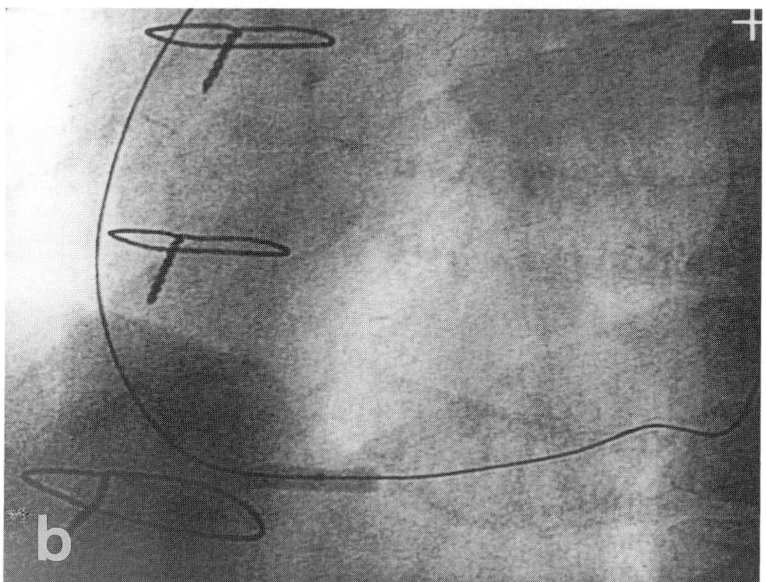

Figure 65

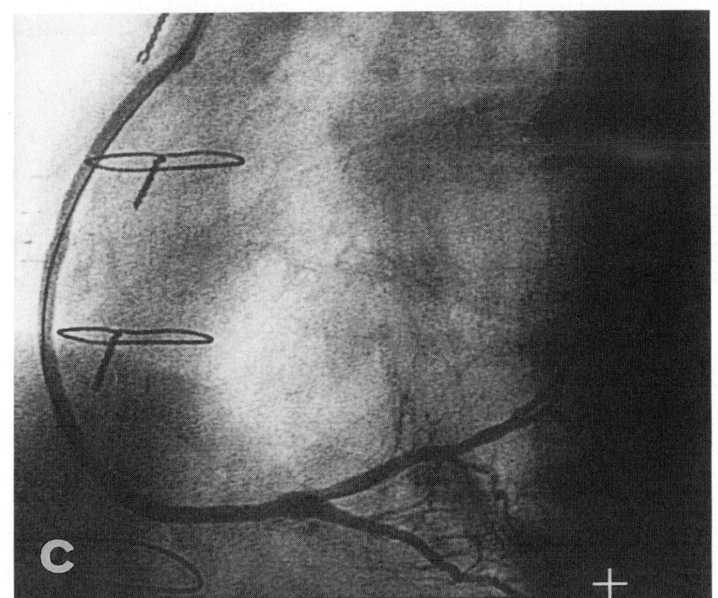
c

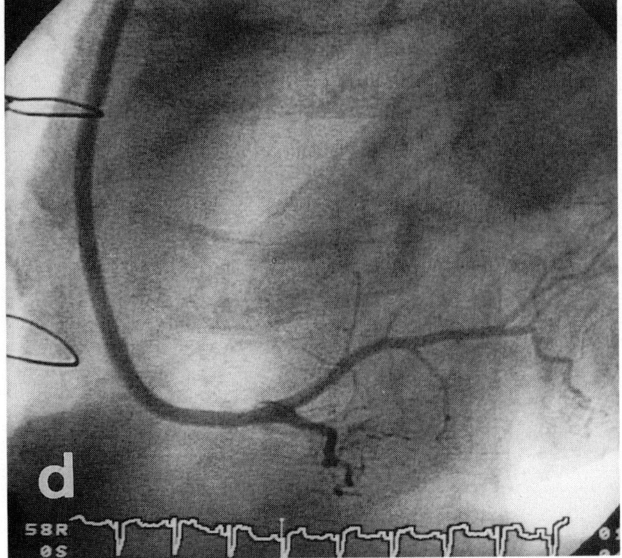
d
58R
0S

Stenoses of the proximal anastomotic site generally respond less favorably to angioplasty, the aortic wall being tough and elastic. However, stenoses of relatively fresh grafts may respond well. In a 64-year-old man, a stenosis of the graft to the LCx (Fig. 66a) was dilated successfully (Fig. 66b). The 5-month follow-up result was good (Fig. 66c).

For venous grafts, large balloons may be required. Balloons up to 6 mm in diameter are available from several manufacturers. The results of angioplasty of graft body stenoses depend on various factors. Short discrete stenoses in fresh grafts (less than a couple of years old) respond well to angioplasty, as in the case of a patient with a stenosis in a 1-year-old graft (Fig. 67a) which was dilated successfully (Fig. 67b). The 3-year follow-up result was excellent (Fig. 67c). Older grafts tend to have more diffuse lesions, and the results of angioplasty are poorer. Additionally, these grafts are often filled with thrombotic and other material, and the risk of distal emobilization is high. Grafts such as the one shown in Figure 68 should not be considered for angioplasty.

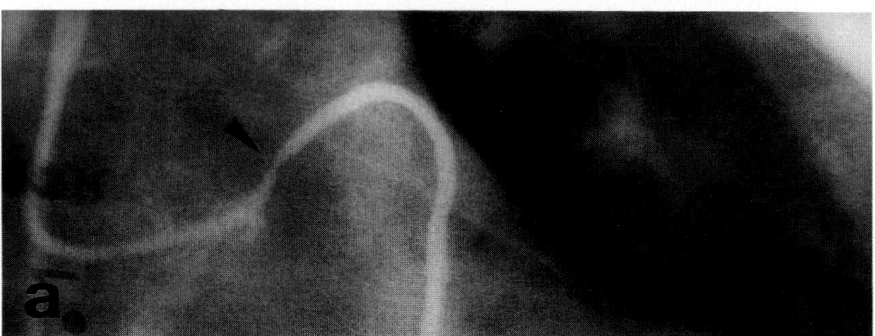

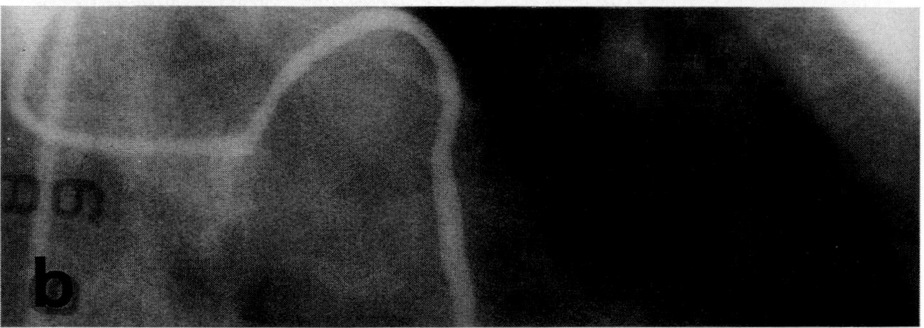

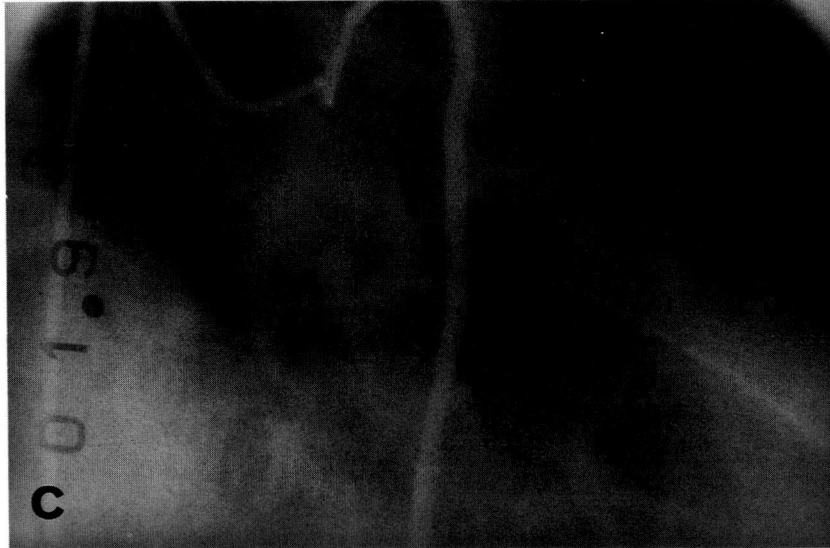

Figure 66

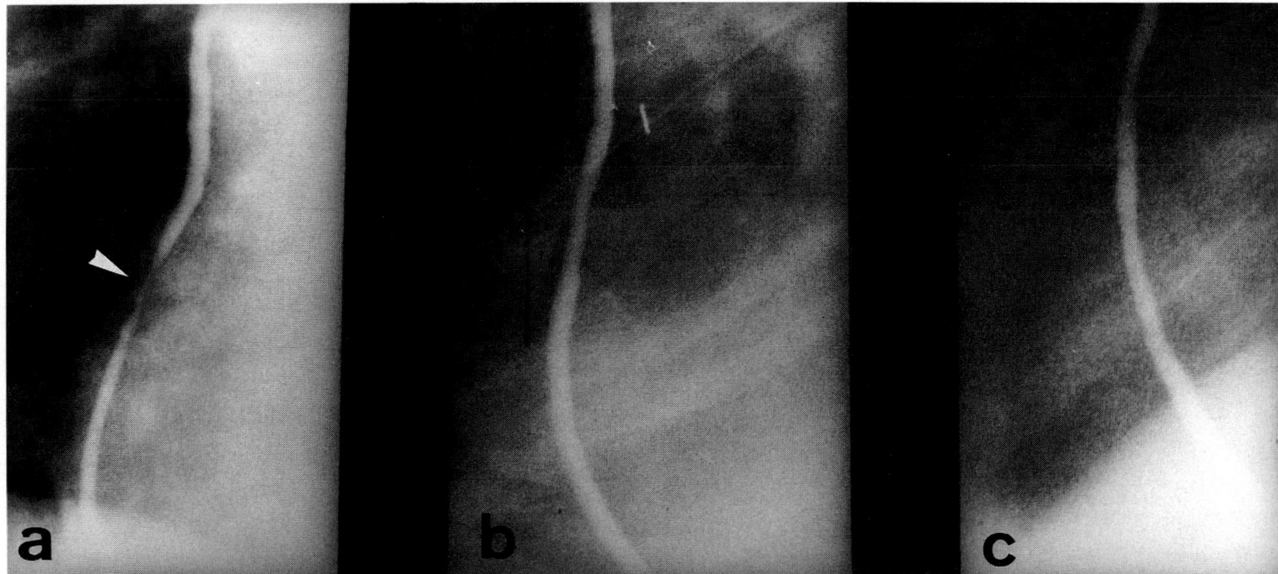

Figure 67

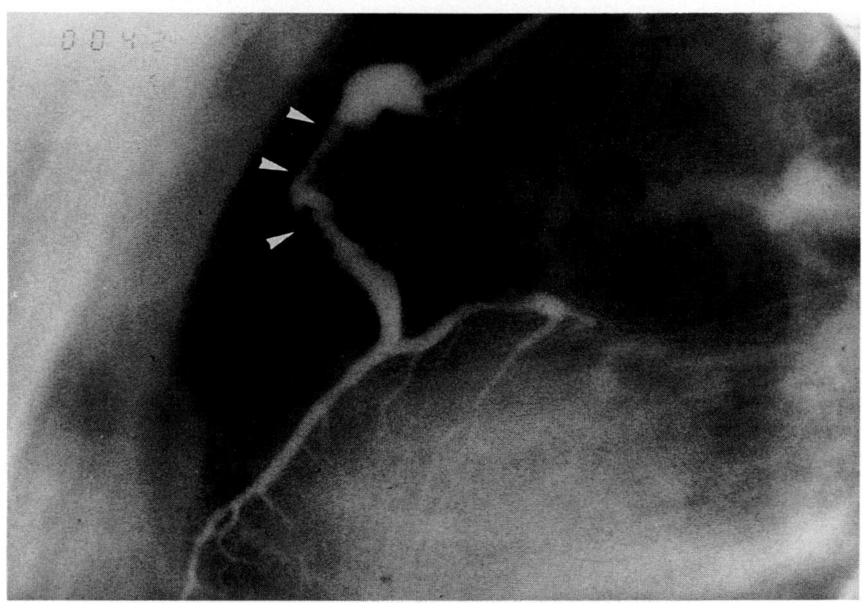

Figure 68

Even occluded grafts can be recanalized in some special circumstances. In a 46-year-old man who had undergone CABG 7 years earlier and presented with unstable angina, the venous graft to the LAD was occluded at the distal anastomosis with minimal residual flow into a small septal branch (Fig. 69a). The distal LAD was supplied by collaterals (Fig. 69b). The graft was recanalized successfully (Fig. 69c), this being associated with the disappearance of collaterals (Fig. 69d). The left ventricular function was preserved (Fig. 69e: diastole, Fig. 69f: systole) despite the temporary occlusion of the graft owing to the collaterals. A 1-year follow-up revealed a restenosis of the dilated segment (Fig. 69g), which was subsequently redilated.

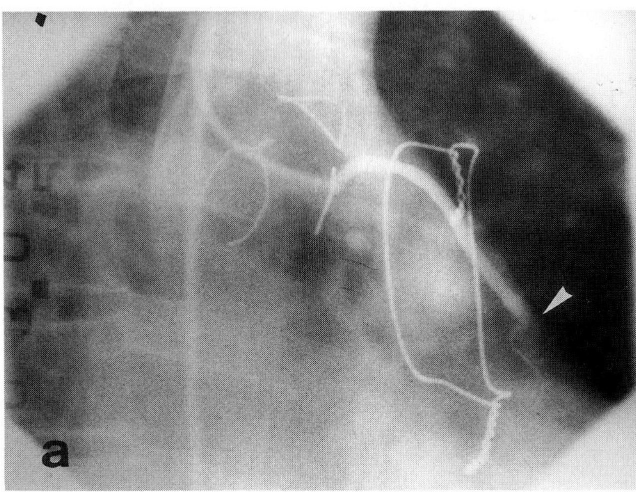

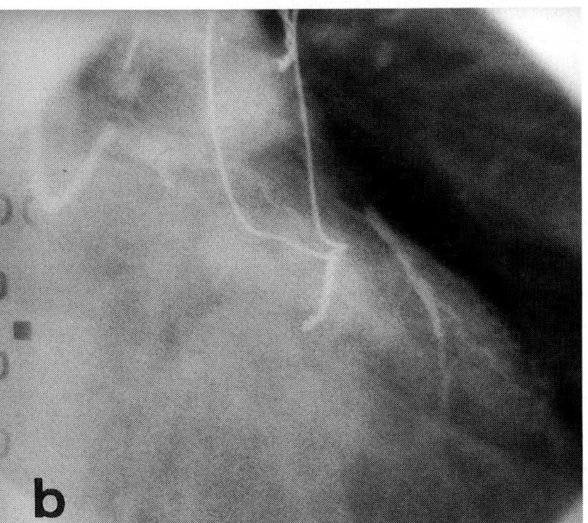

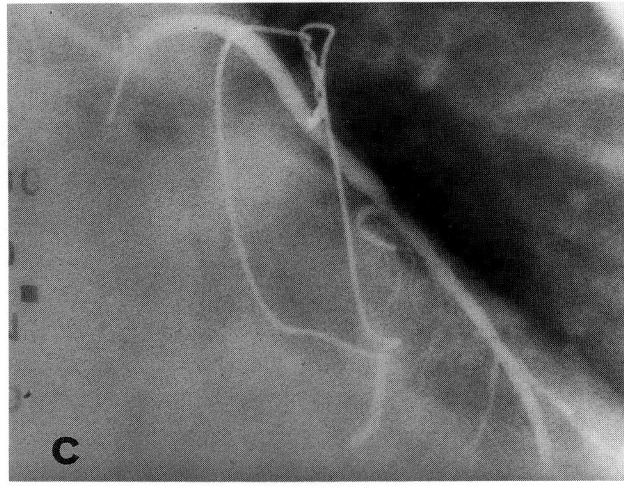

Figure 69

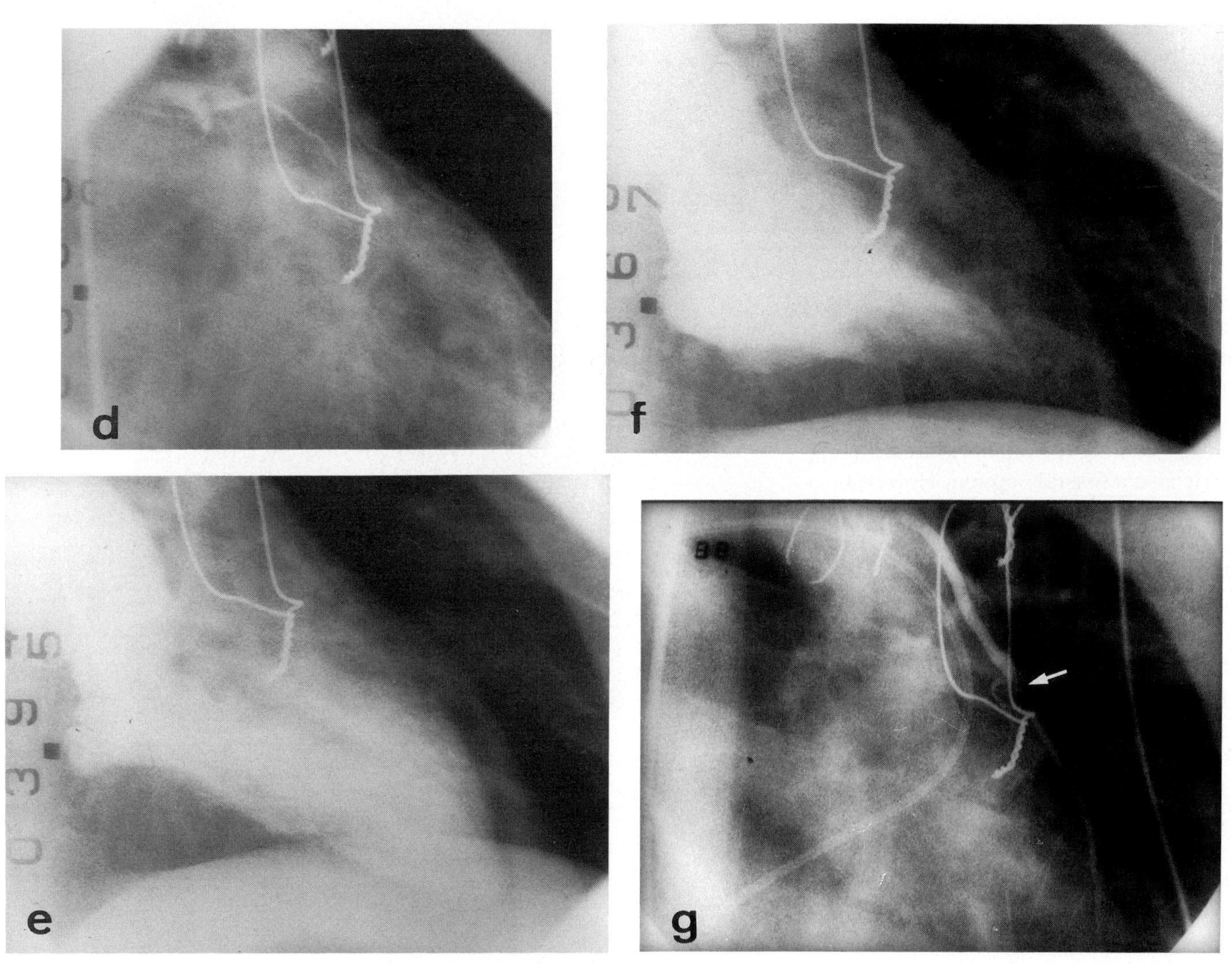
d
f
e
g

Acutely occluded venous grafts may have acceptable long-term results, whereas the long-term results following PTCA of chronically occluded grafts are so poor as to make it a contraindication to an angioplasty attempt. Stenting for venous graft stenoses is also a feasible option. However, the chances of thrombosis may be higher than for native vessels, because of the more sluggish flow in grafts. A 57-year-old man had undergone two CABG operations, 3 years and 6 months earlier, respectively. He presented with class III angina pectoris, despite triple drug therapy. Grafts to the LCx and RCA were closed, and the native vessels showed significant stenoses, with diffusely diseased peripheries. The venous graft to the LAD had a severe stenosis in its body (Fig. 70a). The result after dilatation with a 3.5-mm balloon was poor (Fig. 70b), hence the vessel was stented with a Palmaz-Schatz stent (Johnson & Johnson), with a good angiographic (Fig. 70c) and clinical result.

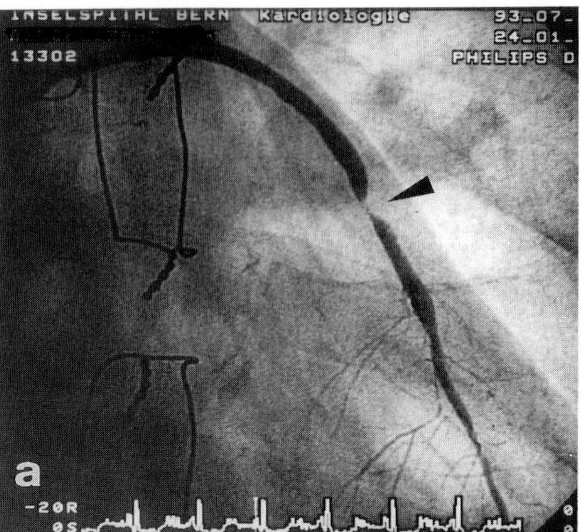

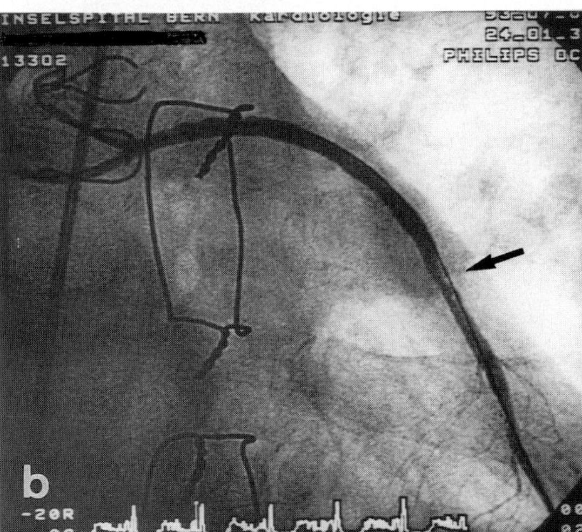

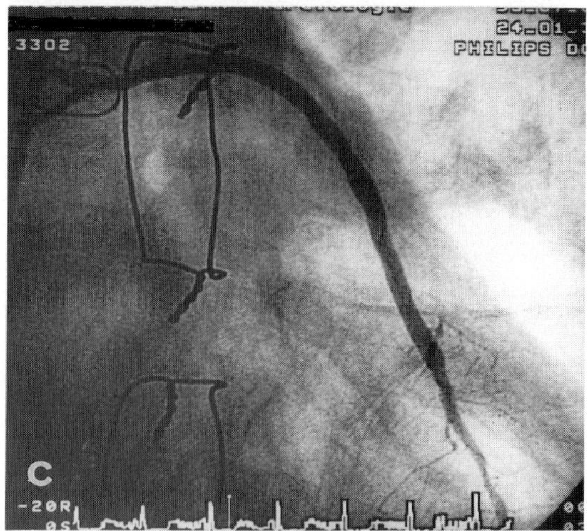

Figure 70

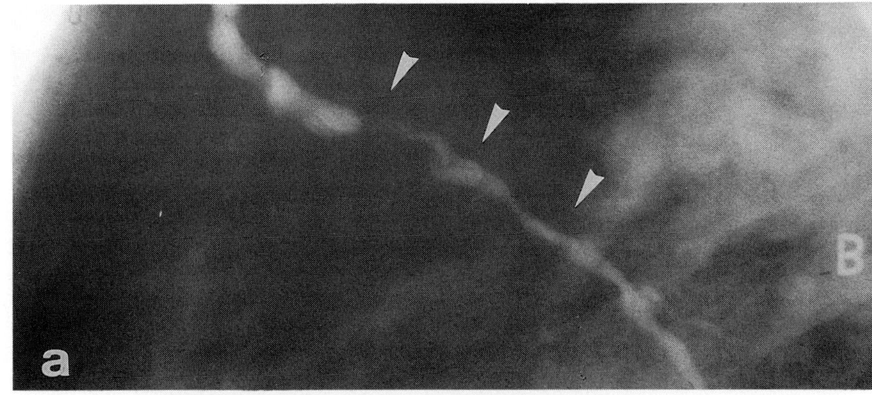

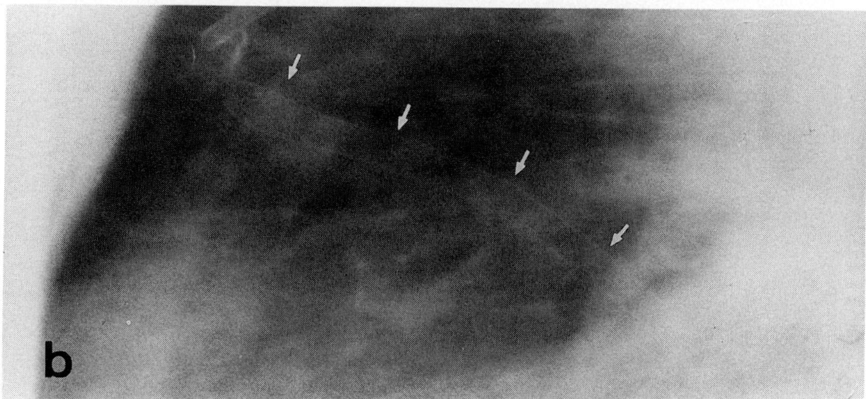

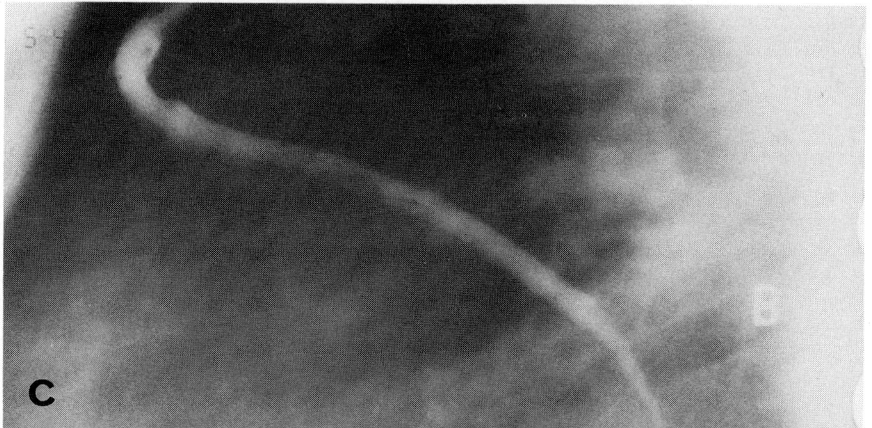

Figure 71

However, stents are no panacea for diffusely diseased old grafts, which are best left alone. This was true in the case of a 60-year-old man with angina due to diffuse stenoses of an 11-year-old graft to the LCx (Fig. 71a). Following an insufficient balloon angioplasty attempt, stenting of the entire length of the graft was carried out, with one 5.5-mm and two 6.0-mm Wallstents (Schneider) (Fig. 71b). However, the flow through the graft remained sluggish (Fig. 71c) and the graft occluded subsequently.

When dealing with patients with prior CABG and diseased grafts, it may sometimes be a better option to dilate the native stenosis for which the graft was implanted in the first place rather than the diseased graft. Such an approach is rational since the restenosis rate after PTCA of the native vessel is lower than that for graft angioplasty. A 45-year-old woman presented with angina 3 months after bypass grafting to the LAD and LCx. Angiography revealed stenoses of the left main coronary artery and the LCx at the insertion of the venous graft (Fig. 72a). The venous graft was diseased, with a significant stenosis in its proximal segment (Fig. 72b). The left main and the LCx arteries were dilated under the protection of the diseased but patent graft. At follow-up 1 week later, the LCx was occluded (Fig. 72c) and the distal vessel saved by the graft (Fig. 72d). The native LCx was redilated. The result 3 months later revealed a normal-looking LCx. The diseased graft was no longer needed, and was indeed occluded (Fig. 72e). A 63-year-

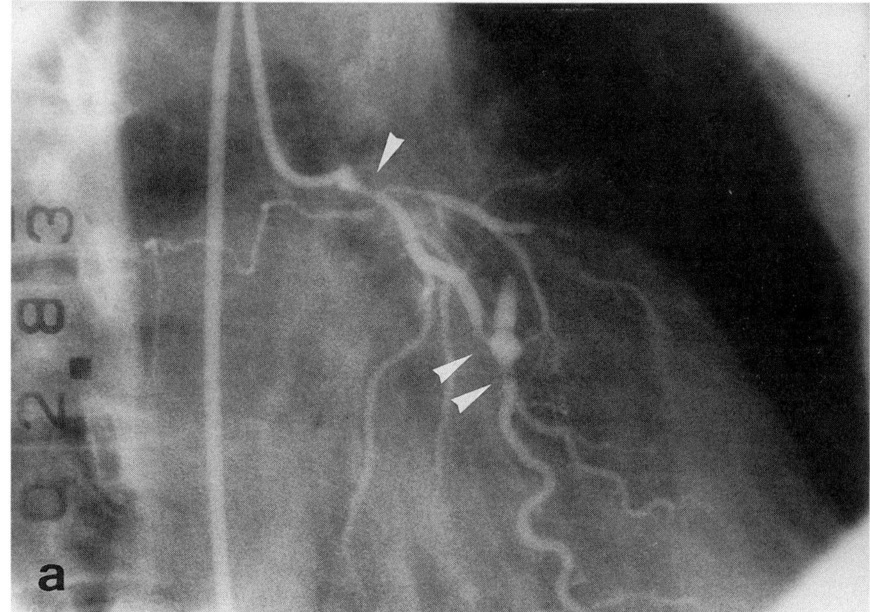

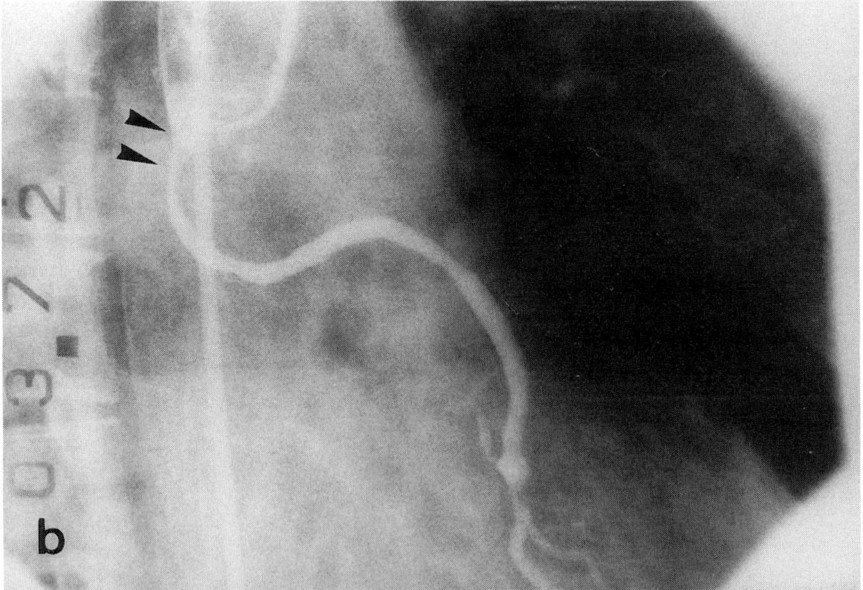

Figure 72

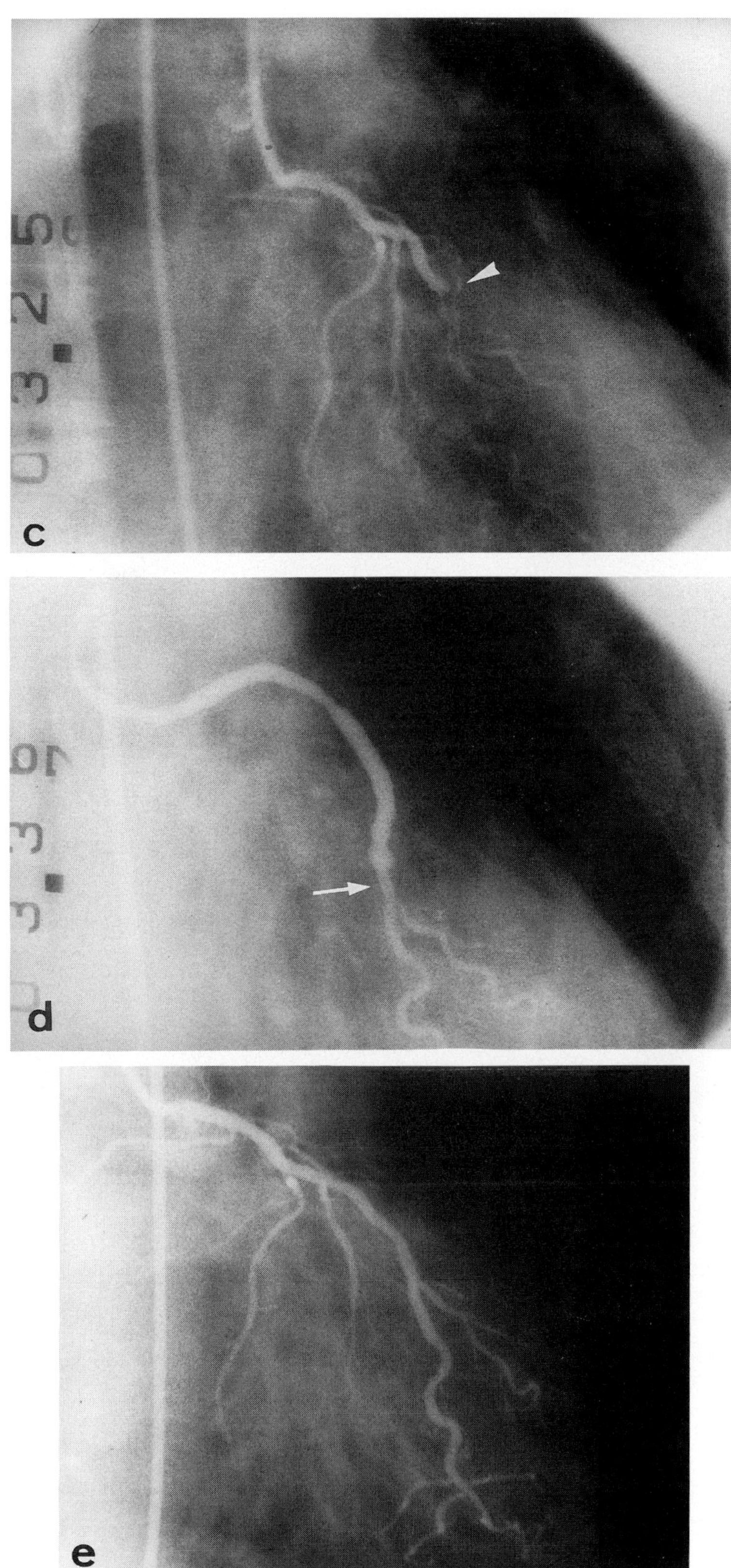

old man with an 8-year-old graft to the LAD had angina. A mild stenosis at the graft insertion site was seen (Fig. 73a, arrowhead) and dilated (Fig. 73b). A stenosis of the LAD proximal to the graft was also seen (Fig. 73a, arrow) but was left alone. The patient returned 20 months later with angina. An angiogram revealed a graft body closure (Fig. 73c,d). The LAD territory was dependent on the stenosed native vessel. This case has to be considered mismanaged in that the native vessel should have been dilated in the first place rather than the graft, since the chances of a native vessel remaining patent are better than those for a graft, as demonstrated here.

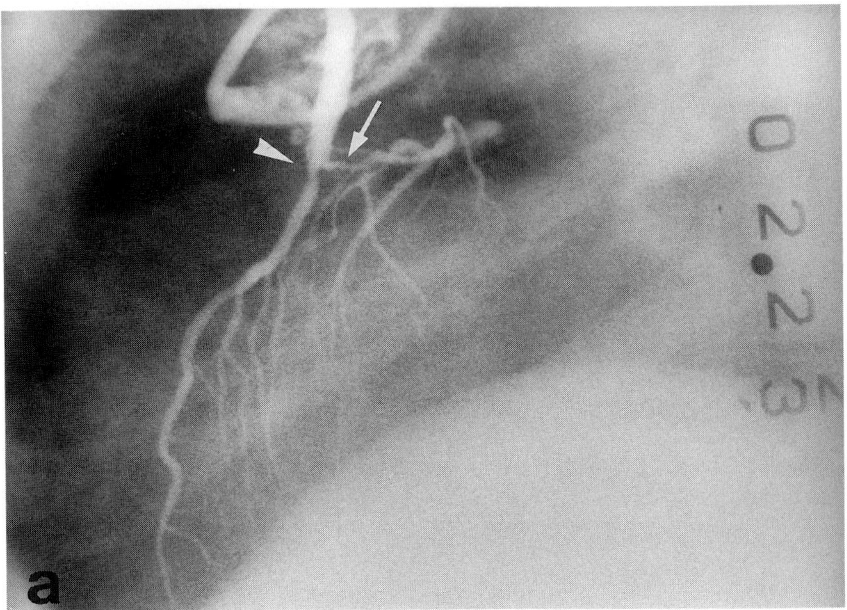

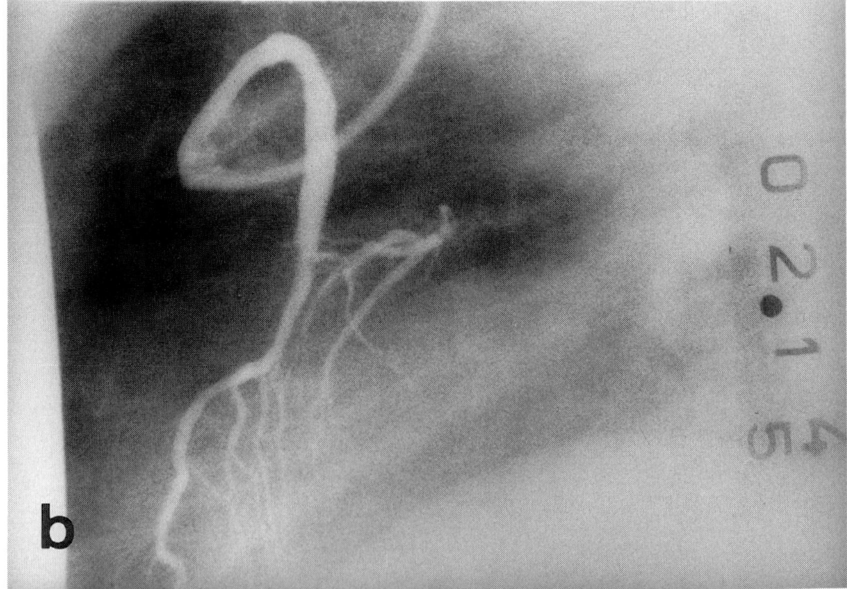

Figure 73

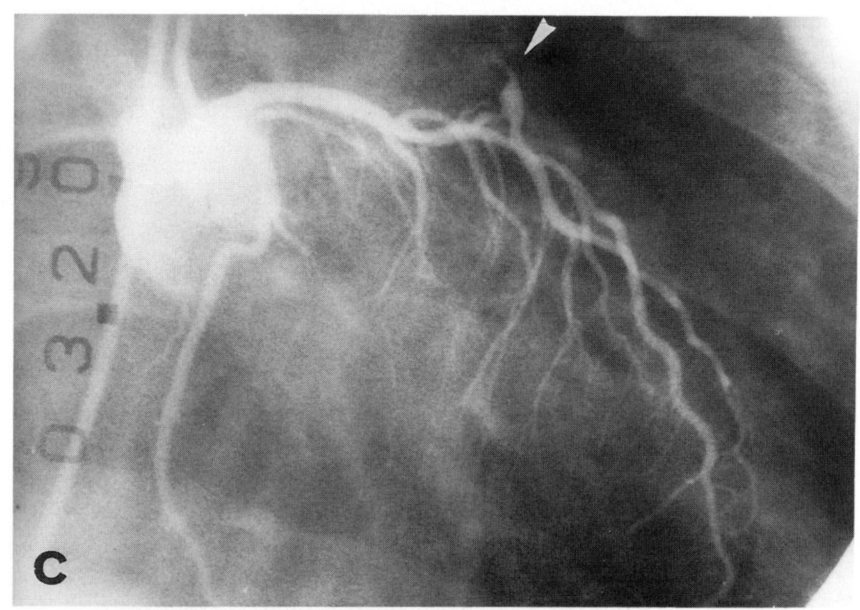
c

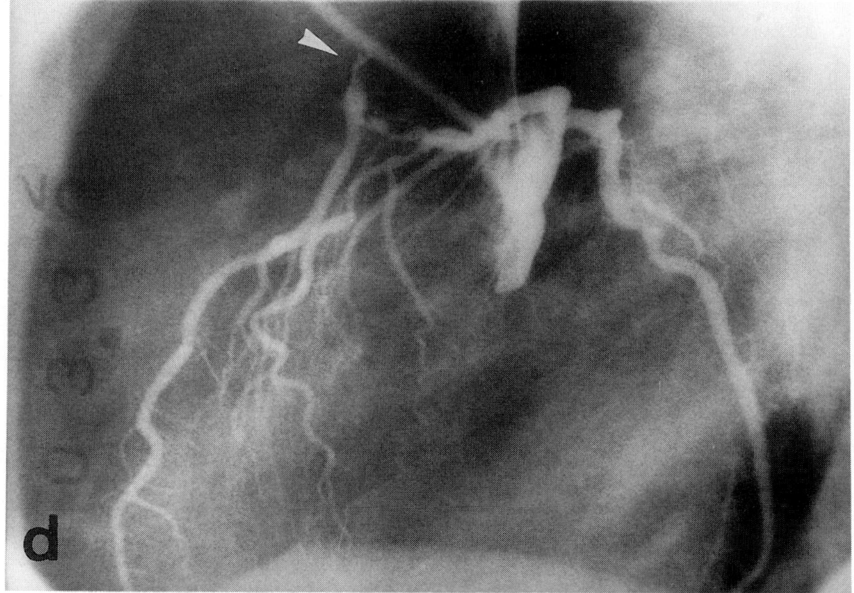
d

Sometimes it may be necessary to dilate the proximal native vessel retrogradely through the graft, as in the case of a 74-year-old man who had undergone CABG to the LAD and LCx for left main stem stenosis, and presented with angina. The angiogram revealed an occluded left main stem and LCx graft. However, the graft to the LAD supplied the LCx retrogradely via a diseased proximal LAD segment (Fig. 74a). This LAD segment was dilated in a retrograde fashion via the venous graft (Fig. 74b), with a good result (Fig. 74c) and relief of the patient's symptoms.

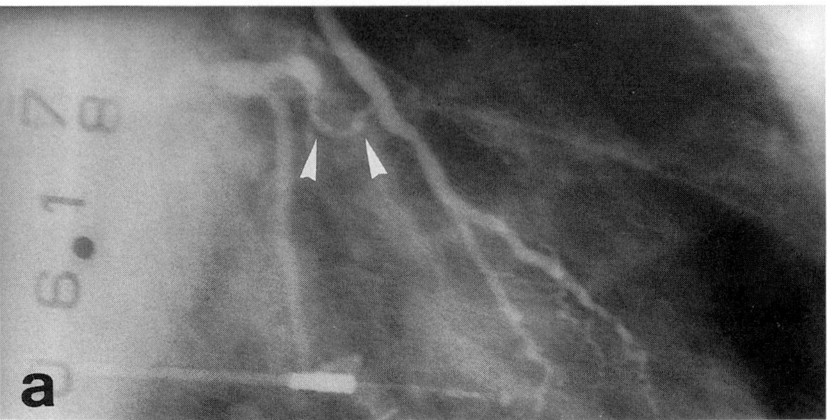

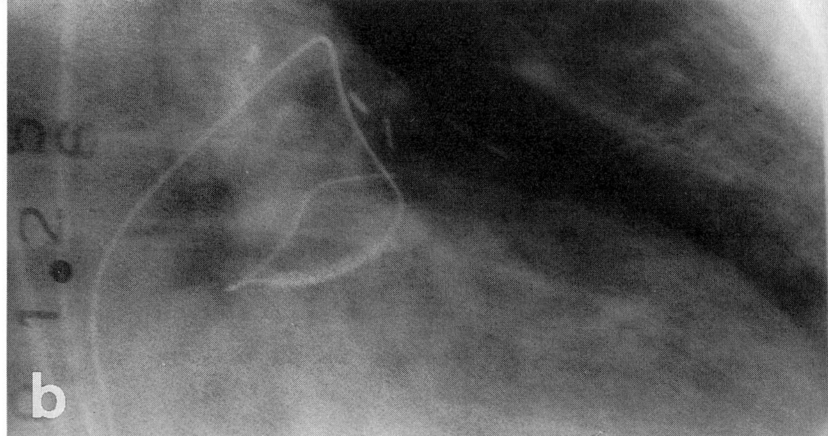

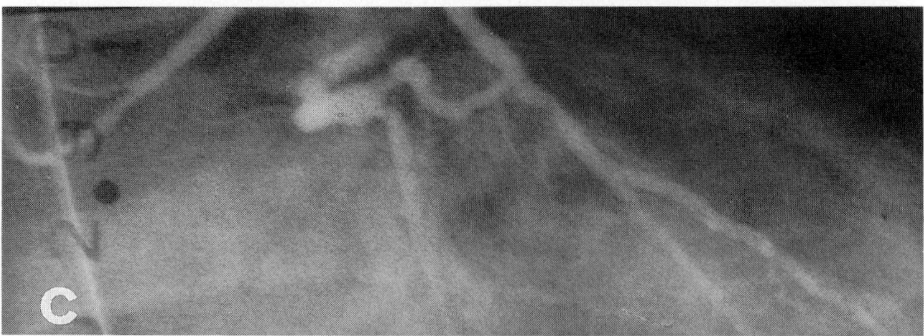

Figure 74

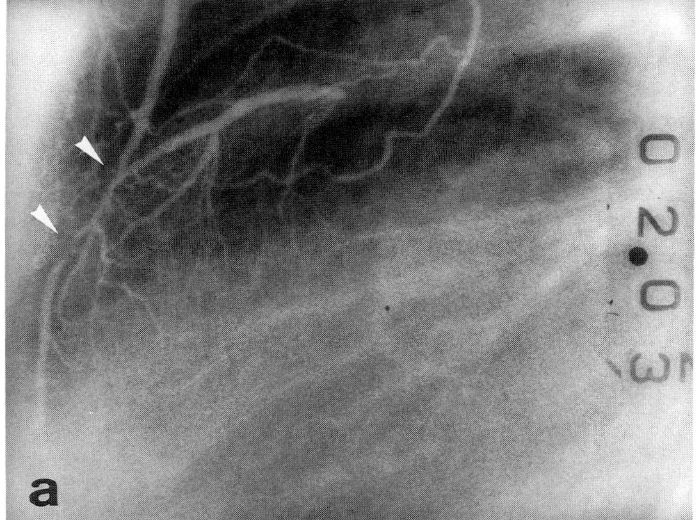

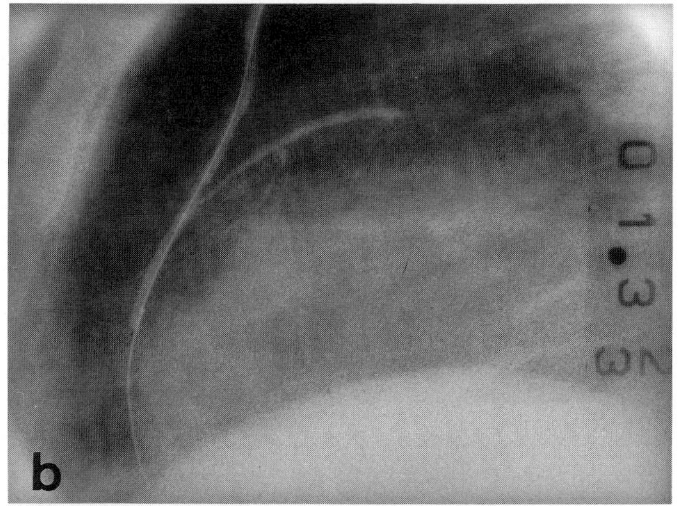

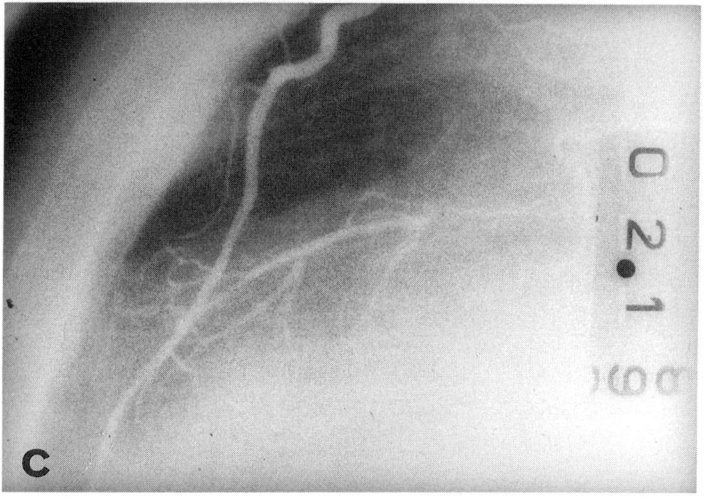

Figure 75

Mammary Artery Grafts

A mammary artery bypass catheter offers good backup support for mammary artery graft angioplasty. Care has to be taken with the guiding catheter, the origin of the mammary artery being friable and prone to dissection. Stenoses at the distal anastomotic site of mammary artery grafts are associated with good immediate and long-term results. A 56-year-old man had undergone CABG 2 months prior with a LIMA graft on the LAD, and presented with persistent symptoms. Angiography revealed a stenosis of the distal anastomotic site and the vessel just distal to the anastomosis (Fig. 75a). Angioplasty was performed with a long balloon (Fig. 75b). The final result was good (Fig. 75c). Long-term results following such distal anastomotic site angioplasty can be expected to be good.

Multiple grafts may need to be dilated in patients following CABG. Such an example is a 49-year-old man with angina 3 months after CABG. Angiography revealed a distal anastomotic site stenosis of the LIMA graft to the LAD (Fig. 76a), which was dilated (Fig. 76b) with a good result (Fig. 76c). Six months later, symptoms recurred. A stenosis of the venous graft to the RCA was detected (Fig. 76d) and dilated (Fig. 76e). The left mammary graft on the LAD was well (Fig. 76f) and remained so at 6-month (Fig. 76g) and 18-month (Fig. 76h) follow-up (demonstrating the anticipated good long-term results after PTCA of the distal anastomotic site of LIMA grafts). The venous graft remained well on control angiograms performed after 6 months (Fig. 76i) and 18 months (Fig. 76j). The ventricular function remained normal (Fig. 76k: diastole, Fig. 76l: systole).

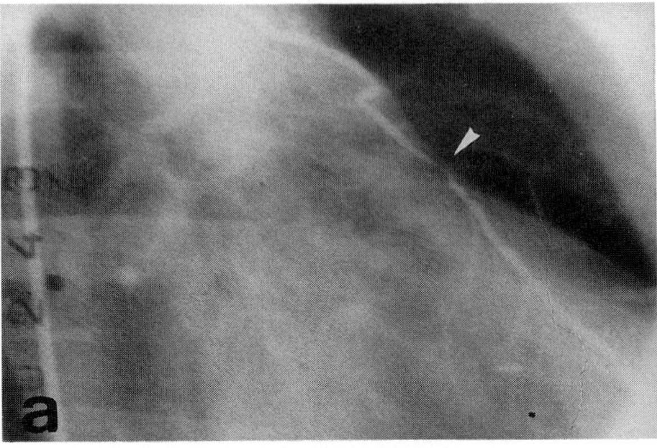

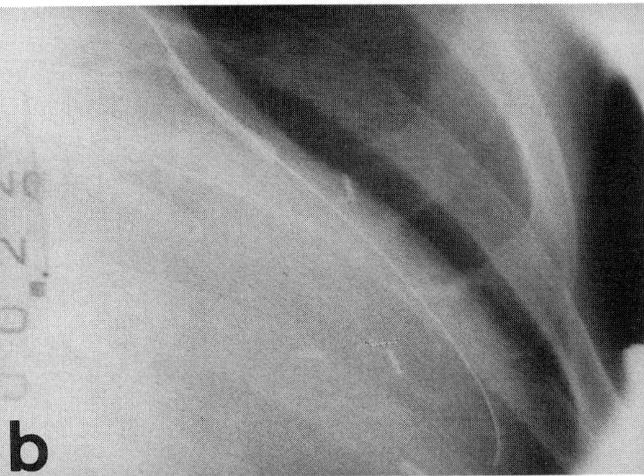

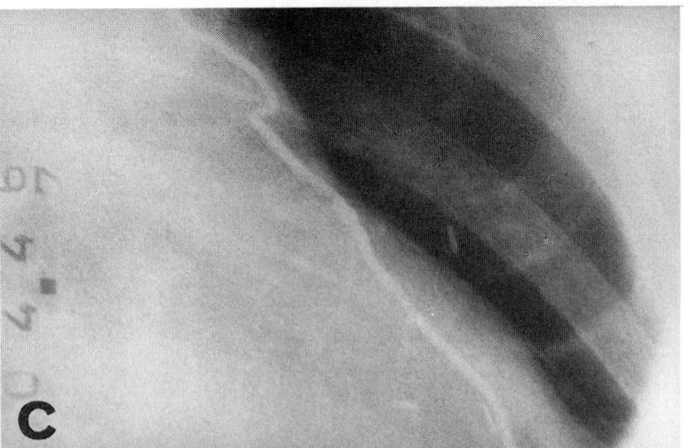

Figure 76

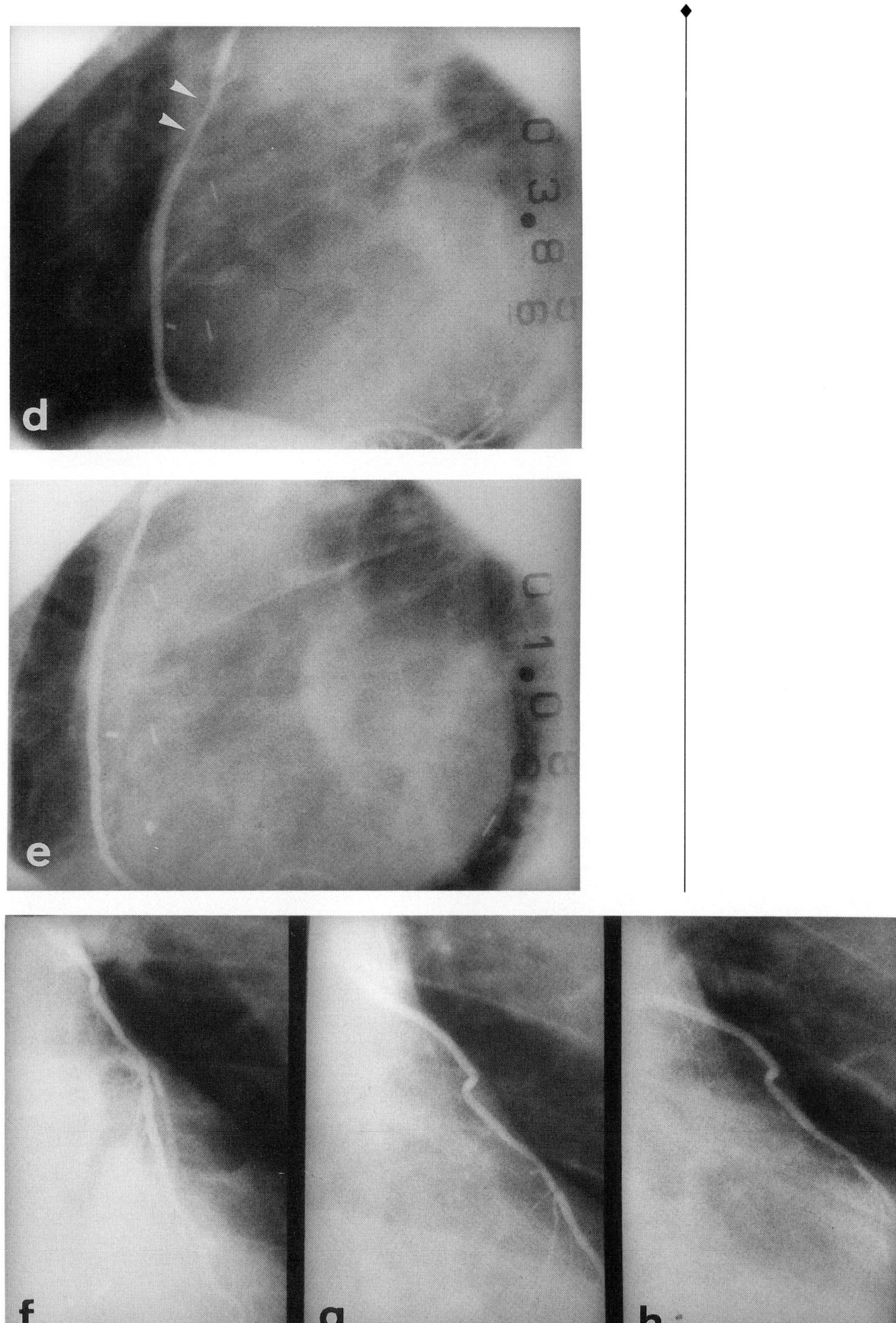
d
e
f
g
h

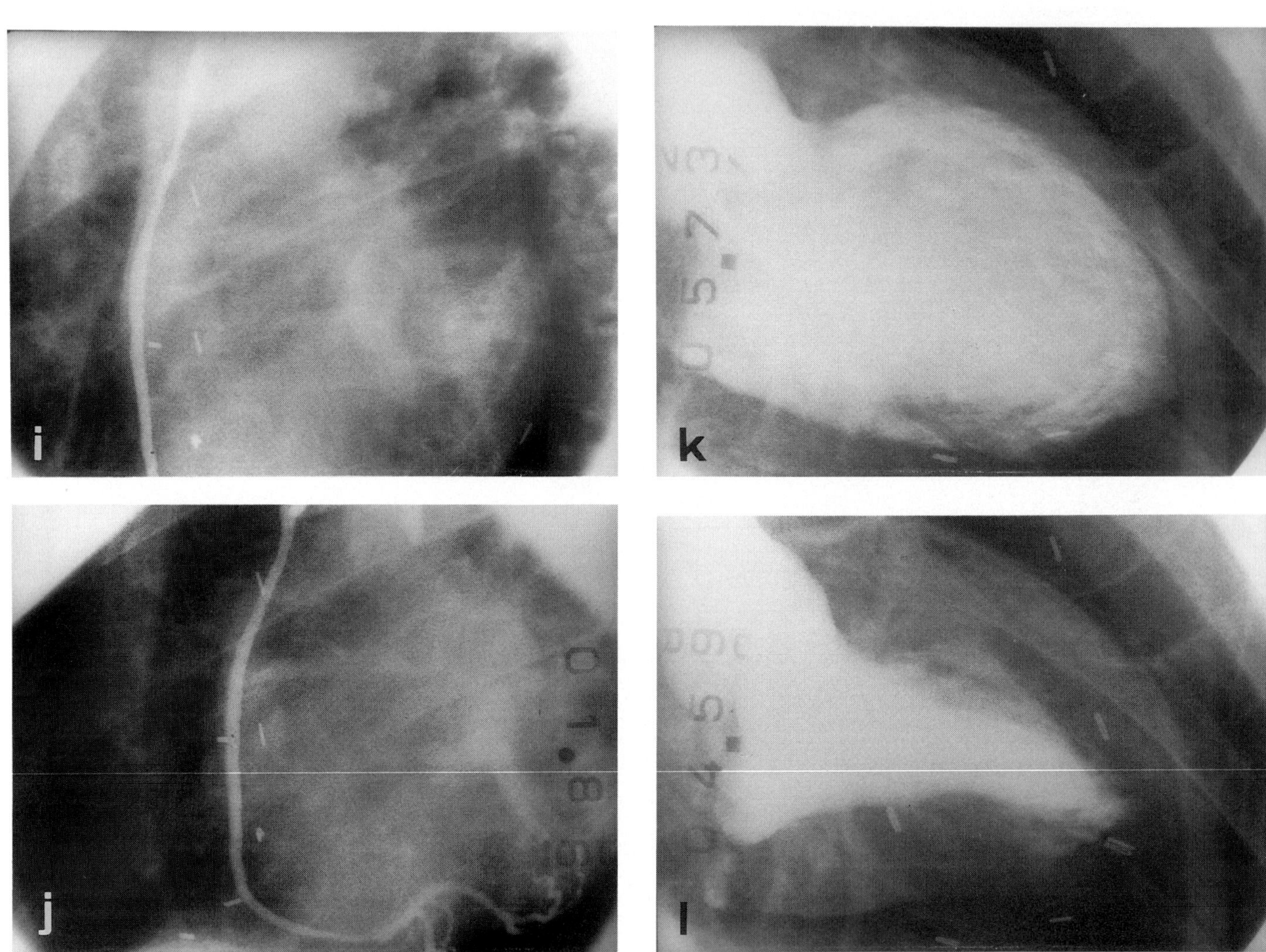

Figure 76 (Continued)

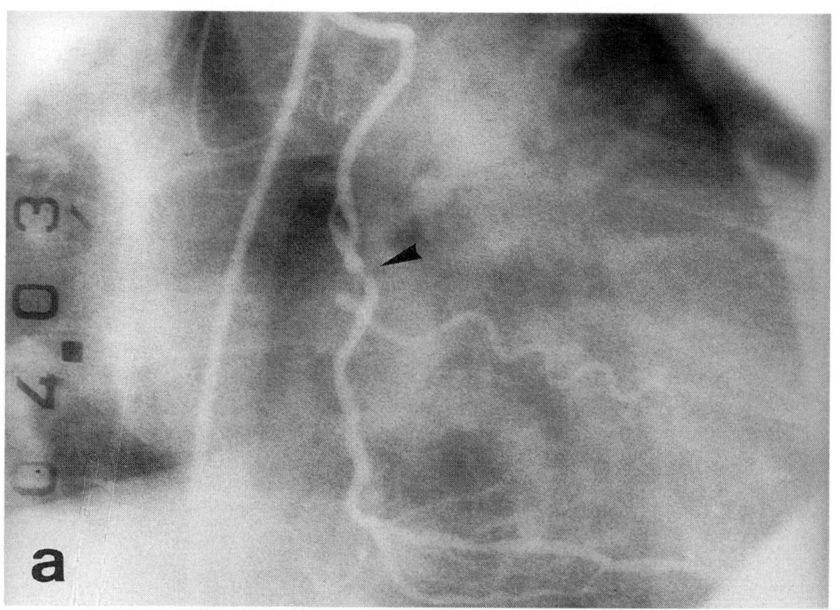

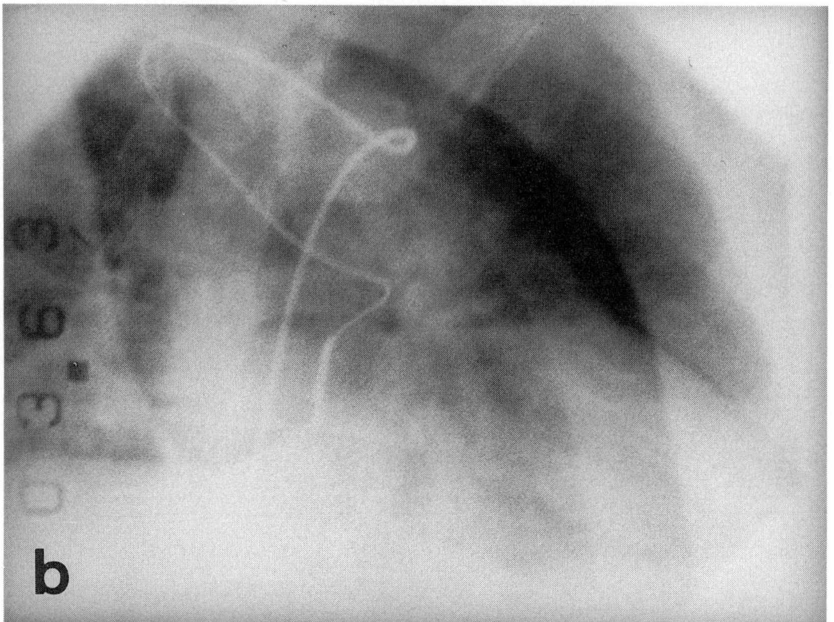

Figure 77

Another example is a 40-year-old man who had undergone CABG with a LIMA to the LAD and a right mammary graft to the RCA. He presented 3 months after surgery with a stenosis of the distal anastomotic site and the native RCA just distal to the anastomosis (Fig. 77a). These lesions were dilated via the graft despite the somewhat intricate access to this right internal mammary artery (Fig. 77b). The result was good (Fig. 77c). The patient presented once again 7 months later with angina. The right mammary graft was well (Fig. 77d). However, there was now a stenosis of the anastomotic site of the LIMA on the LAD (Fig. 77e) which was dilated successfully (Fig. 77f).

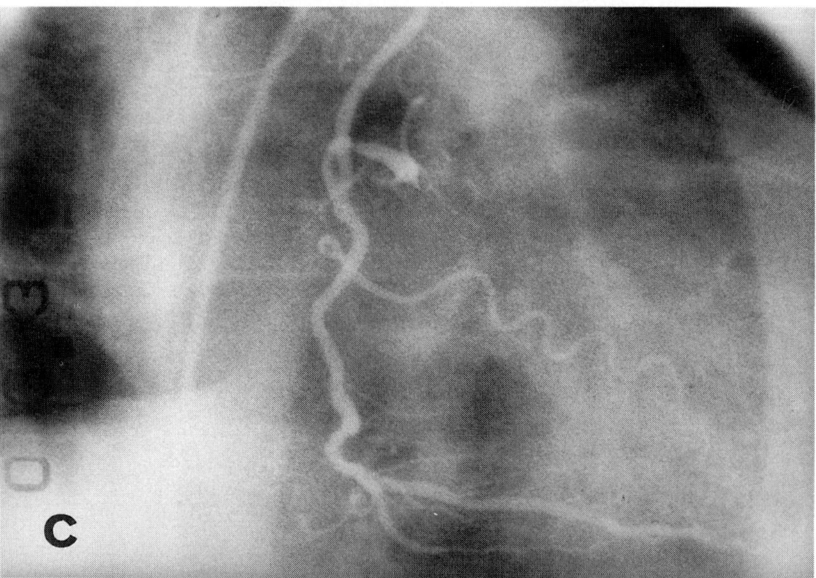

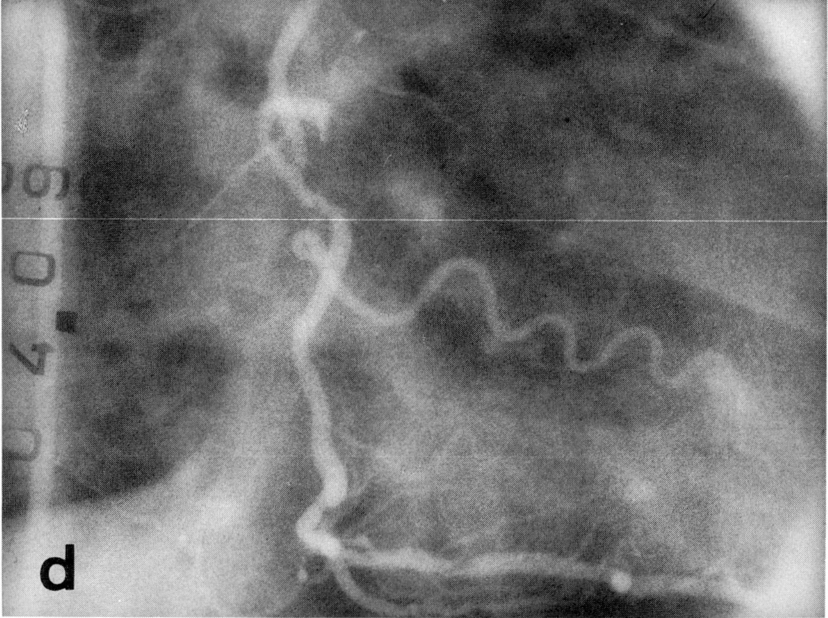

Figure 77 (Continued)

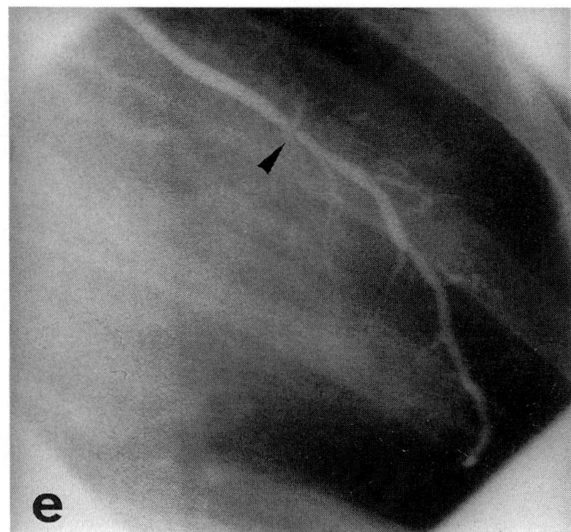
e

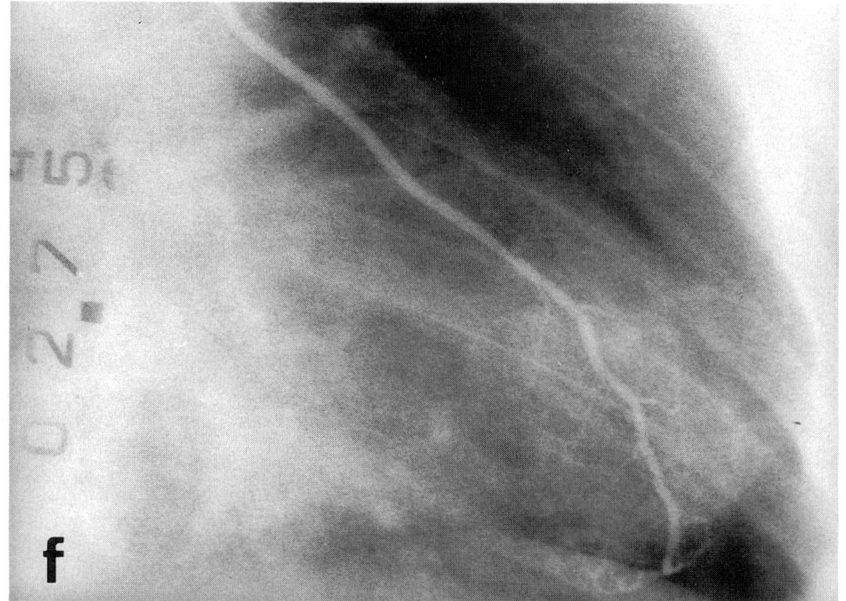
f

Occasionally, angioplasty of distal stenoses of a coronary artery may have to be performed through the mammary artery graft. Foreshortened versions of mammary guiding catheters are available to allow for the increased distance the guidewire and balloon have to travel to reach the target lesion. A 59-year-old man presented 2 years after CABG, including a LIMA graft to the LAD, with a stenosis of the distal LAD (Fig. 78a). Since the proximal LAD was occluded, the lesion was dilated via the graft. The final result was good (Fig. 78b).

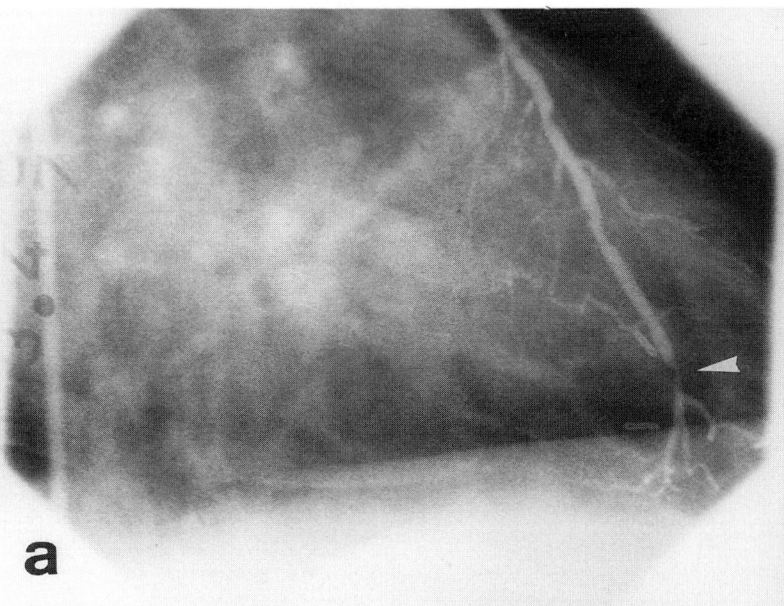

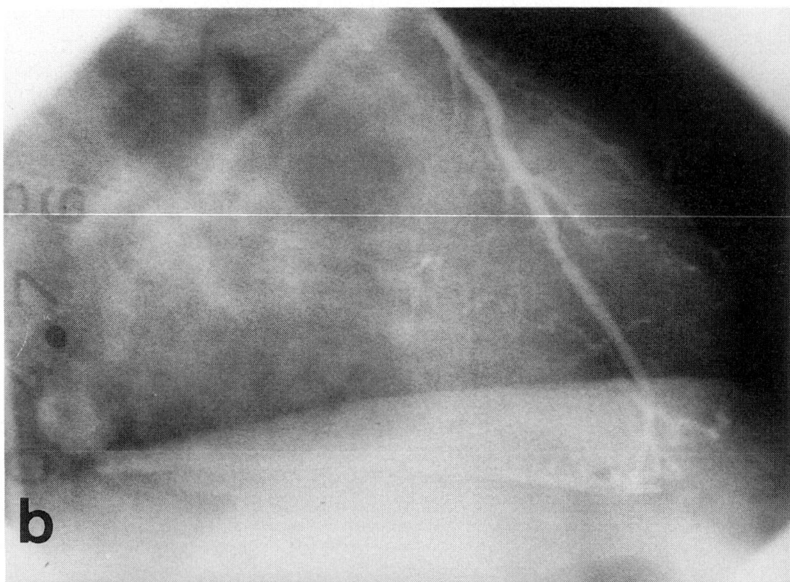

Figure 78

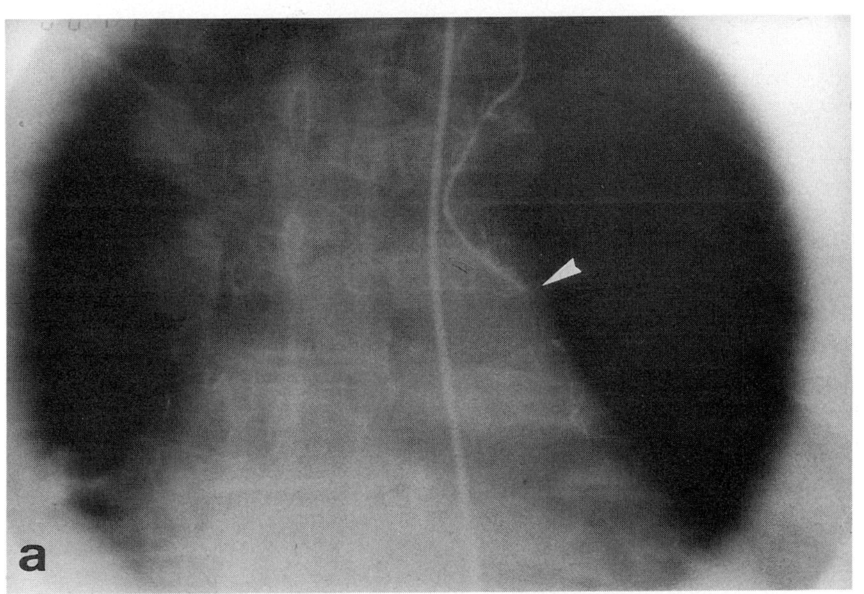

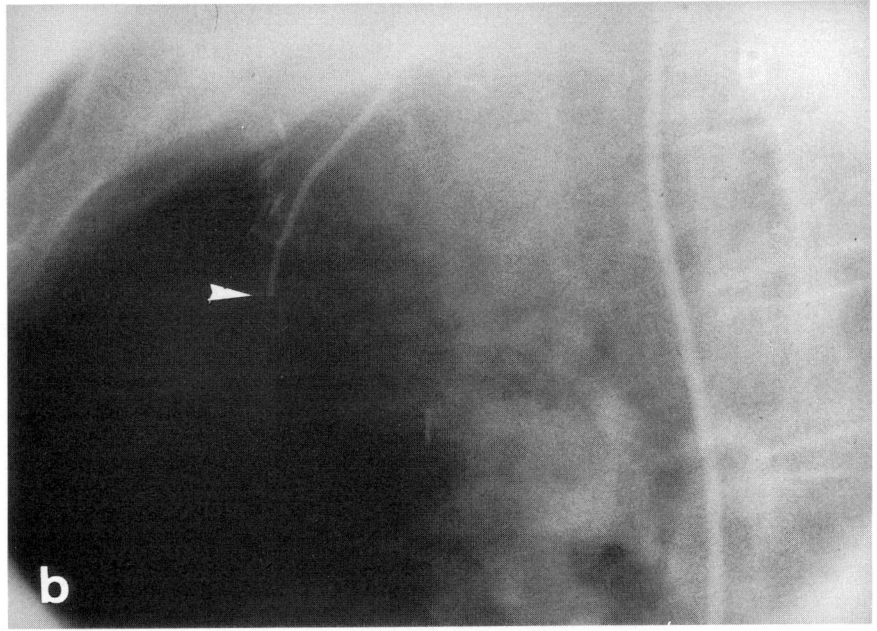

Figure 79

Angioplasty of occluded mammary bypass grafts is also feasible and should probably be attempted in selected patients. A 59-year-old man presented with recurrence of symptoms 4 months after CABG. Angiography revealed an occluded LIMA graft (Fig. 79a: RAO, Fig. 79b: lateral view). The occlusion was crossed with a Magnum wire backed with a Magnarail probing catheter (Fig. 79c). After passage of the wire alone, distal flow was established and revealed a diseased distal LAD (Fig. 79d), which was probably the cause for the occlusion of the LIMA graft soon after surgery. The distal LAD disease had not been apparent from the film taken before bypass grafting, since it had been subtended by collaterals exclusively. Angioplasty of the distal LAD was performed through the LIMA graft, along with angioplasty of the graft itself (Fig. 79e). The final result was good (Fig. 79f). A 3-month follow-up revealed a patent graft (Fig. 79g) and a good distal LAD (Fig. 79h).

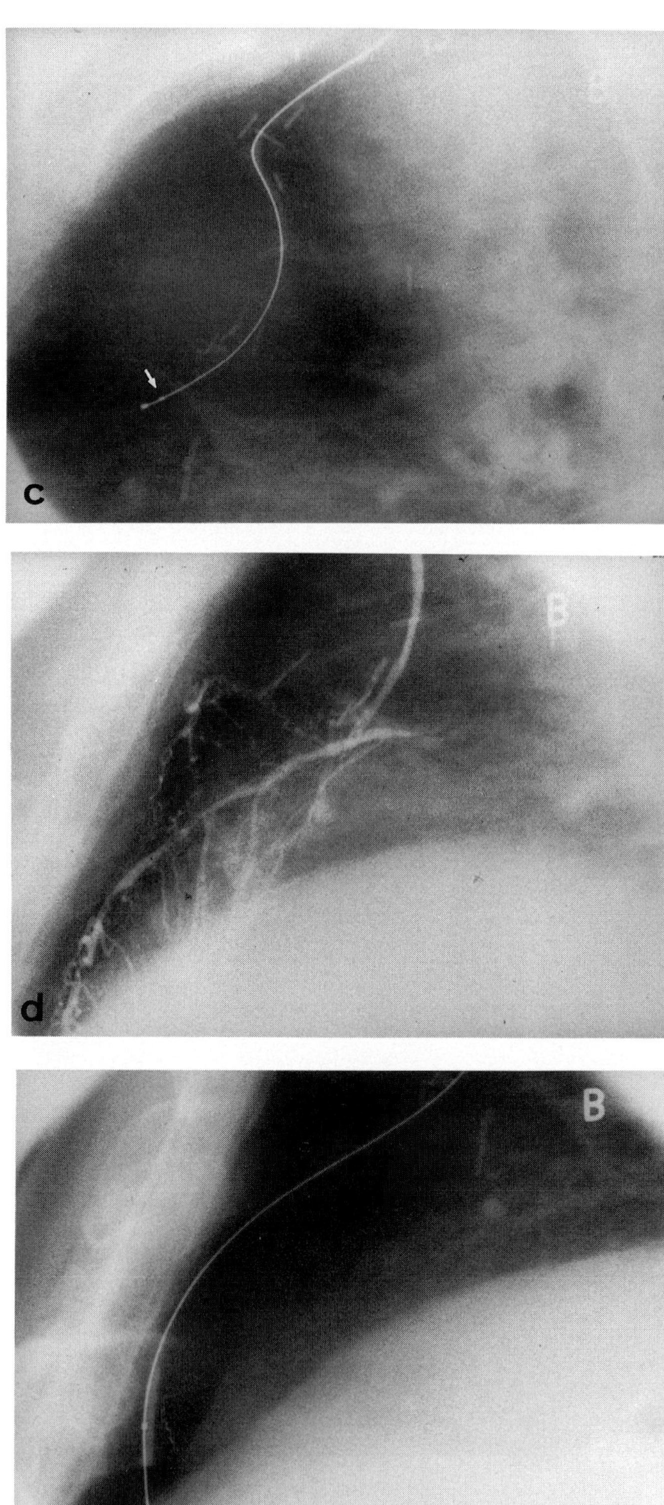

Figure 79 (Continued)

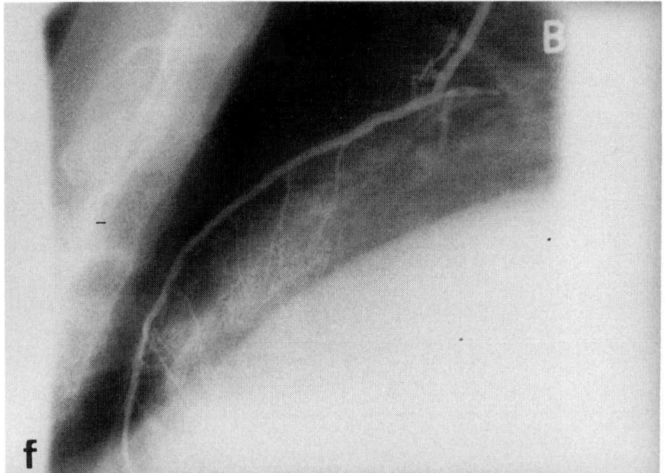
B
f

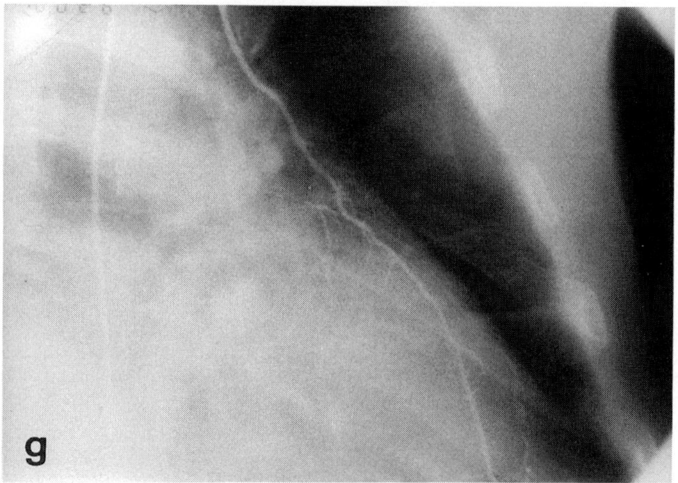
g

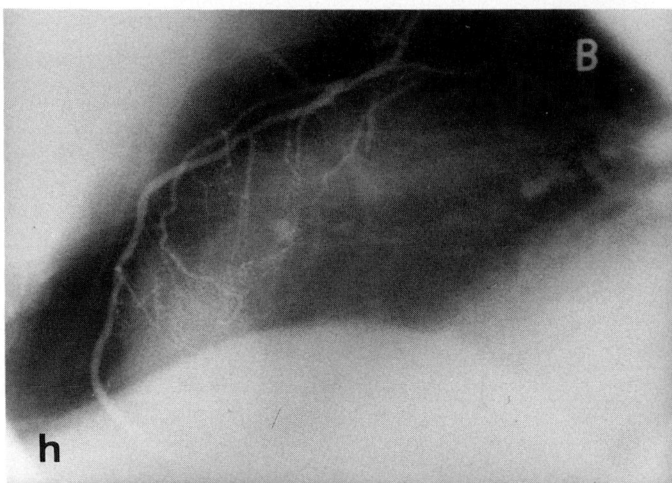
B
h

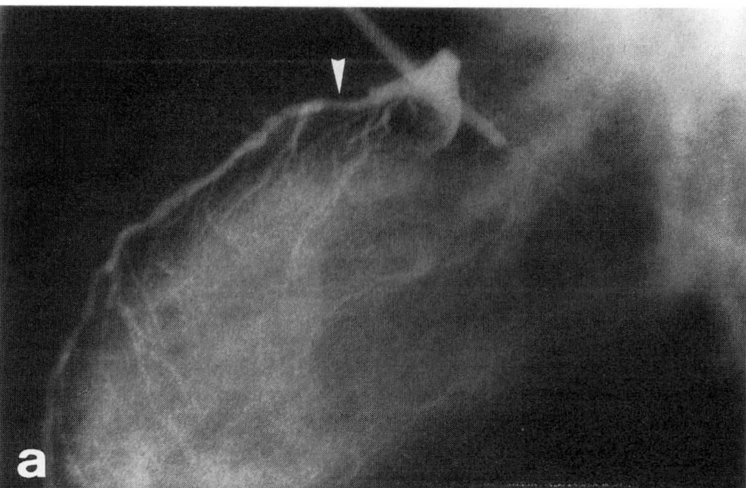

Sometimes, angioplasty may be required for correcting a surgical error. A 46-year-old man underwent CABG for a borderline stenosis of the proximal LAD (Fig. 80a). Two years later angina recurred. An angiogram revealed that the proximal stenosis had remained the same or even regressed. However, there was now a stenosis in the mid LAD at the site of insertion of the venous graft (Fig. 80b). The graft itself was occluded. The stenosis was dilated (Fig. 80c), with a good result (Fig. 80d). Two-year (Fig. 80e) and 5-year (Fig. 80f) follow-up revealed a good long-term result. In this patient CABG had been unnecessary, and only caused an iatrogenic stenosis. A more

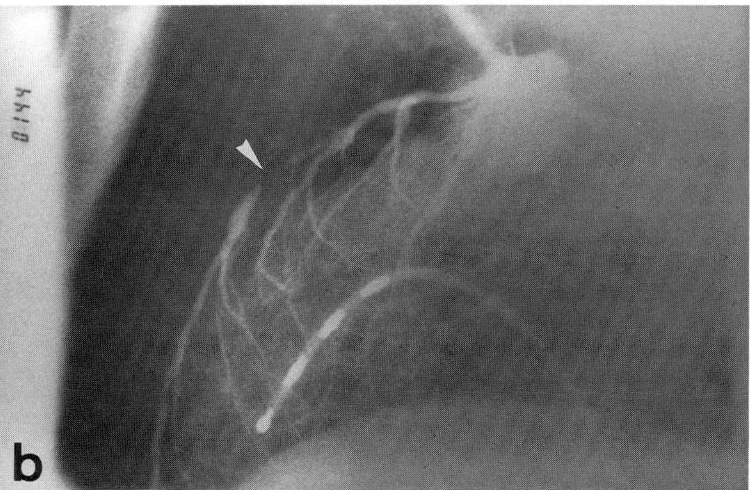

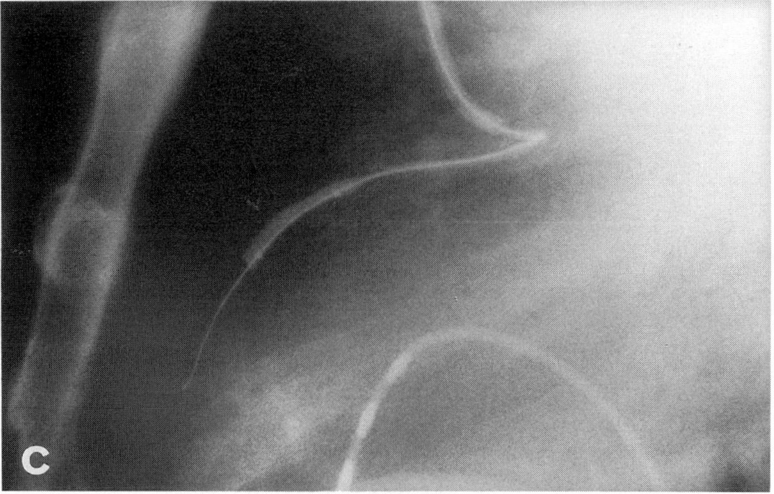

Figure 80

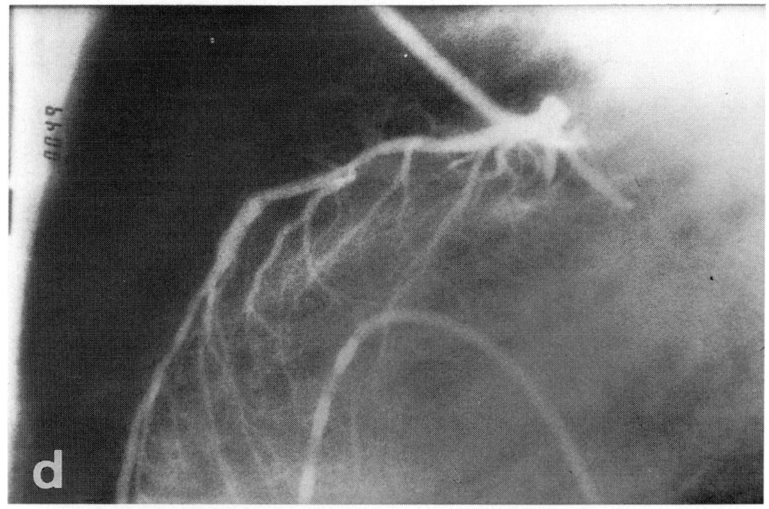
d

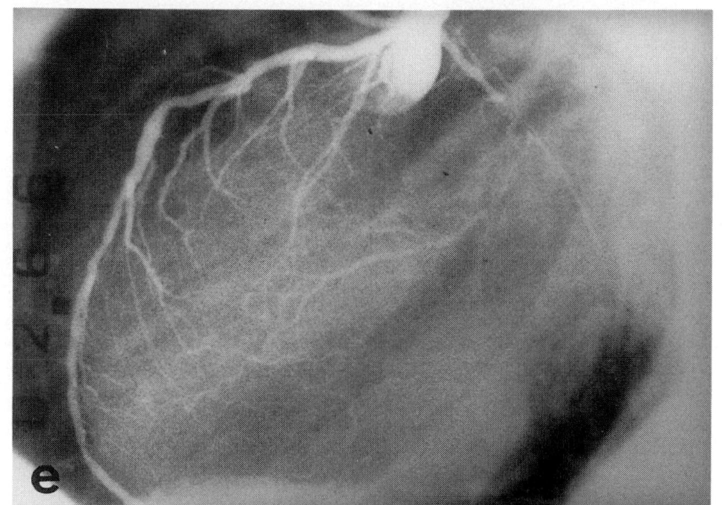
e

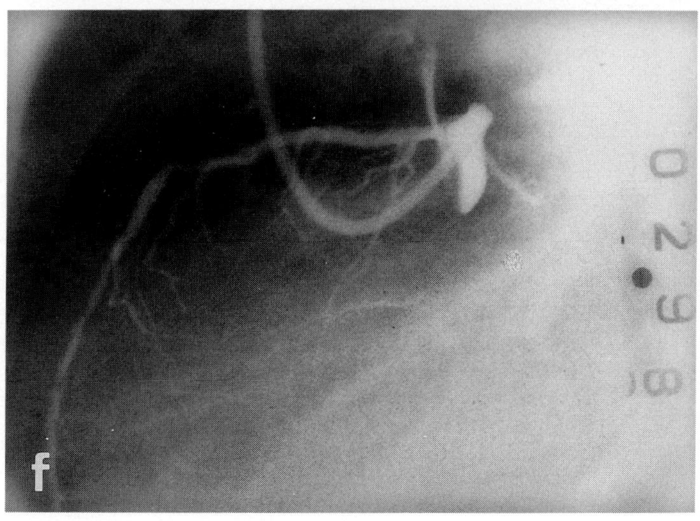
f

serious example is that of a 57-year-old woman who received a graft to her LAD which was erroneously placed proximal to the stenosis (Fig. 81a). The patient's symptoms persisted, and the lesion was successfully dilated (Fig. 81b), with a good result (Fig. 81c) and relief of angina.

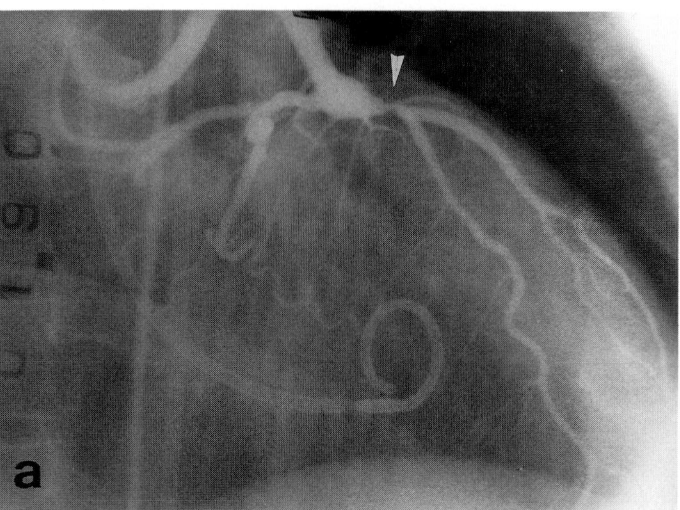

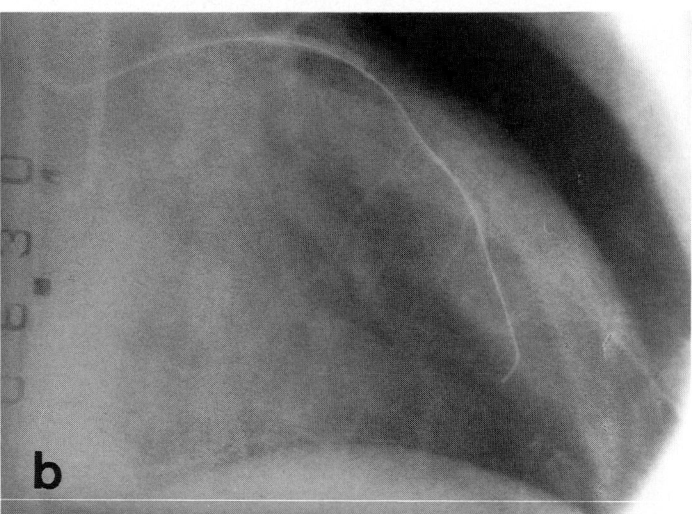

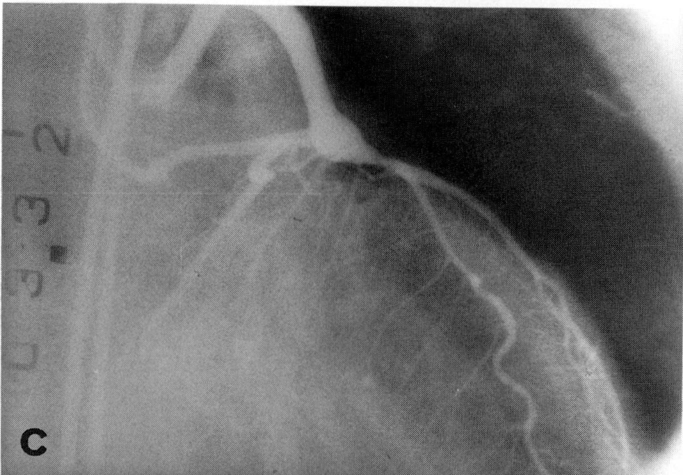

Figure 81

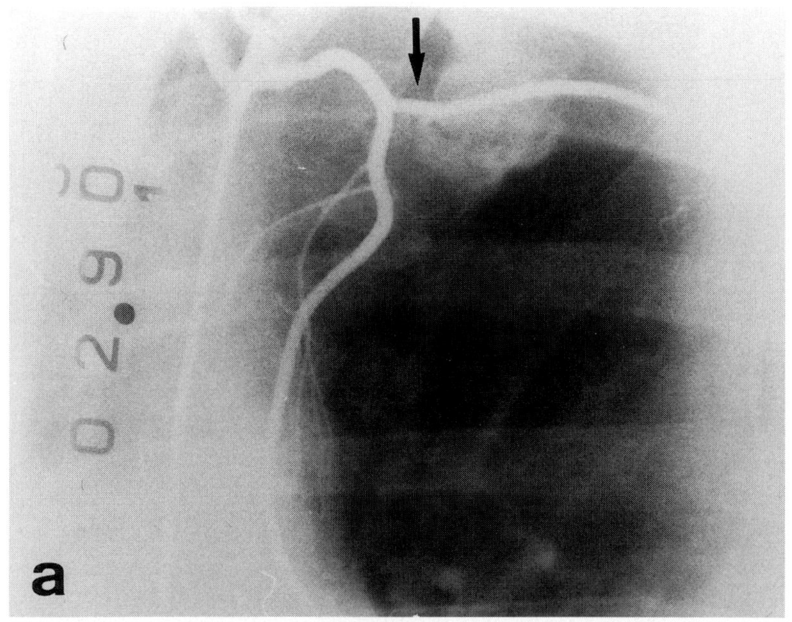

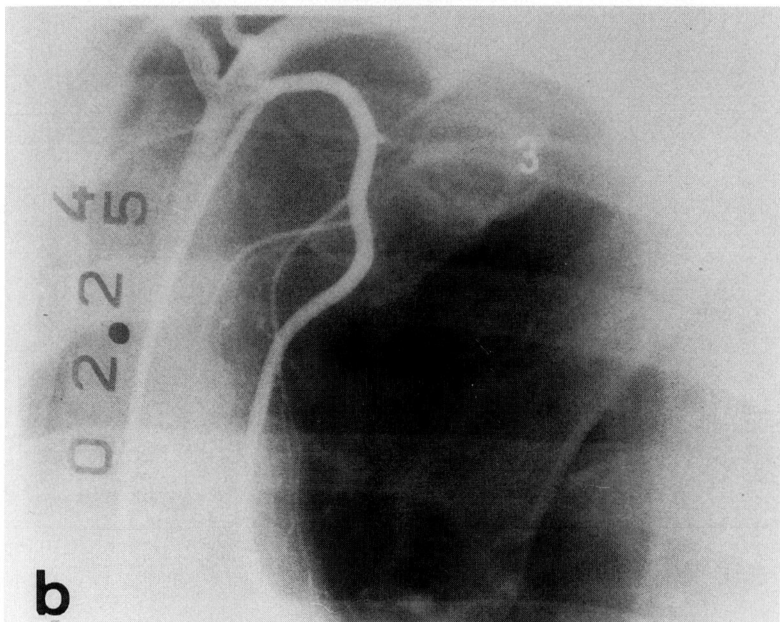

Figure 82

Rarely, a major unligated side branch of a mammary artery graft can cause ischemia by a steal phenomenon. A 58-year-old man had ongoing chest pain with a positive stress test 6 months following CABG. No significant graft stenoses were detected. However, a large side branch of the LIMA graft to the LAD was seen (Fig. 82a). This was closed by coil embolization (Fig. 82b) and resulted in relief of symptoms and a normalizing of the stress test. This case also emphasizes the need for evaluating the mammary arteries and their side branches prior to CABG.

2.5 ANGIOPLASTY FOR RESTENOSIS

Restenosis rates of 30 to 40% continue to plague the procedure. This rate remains unchanged for subsequent PTCAs, so that occasional patients will have several procedures. A 44-year-old man presented with a stenosis of the proximal LAD (Fig. 83a) which was dilated successfully (Fig. 83b). Seven months later he presented with restenosis (Fig. 83c). Reangioplasty was performed with a good result (Fig. 83d). Five months later an angiogram performed for recurrence of symptoms revealed a severe restenosis, with near-total occlusion of the vessel supplied by ipsi- and contralateral collaterals (Fig. 83e), which was redilated (Fig. 83f). The patient remained asymptomatic. A repeat angiogram performed 18 months later showed a good long-term result (Fig. 83g). The left ventricle was normal (Fig. 83h: diastole, Fig. 83i: systole) despite the three interventions and intercurrent functional occlusion.

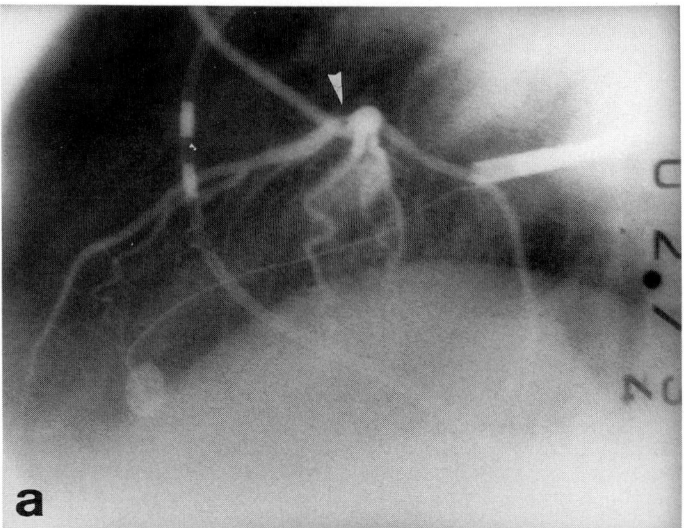

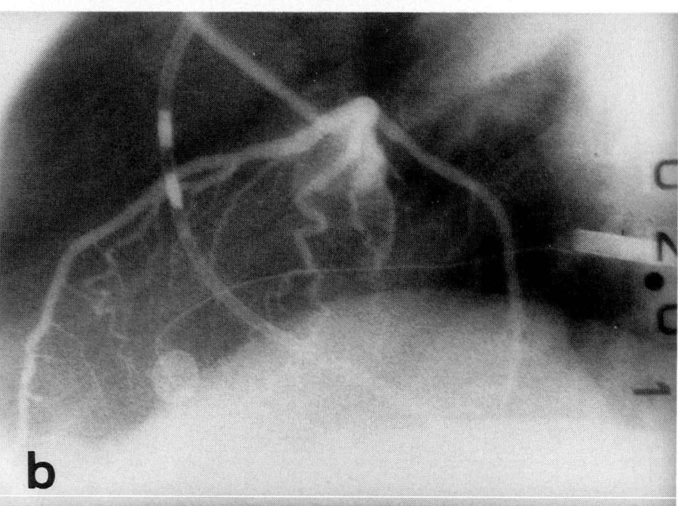

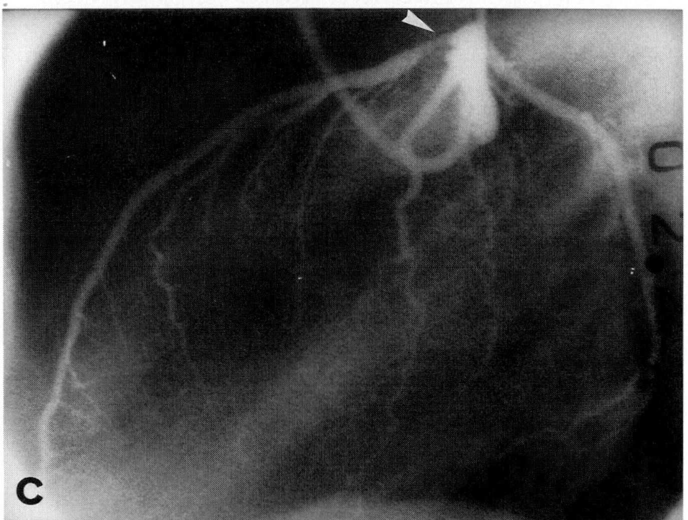

Figure 83

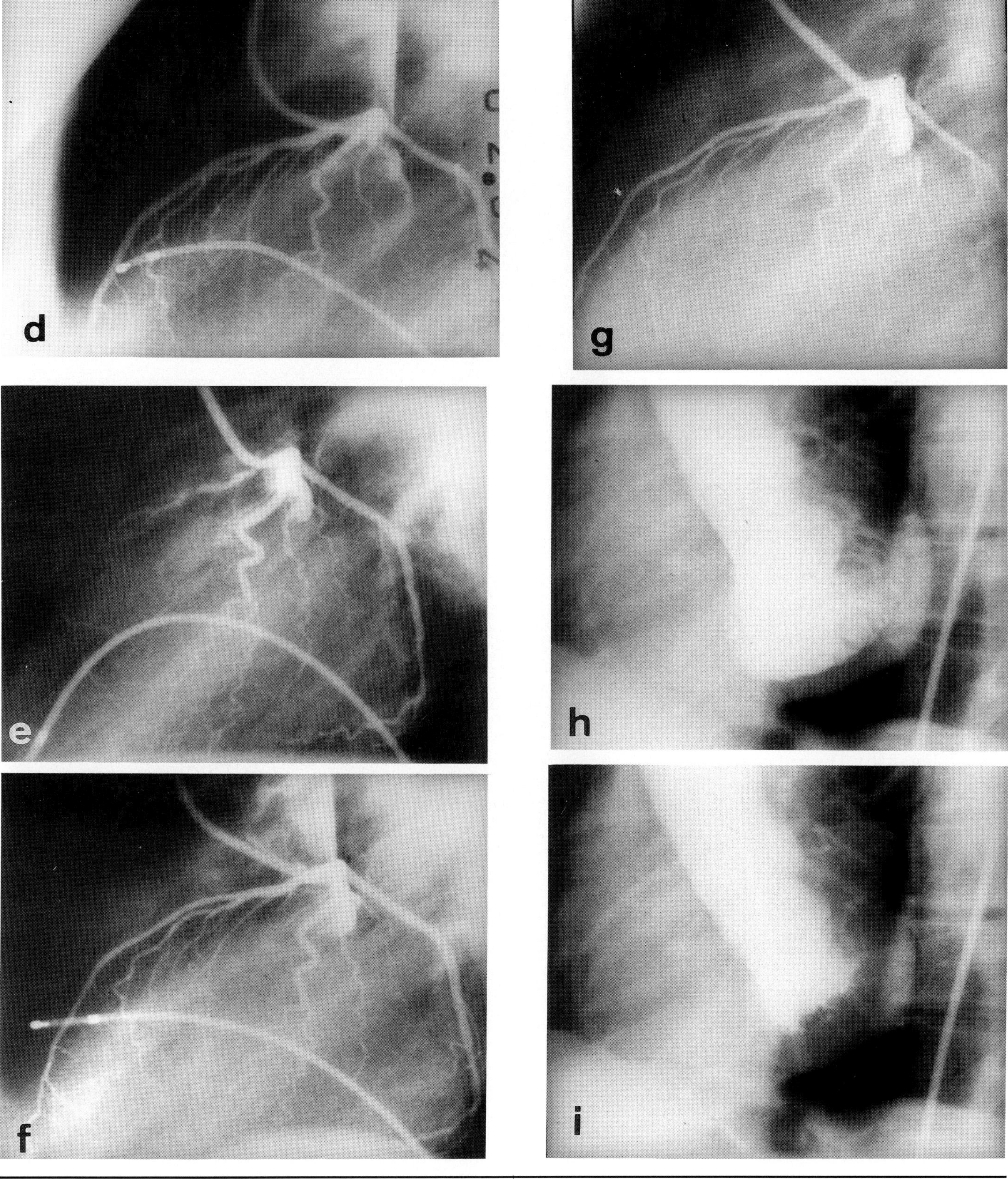
d
e
f
g
h
i

However, the problem of restenosis can occasionally frustrate all efforts. A 64-year-old man underwent PTCA for a short discrete stenosis of the RCA (Fig. 84a) with a good result (Fig. 84b). A second PTCA became necessary 5 months later for restenosis (Fig. 84c), which was performed with a good result (Fig. 84d). Six months later, symptoms recurred, and a stress test was positive for ischemia. Re-restenosis of the RCA (Fig. 84e) was detected and dilated (Fig. 84f), with clinical recovery. Seven months later, symptoms and restenosis recurred (Fig. 84g). The left coronary system was normal (Fig. 84h). The patient refused another PTCA attempt. Alternative devices were not available at that time, and he was referred for CABG. As demonstrated in this example, it is often impossible to state which lesion will restenose. This is further exem-

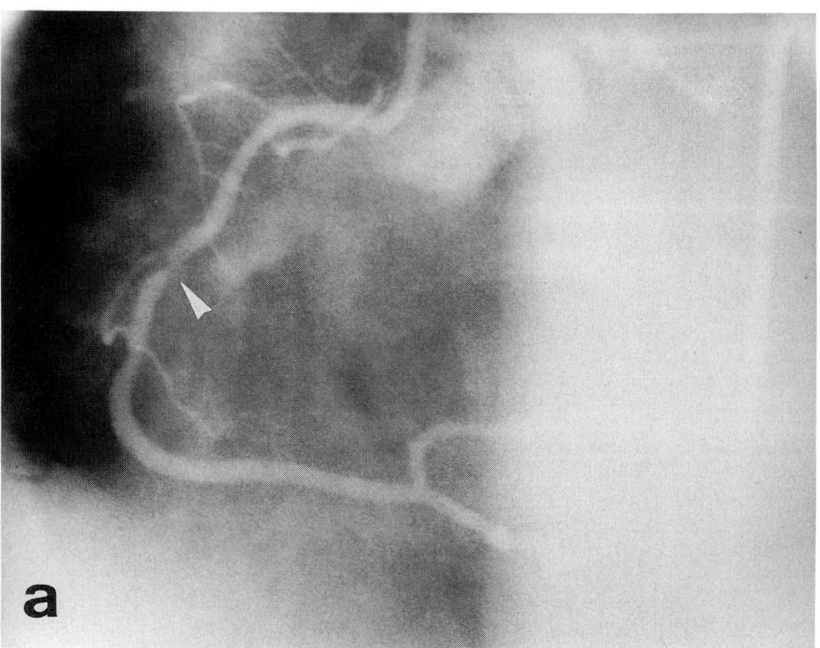

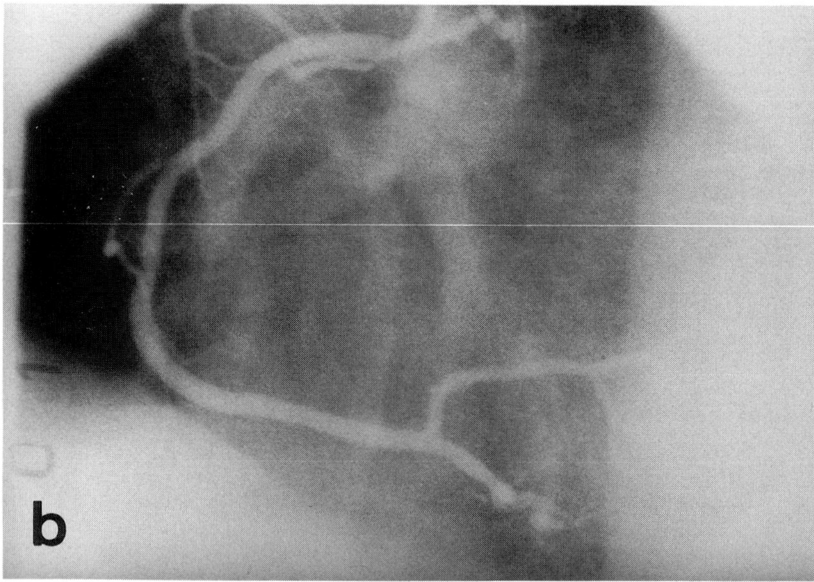

Figure 84

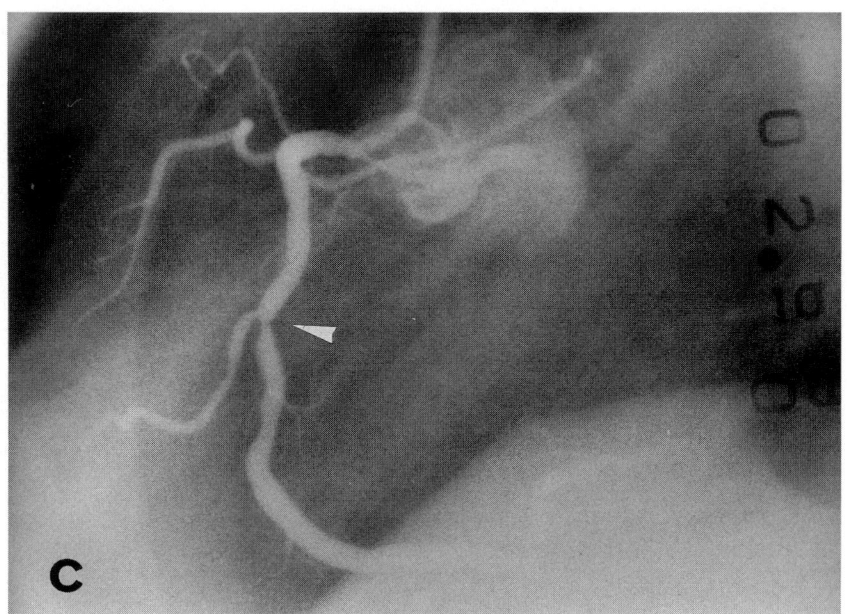
c

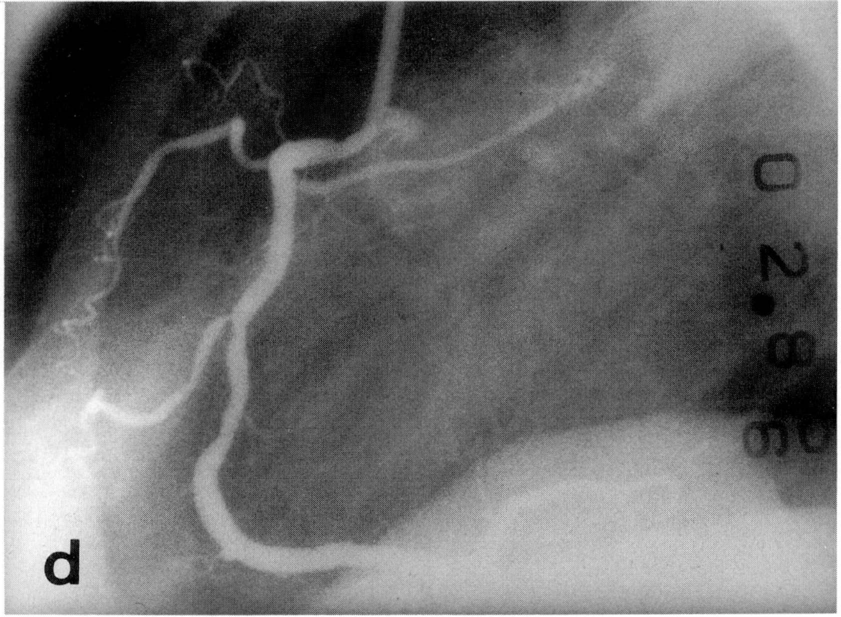
d

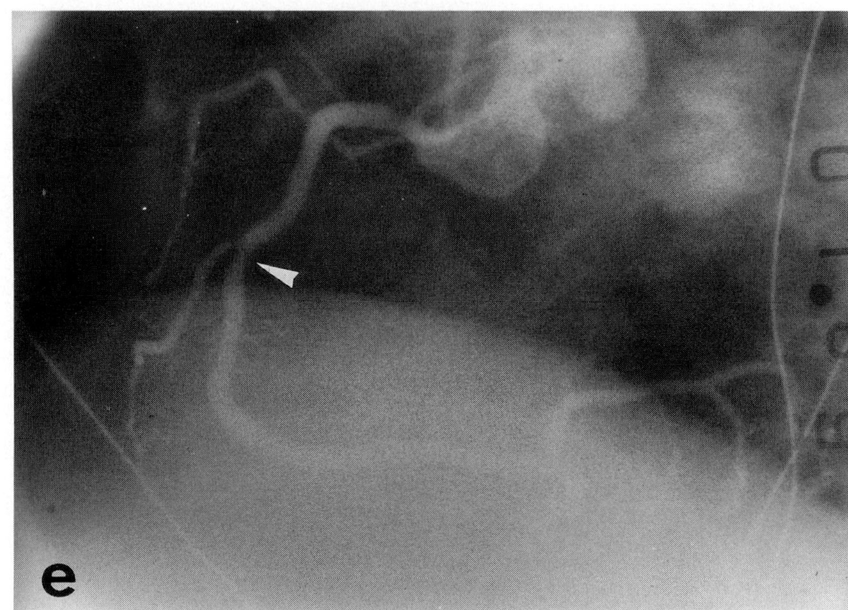

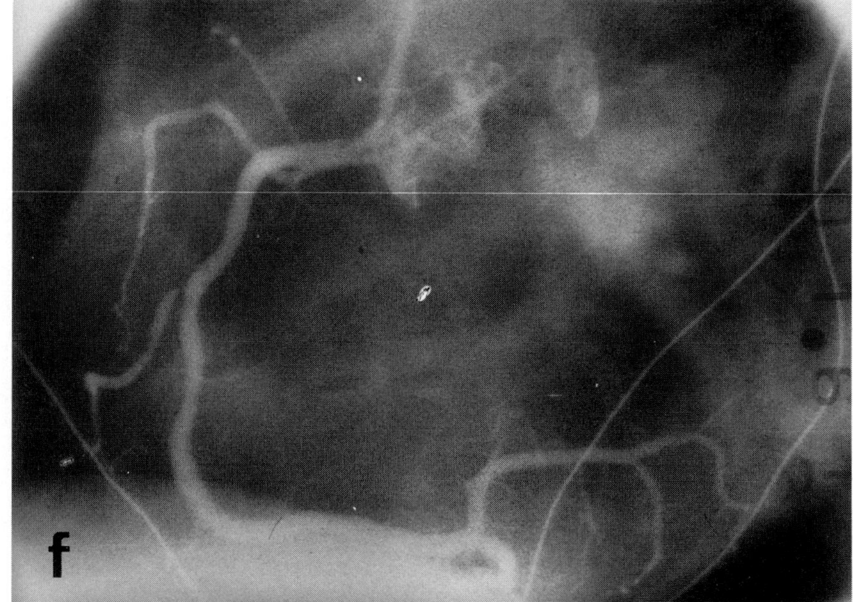

Figure 84 (Continued)

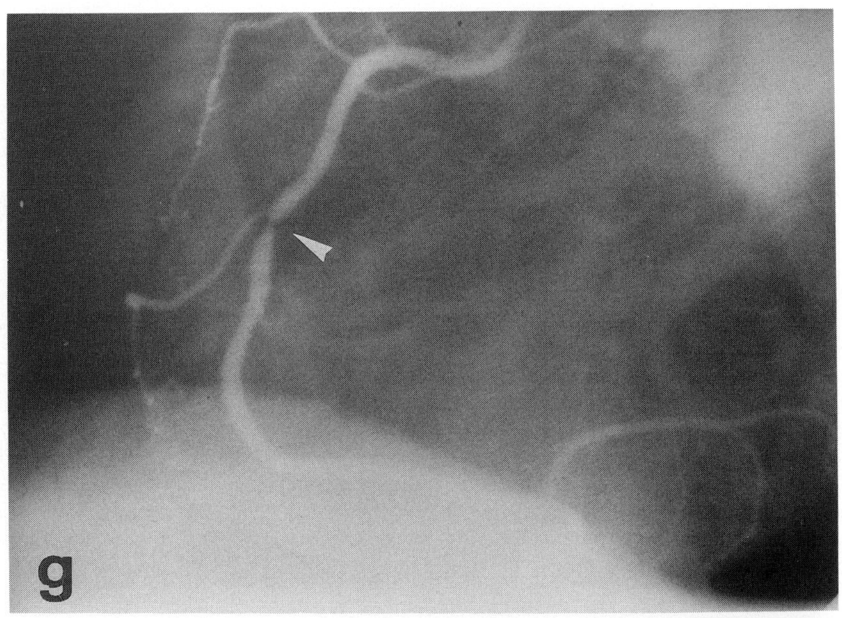
g

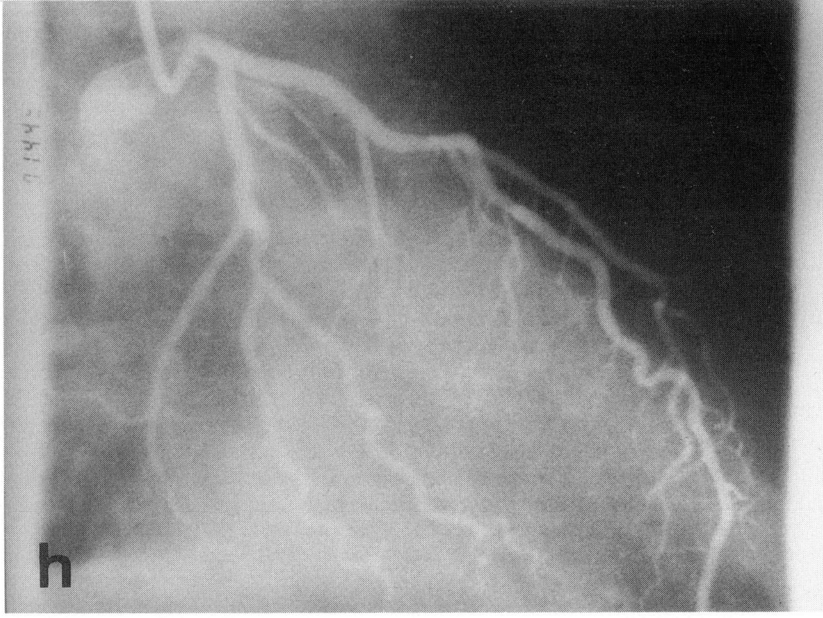
h

plified by a case with a tandem stenosis of the LAD (Fig. 85a). The proximal lesion (double arrowhead) was much less severe than the distal one (single arrowhead). The lesions were dilated with a 3.0-mm balloon with a good result (Fig. 85b). One year later angina recurred. A restenosis was seen of the proximal lesion (which was the less severe one to start with), while the distal lesion result was good (Fig. 85c). Repeat PTCA was performed, with a good result (Fig. 85d). A 3-month follow-up revealed no evidence of restenosis (Fig. 85e).

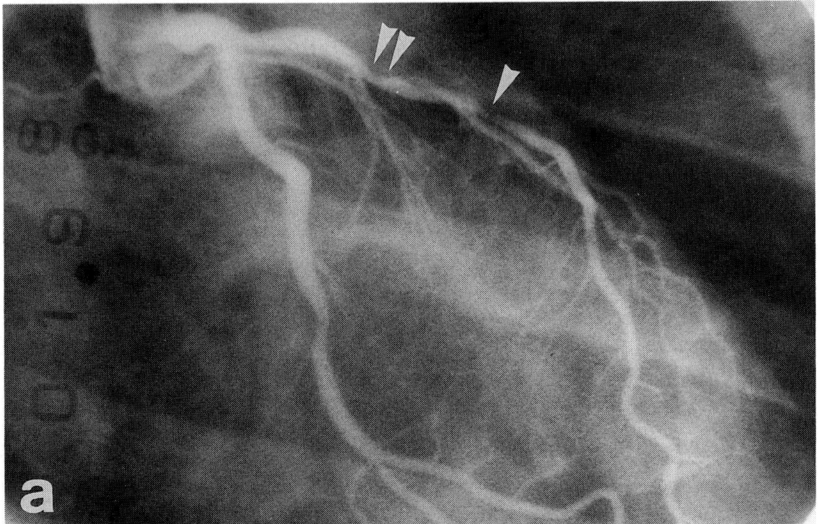

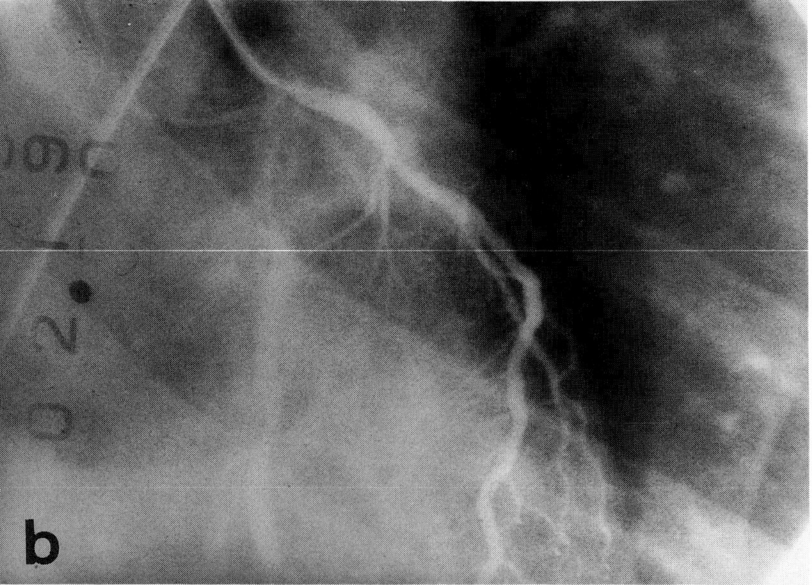

Figure 85

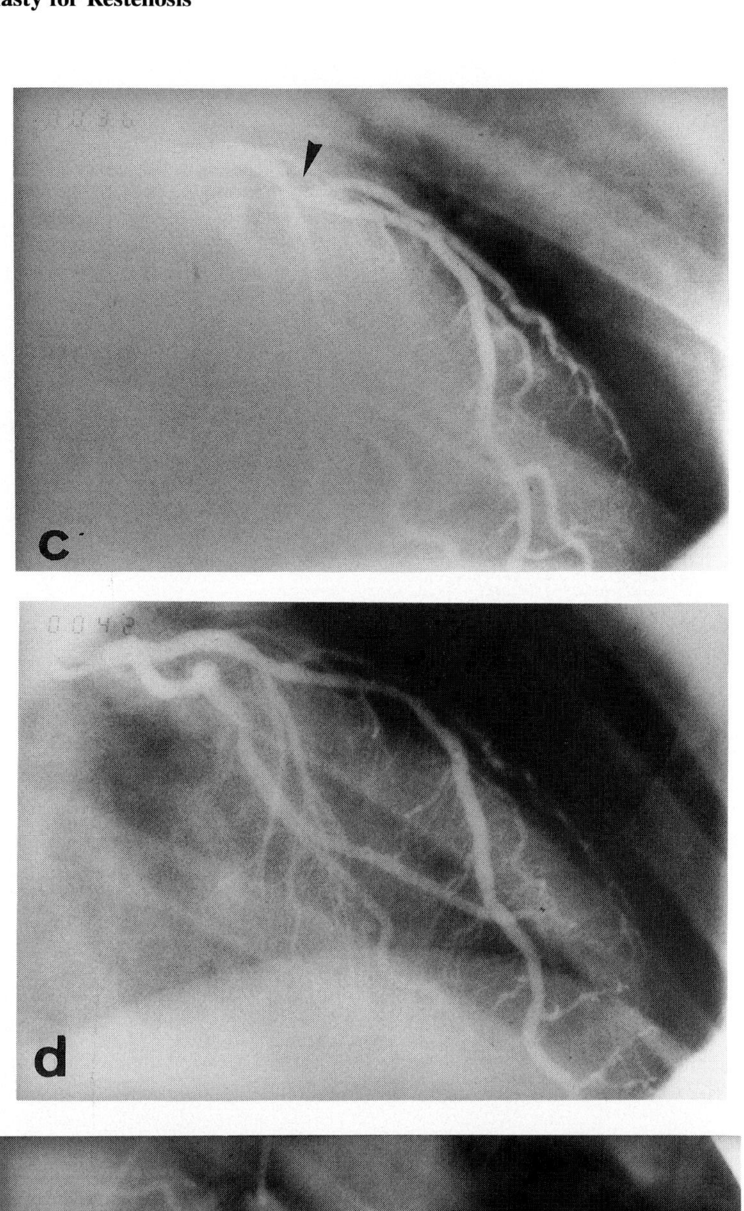
c
d

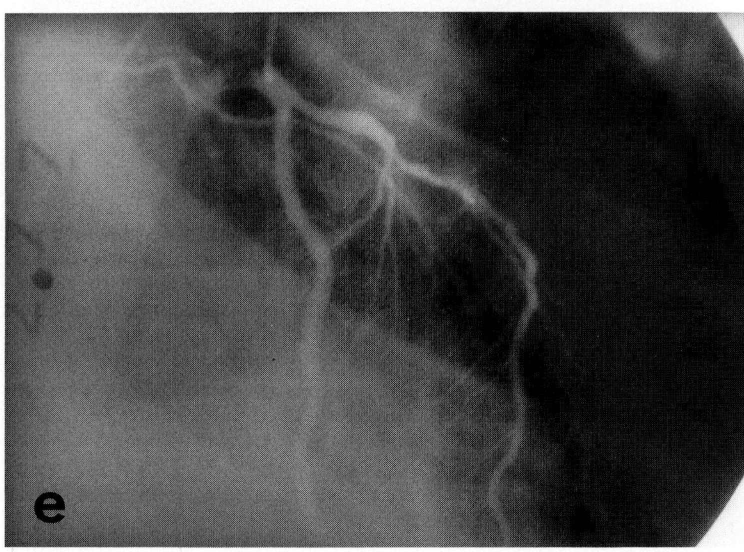
e

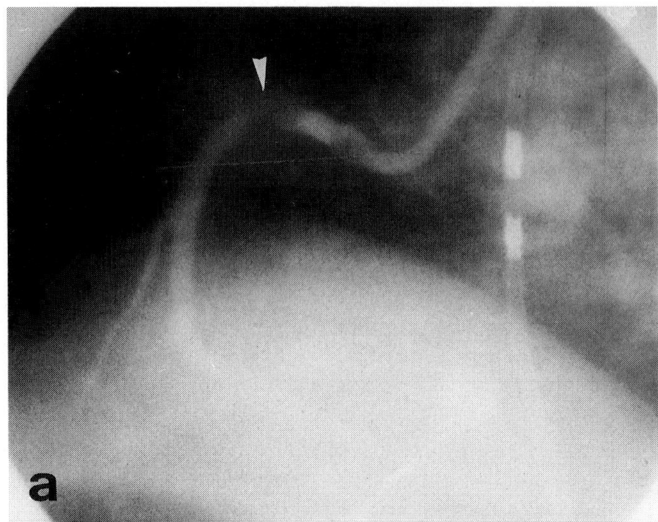

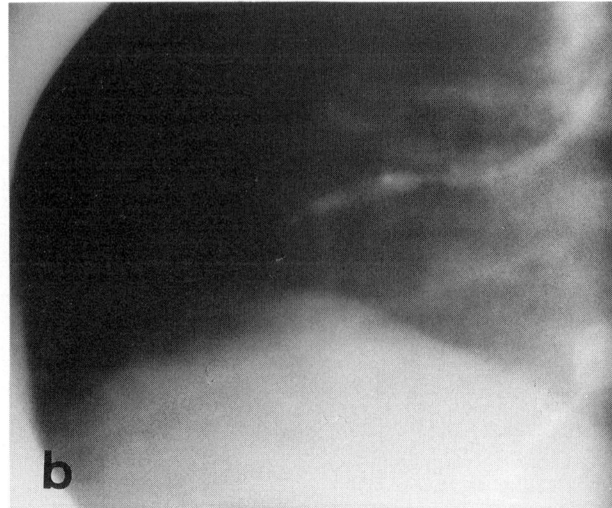

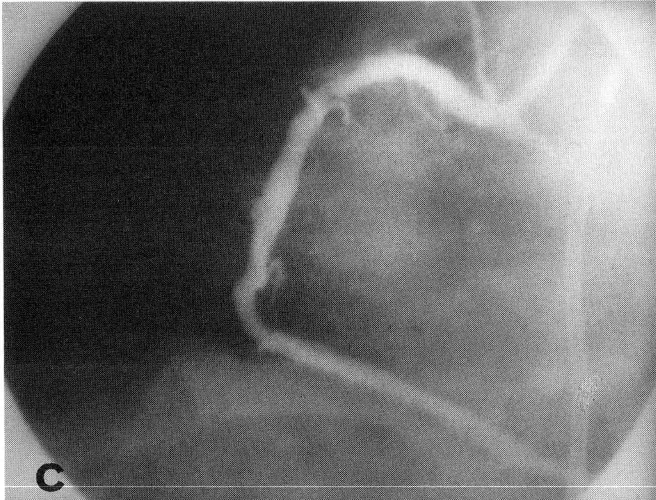

However, the recurrence of symptoms after angioplasty need not always be due to restenosis, as demonstrated by an amusing story. A heart surgeon with double-vessel disease came for angioplasty to Andreas Gruentzig in 1982, much to the dismay of his surgical colleagues. The RCA stenosis (Fig. 86a) was dilated (Fig. 86b), with a good result (Fig. 86c). A few days later, an LAD stenosis (Fig. 86d) was also dilated (Fig. 86e), with a good result (Fig. 86f). Ten months later symptoms recurred. The surgeon was annoyed, since he suspected restenosis and feared taunts from his colleagues, who had warned him not to have this "crazy procedure" in the first place. He slipped out the back door (as he put it) to see Gruentzig. Angiography revealed good results of the LAD (Fig. 86g) and RCA (Fig. 86h, arrow) lesions. However, a new lesion was present in the mid RCA (Fig. 86h, arrowhead), which was dilated (Fig. 86i) with a good result (Fig. 86j).

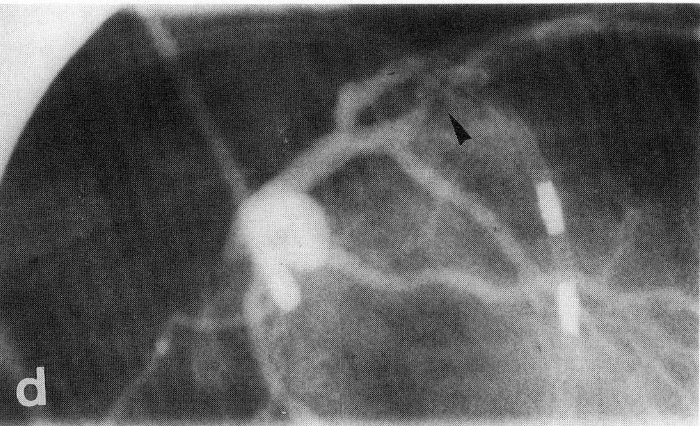

Figure 86

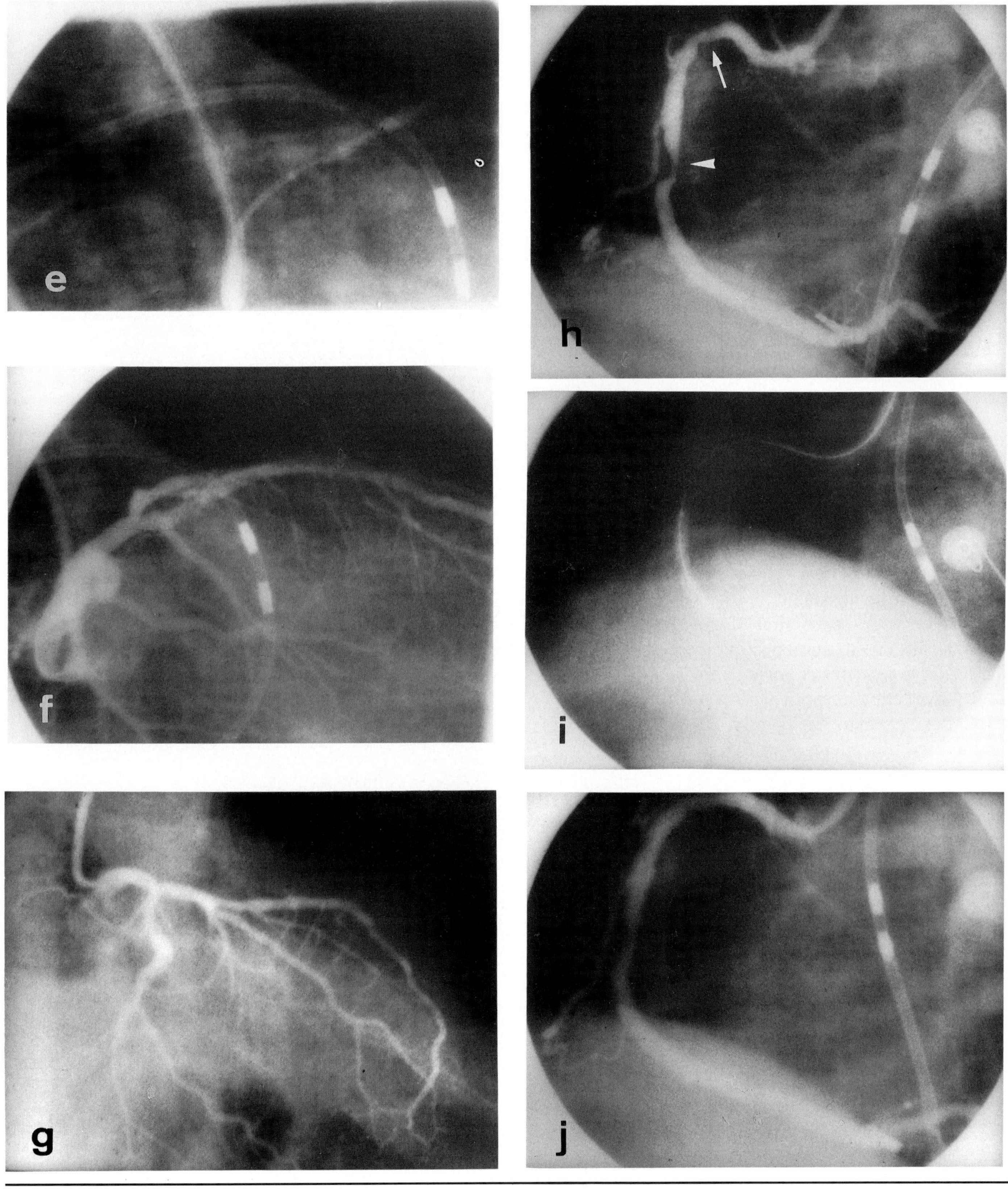
e
f
g
h
i
j

2.6 ANGIOPLASTY FOR UNSTABLE ANGINA

This condition is associated with an unstable plaque, with rupture and thrombosis of the lesion. Results of angioplasty in such a situation are gratifying. However, there is a higher incidence of acute occlusion, especially in conjunction with a suboptimal angioplasty result, due to thrombosis at the site of the lesion. Results may be improved by pretreating with heparin for a few days prior to angioplasty. The angioplasty procedure is essentially the same as for stable angina, except that prolonged and generous heparinization before and after the procedure is recommended. Intravenous administration of a million units of urokinase during angioplasty may also be em-

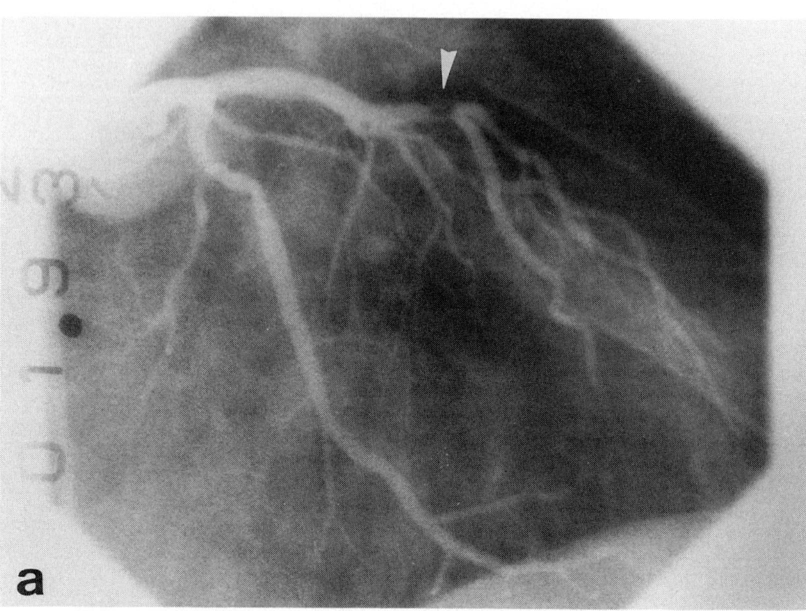

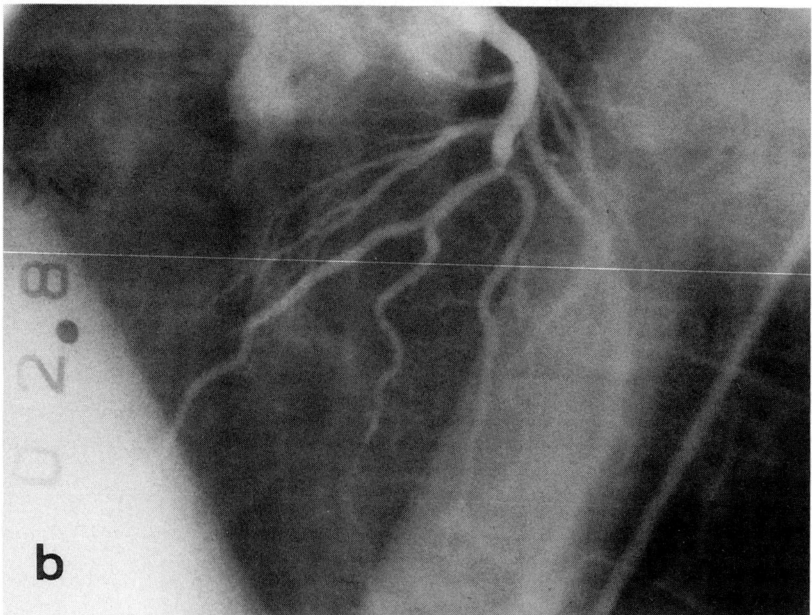

Figure 87

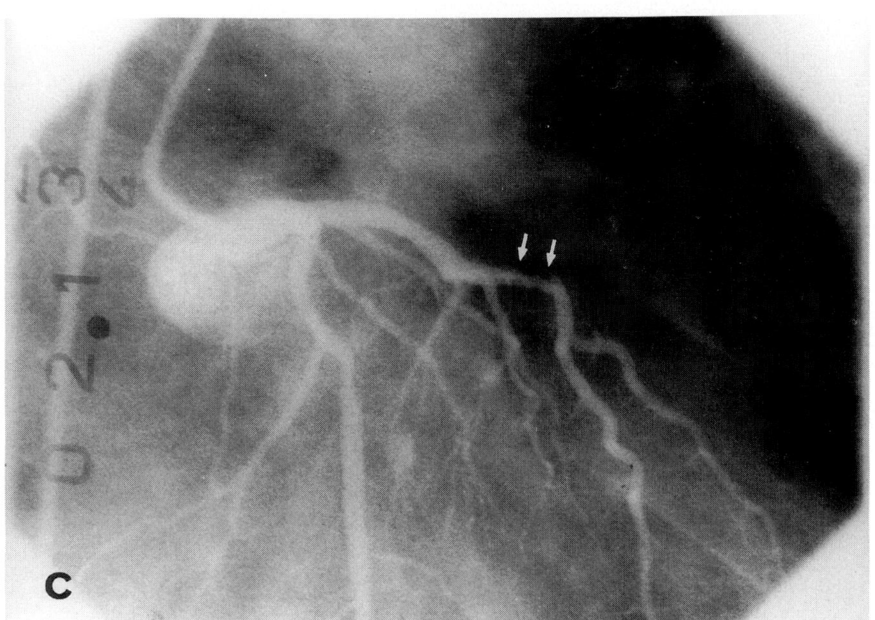

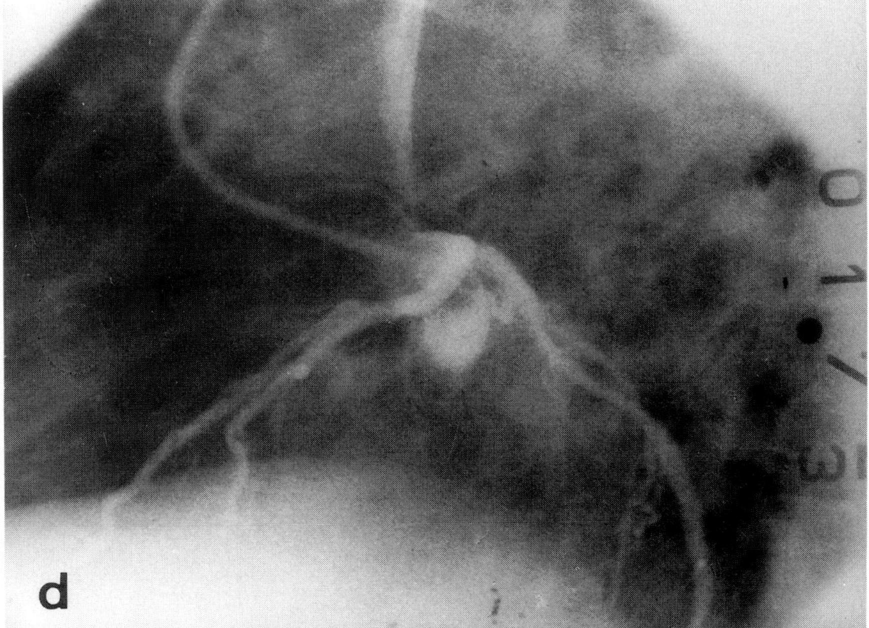

ployed as an adjunctive method of reducing thrombosis, although its efficacy is unproved. A 53-year-old man presented with unstable angina and an eccentric thrombotic lesion in the mid LAD (Fig. 87a) which was not evident in the LAO cranial view (Fig. 87b). PTCA was performed, which resulted in occlusion of the diagonal branch of the LAD and some residual haziness in the region of the lesion (Fig. 87c,d). One million units of urokinase were administered intravenously. The patient suffered only a small infarction, with a minimal CPK rise. This case demonstrates some of the complications of angioplasty of a thrombotic lesion: the common persistence of residual irregularities, and occasional side branch occlusions due to a displacement of the thrombotic material.

A residual elastic thrombus at the dilated site is a frequent finding with unstable angina, and this may provide the nidus for acute occlusion. This can be treated by stenting. Use of half a Palmaz-Schatz stent for a short lesion in this setting is especially attractive, since it achieves an excellent angiographic result, and the shorter stent may be associated with a lesser tendency to thrombosis (see Section 3.5). Sometimes dilating with a larger balloon may solve the problem. A 59-year-old male with unstable angina underwent angioplasty for a thrombotic RCA lesion (Fig. 88a). After an initial good result, the vessel closed over a 15-minute period (Fig. 88b). The lesion was redilated with a larger balloon, with a good result (Fig. 88c). A 1-year follow-up revealed no restenosis (Fig. 88d). Using a larger balloon might result in further plastering of the thrombus against the vessel wall, resulting in a reduced tendency to thrombosis and acute closure.

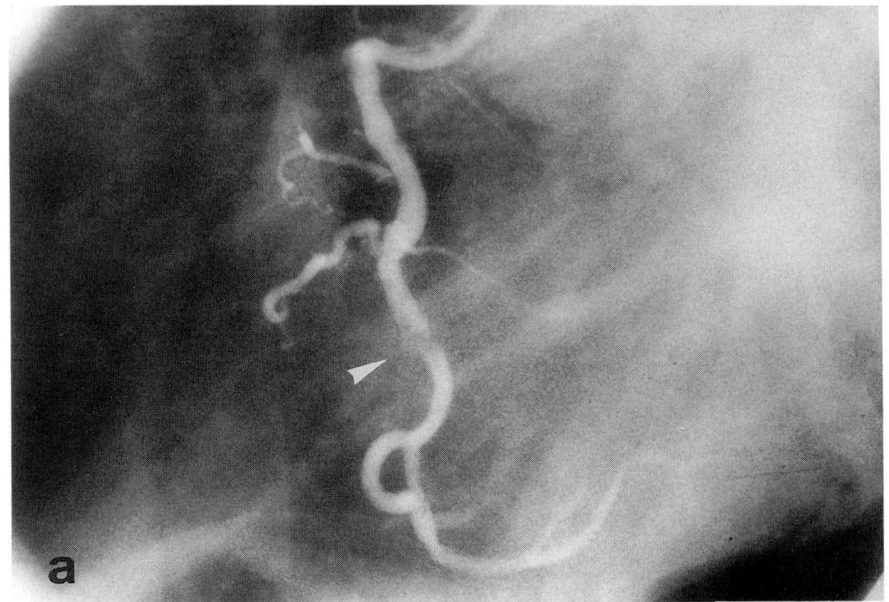

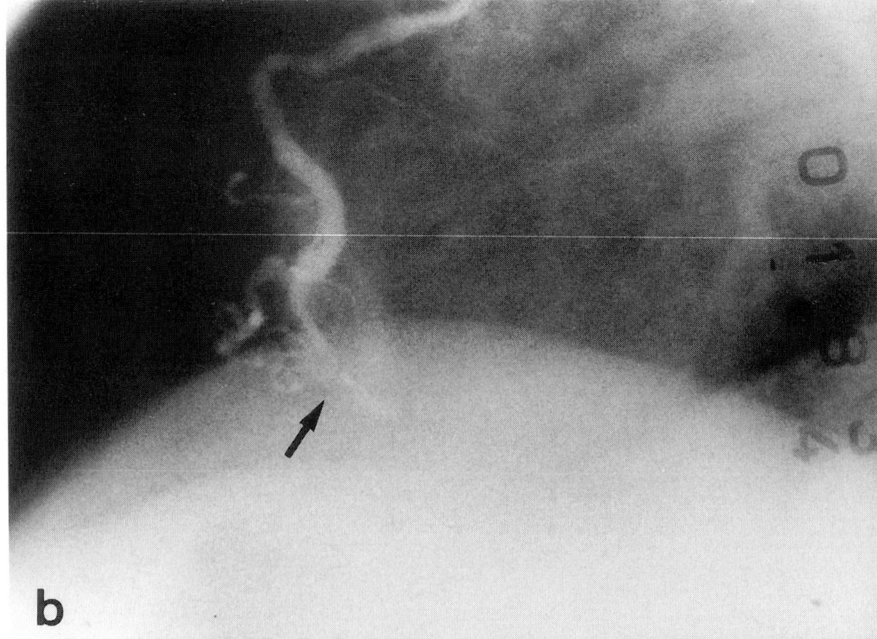

Figure 88

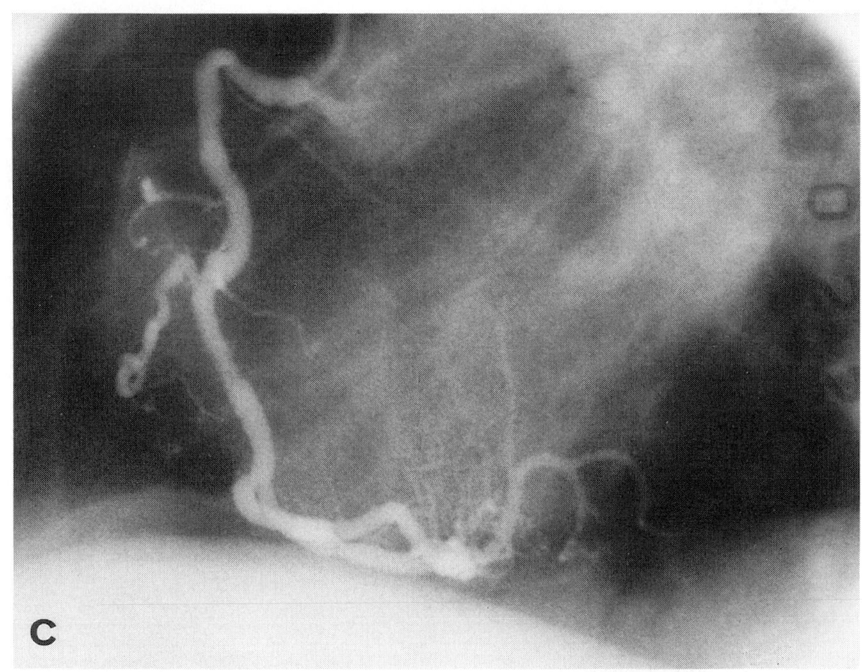
c

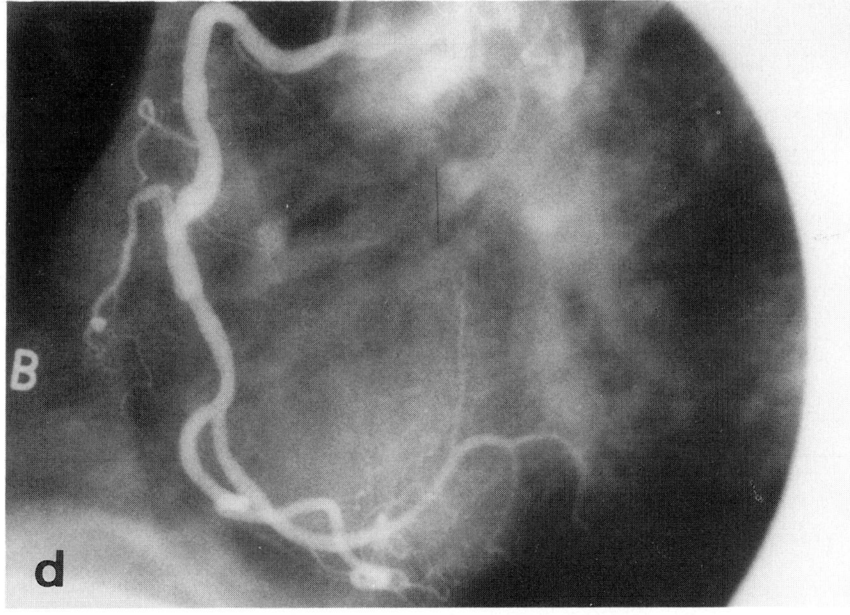
B
d

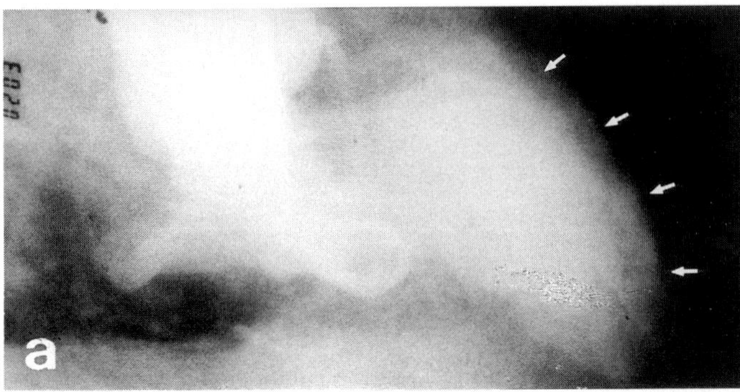

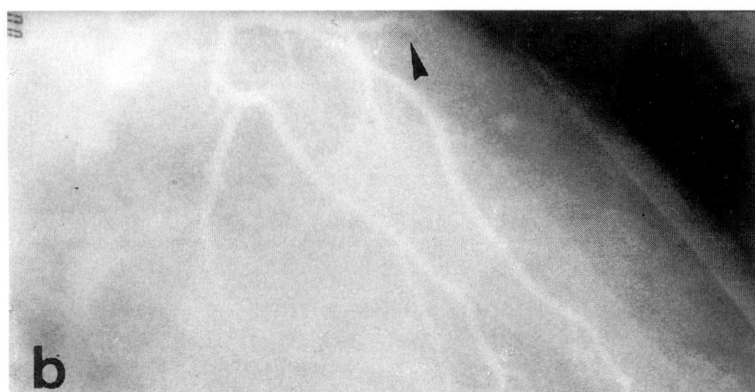

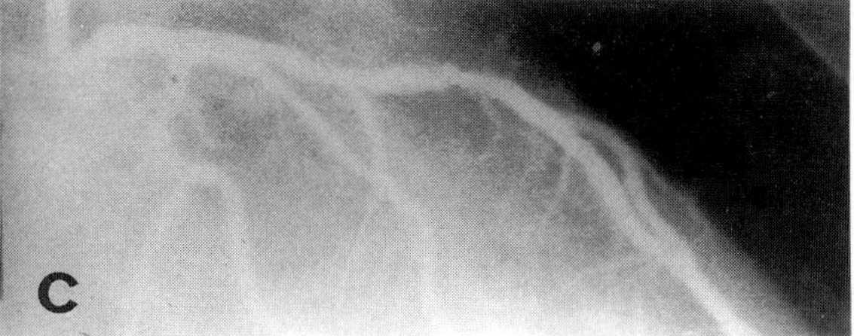

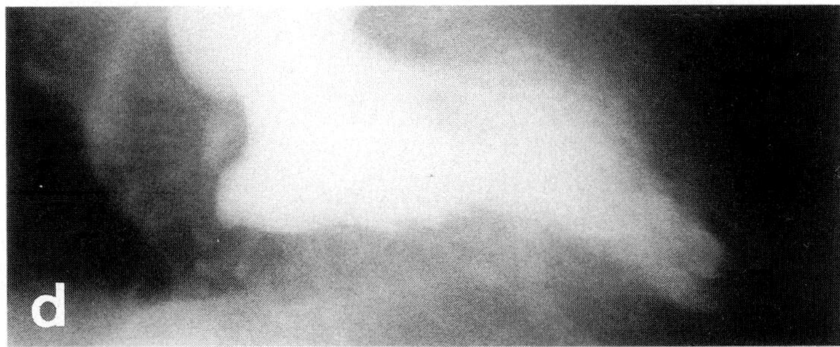

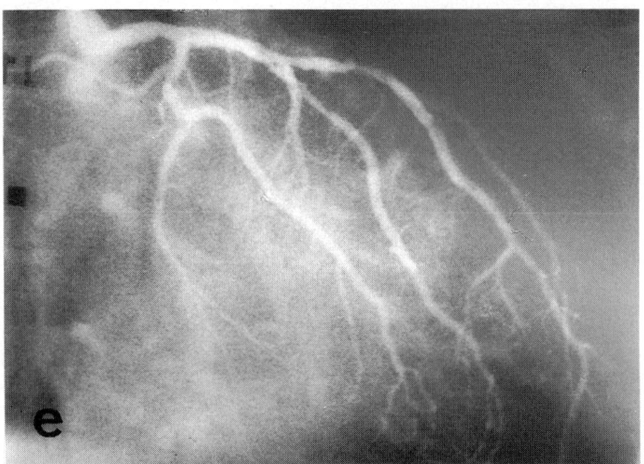

Figure 89

2.7 ANGIOPLASTY FOR ACUTE INFARCTION

Primary PTCA constitutes an excellent therapy for acute myocardial infarction. It has been shown to be superior to thrombolytic therapy in obtaining vessel patency, improving survival, and reducing recurrent ischemia. However, the logistics involved in performing such procedures at all times limit its applicability. Prolonged heparinization and intravenous urokinase are useful adjunctive measures to angioplasty in this setting. Half a Palmaz-Schatz stent for a residual irregularity due to a thrombus is also a suitable

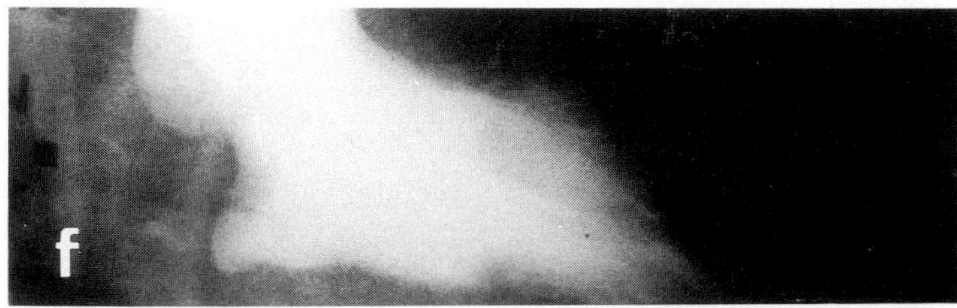

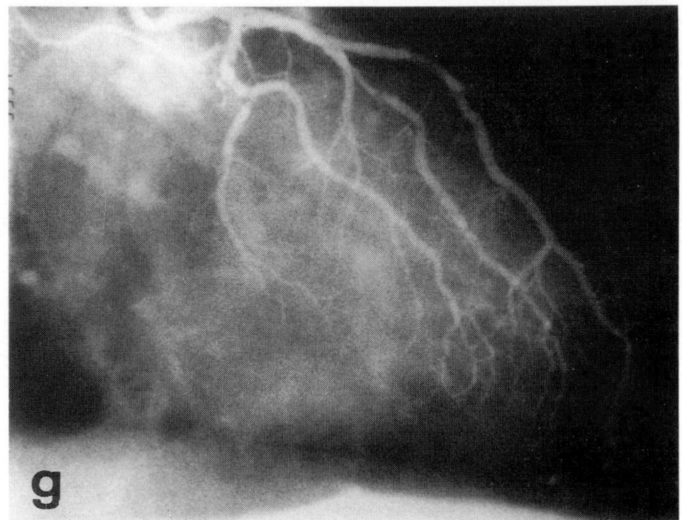

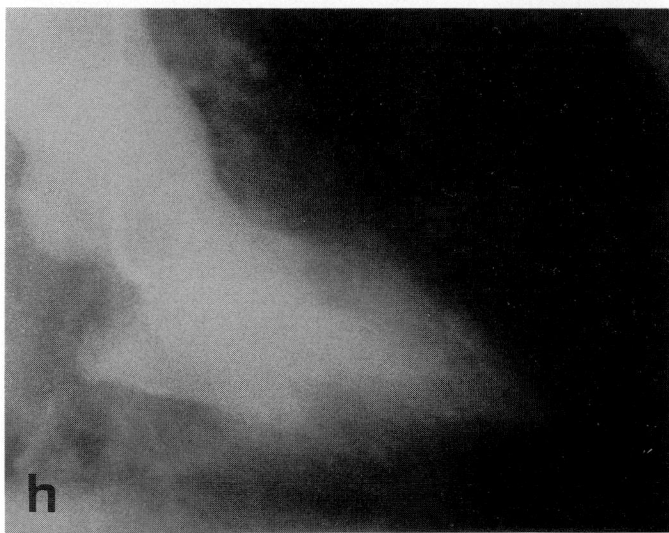

therapy, as in the case of unstable angina (see above). A patient with an acute anterior wall myocardial infarction (Fig. 89a: systole) due to an occluded LAD (Fig. 89b) underwent successful recanalization of the vessel. A follow-up evaluation after 1 week (Fig. 89c) revealed a patent LAD, with improvement of the anterior wall function (Fig. 89d: systole). The result was maintained at 7-month follow-up (Fig. 89e), with further improvement of the left ventricular function (Fig. 89f: systole). A repeat evaluation at 3 years showed an excellent long-term angioplasty result (Fig. 89g), with near-normal left ventricular function at rest (Fig. 89h).

Coronary angiography in a 46-year-old man with acute myocardial infarction revealed a subtotal occlusion with a thrombus in the LAD (Fig. 90a). Postangioplasty, a radiolucency persisted in the region of the lesion, with sluggish distal flow (evident by the poor distal opacification of the LAD, whereas the LCx is fully opacified) (Fig. 90b). The lesion was recrossed, and a prolonged inflation made with the same balloon, with a good result (Fig. 90c). A 1-year follow-up revealed a good long-term result (Fig. 90d).

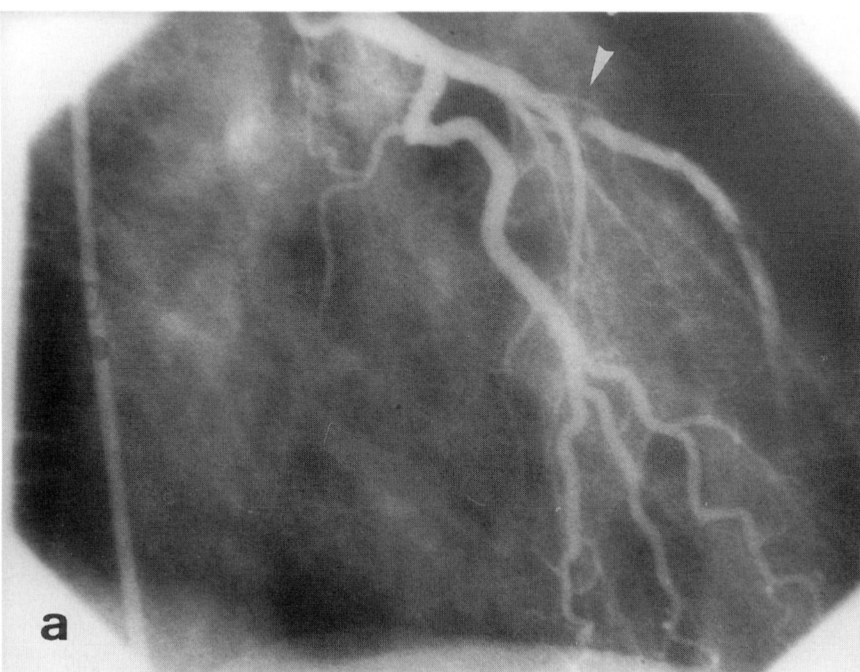

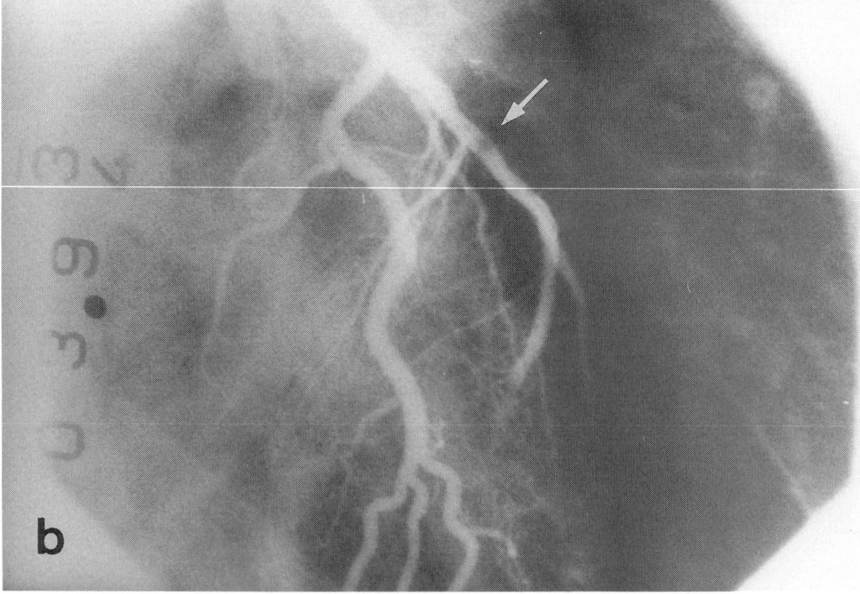

Figure 90

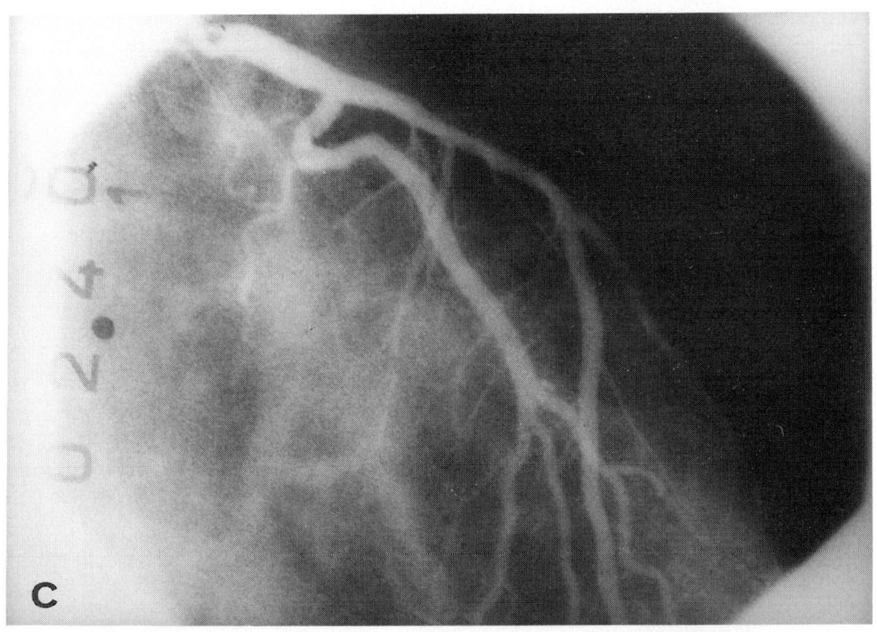

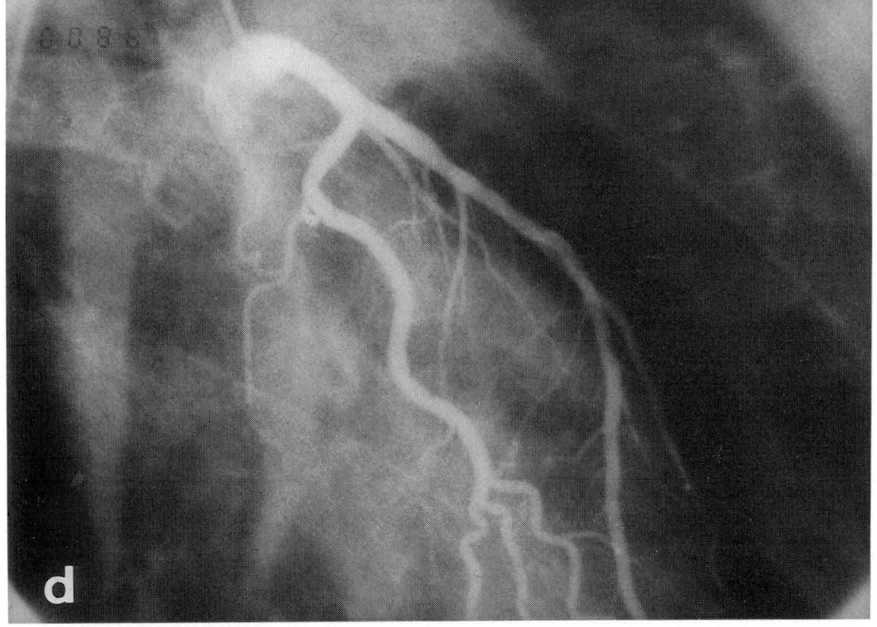

However, even more than angioplasty for stable angina, PTCA in the setting of an acute myocardial infarction is associated with the risk of restenosis. A 59-year-old male suffered an inferior wall myocardial infarction due to RCA occlusion (Fig. 91a). The vessel was dilated successfully (Fig. 91b). Angiography performed 1 week after the procedure revealed a good result (Fig. 91c). However, angina occurred 7 months later, with restenosis (Fig. 91d). Reangioplasty was performed successfully (Fig. 91e), and the patient remained asymptomatic after this.

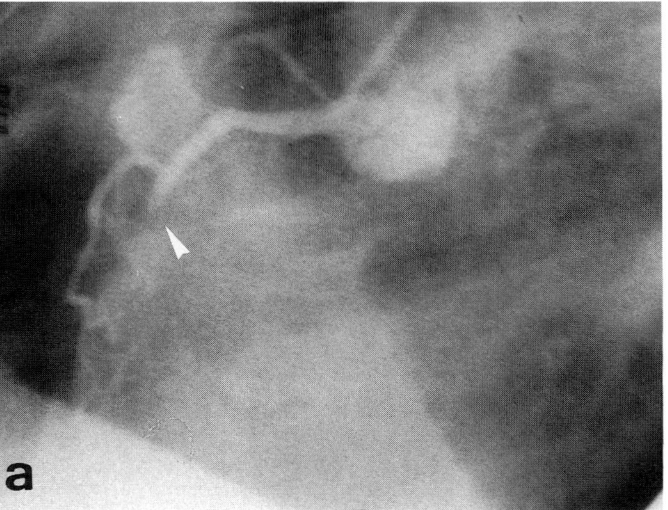

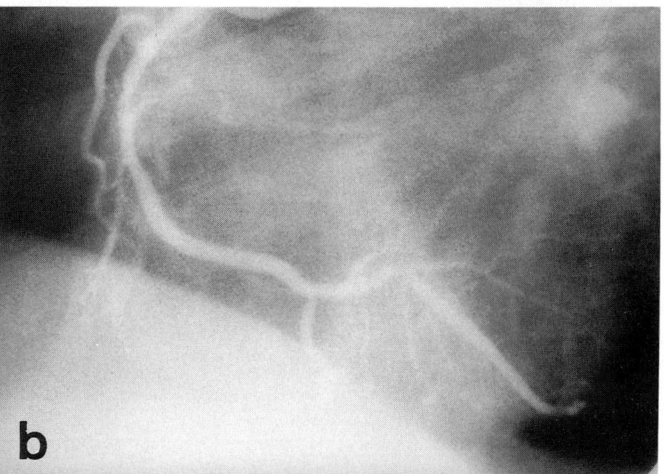

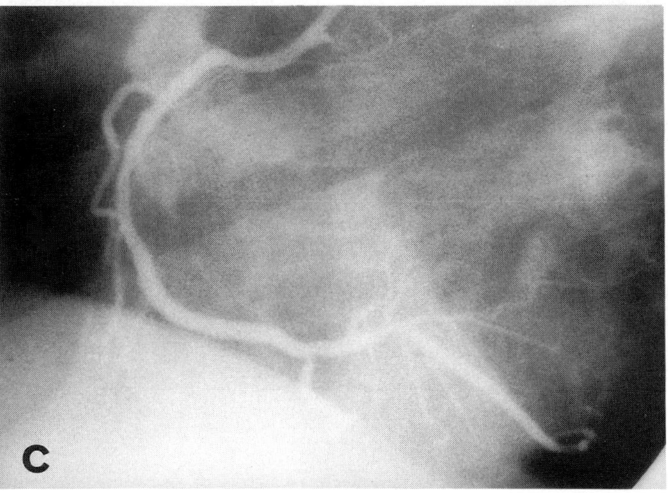

Figure 91

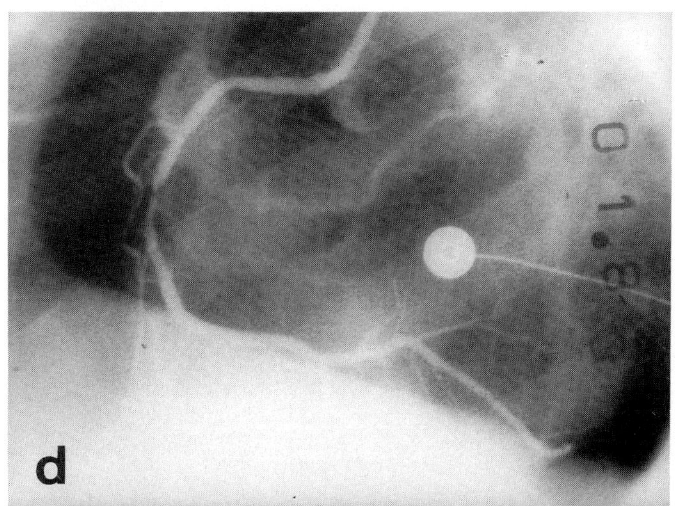
d

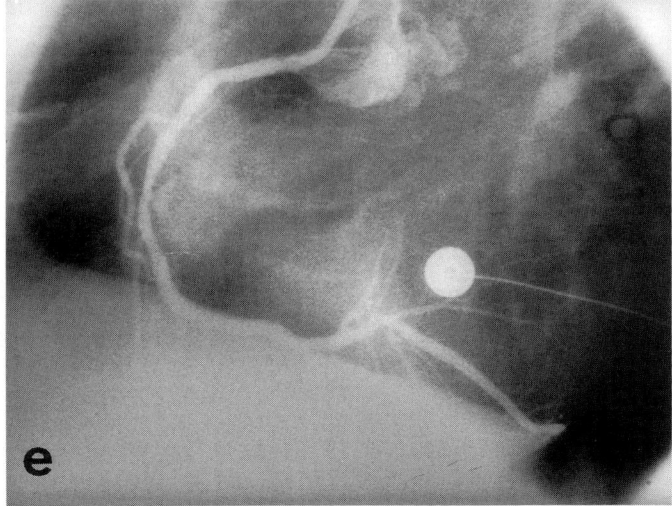
e

3
Complex Lesions

3.1
LONG STENOSES

The length of most balloon catheters is 20–25 mm. If a lesion is too long to be covered by a single balloon inflation, it is advisable to utilize a long balloon (30–60 mm). Such a balloon covers long stenoses and obviates the need for multiple inflations. However, tapered long balloons may be required for rapidly tapering arteries to avoid disproportionate dilation of the distal part of the vessel. In the absence of a long balloon, long lesions must be addressed by serial dilations, starting distally, and progressing proximally, with overlapping areas of inflation.

Long balloons can be very useful for rapid PTCA of long stenoses. A 48-year-old man with a long stenosis of the LAD (Fig. 92a) was treated with a single inflation of a 3.0-mm-long balloon, which adequately covered the entire length of the stenosis (Fig. 92b,c), and yielded a good immediate (Fig. 92d) and 5-month follow-up result (Fig. 92e). However, long balloons have all the disadvantages of normal-sized balloons and may cause more dissections, especially in curved ves-

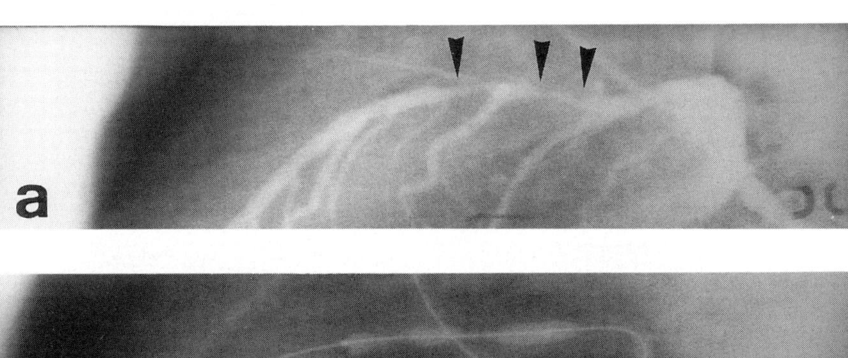

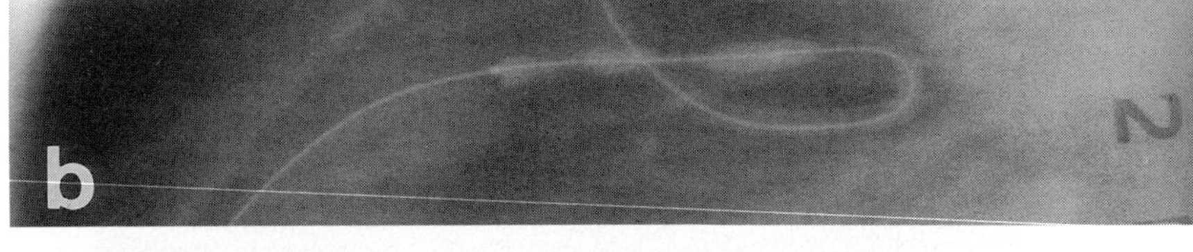

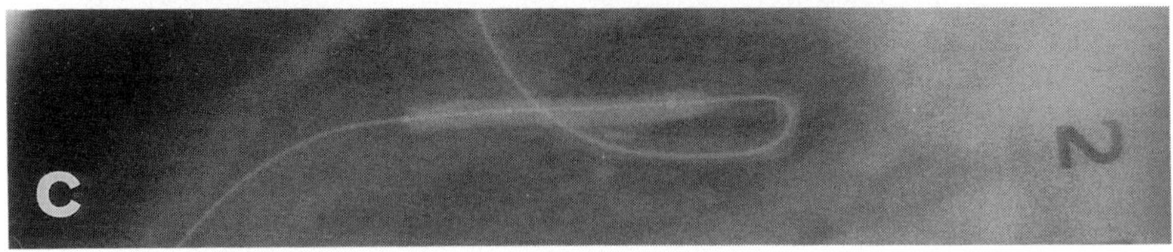

Figure 92

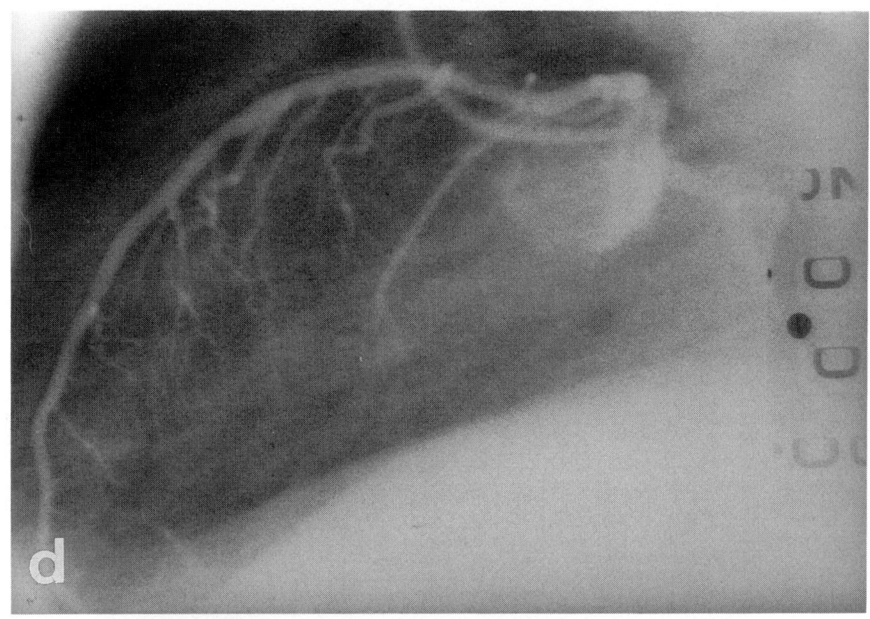
d

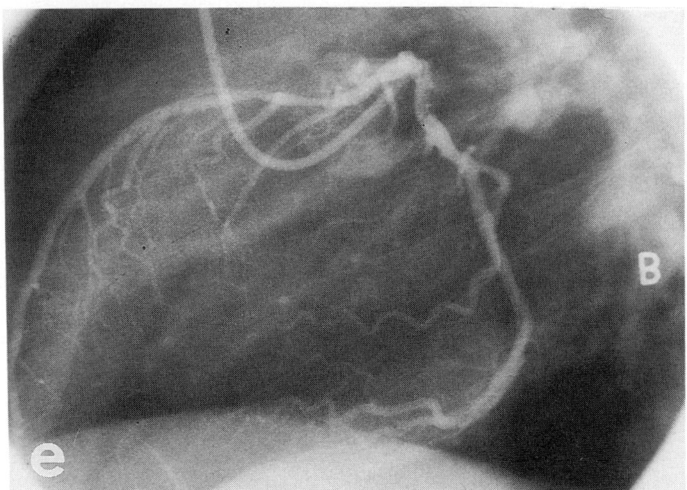
B
e

sels. A 66-year-old woman with a long stenosis of the LAD (Fig. 93a) was treated with a long balloon (Fig. 93b). However, the result was a long dissection (Fig. 93c) extending over the entire length of the stenosis. Such long dissections are difficult to treat. Prolonged balloon inflations may be preferred since stenting requires serial stents. This remains an option but it is better suited for wide proximal vessels, due to the increased risks of thrombosis of multiple stents in small vessels.

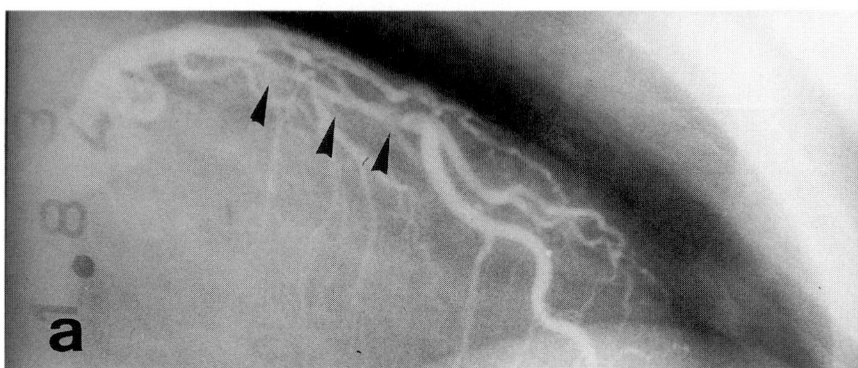

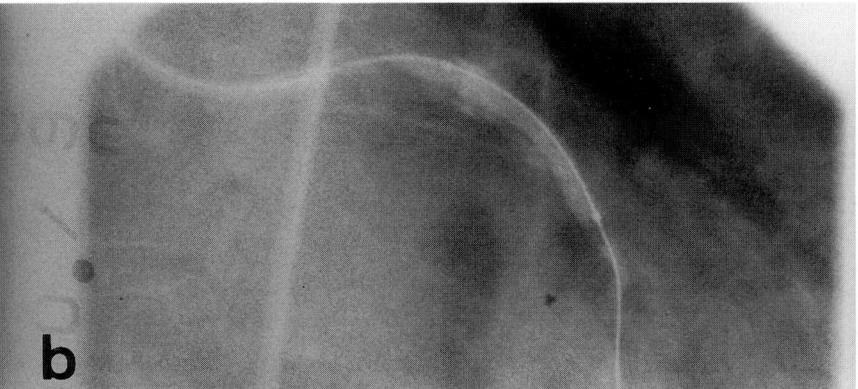

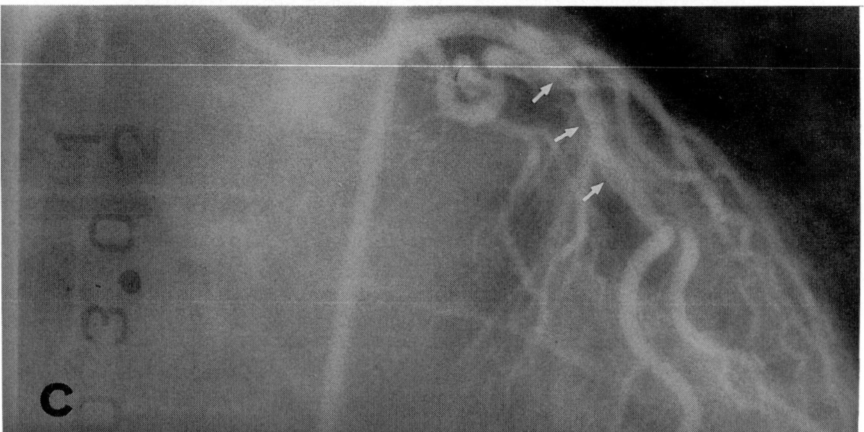

Figure 93

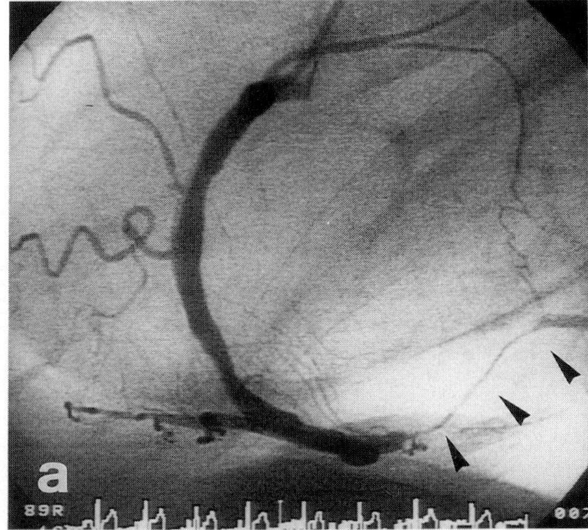

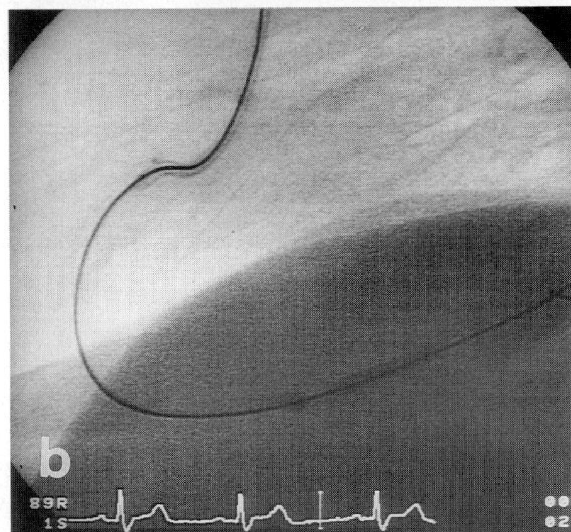

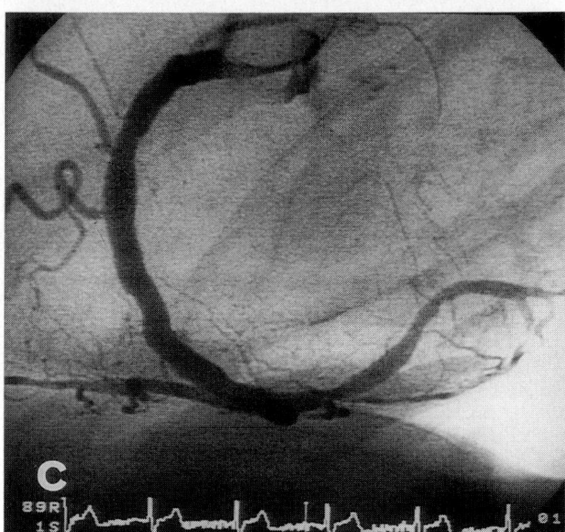

Figure 94

An interesting finding was observed during PTCA of a long lesion in the posterolateral branch of the RCA in a 56-year-old man (Fig. 94a). The tight stenosis was crossed using a Magnum wire. Since the Magnarail balloon catheter was available only in a 20-mm length at that time, it was decided to carry out serial dilatations of the long lesion. However, after a first proximal balloon inflation (Fig. 94b), the result was good, the remainder of the "long" lesion having disappeared (Fig. 94c). It had been due to poor filling rather than an anatomical narrowing. This is an uncommon occurrence, but its possibility has to be kept in mind.

3.2 TANDEM AND SERIAL LESIONS

Lesions situated in a tandem manner can sometimes cause technical difficulties, especially if a tight proximal lesion impairs manipulation of the guidewire for crossing the distal lesion. In general, the distal lesion should be dilated first so that one can take advantage of the ideal balloon profile while crossing both lesions. However, if the proximal lesion is so tight as to impair visibility or manipulation of the guidewire or balloon, it has to be dilated first. A single long balloon can be used if the stenoses are adjacent. If, however, the lesions are widely separated or if the vessel tapers rapidly between the stenoses, a normal balloon is preferable. A compliant balloon can be a compromise if vessel size differs, using low pressures and hence a smaller size in the distal stenosis, and a higher pressure with the ensuing increased balloon diameter for the proximal one. This approach, however, may cause problems in case of a tough distal lesion requiring high pressures.

Serial lesions in general yield less satisfactory procedural success rates

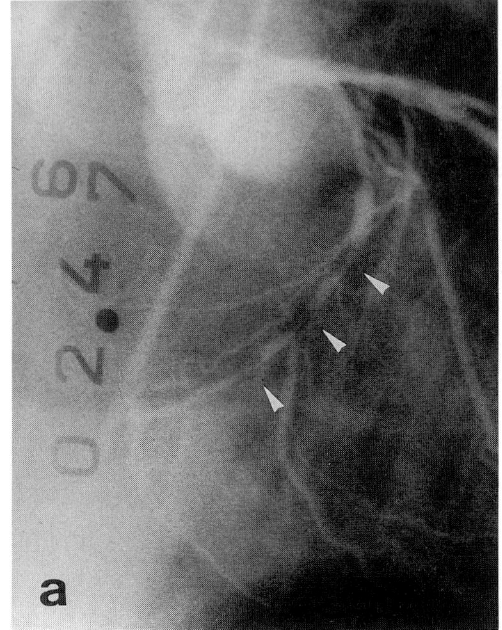

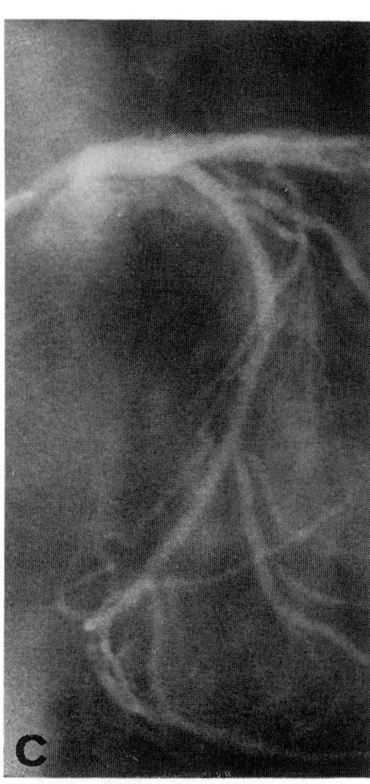

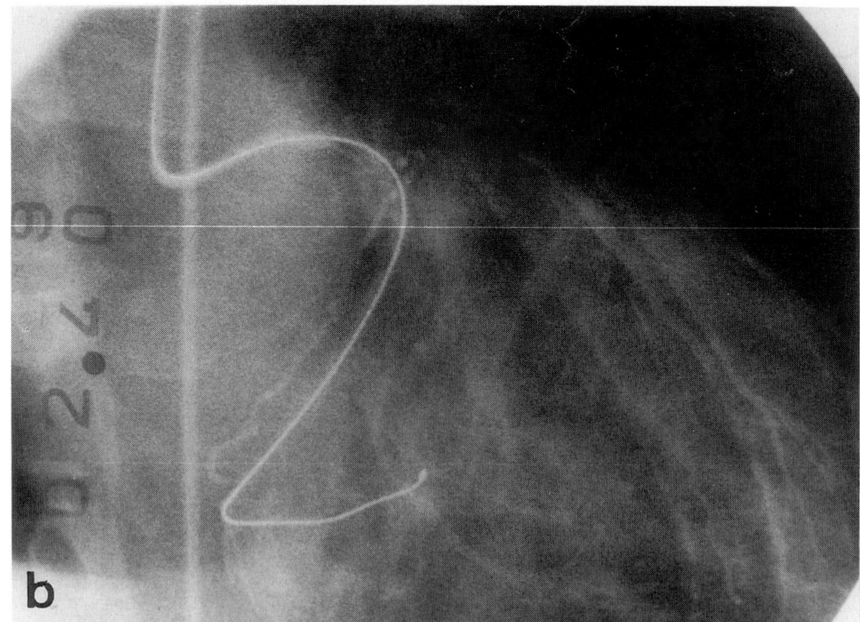

Figure 95

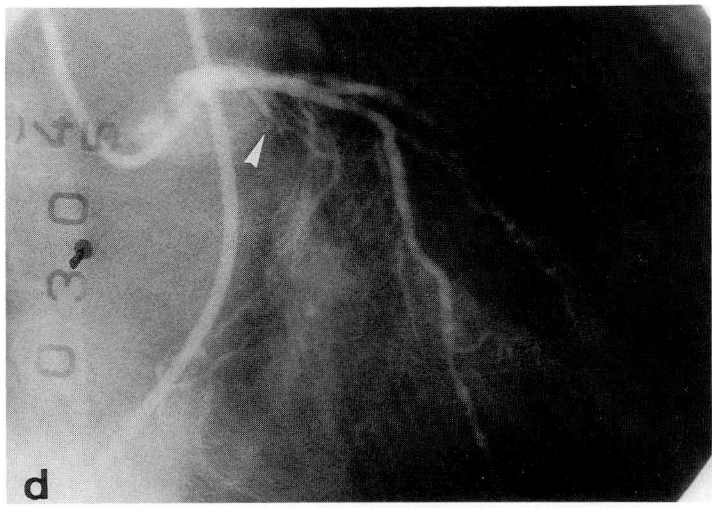

Figure 95 (Continued)

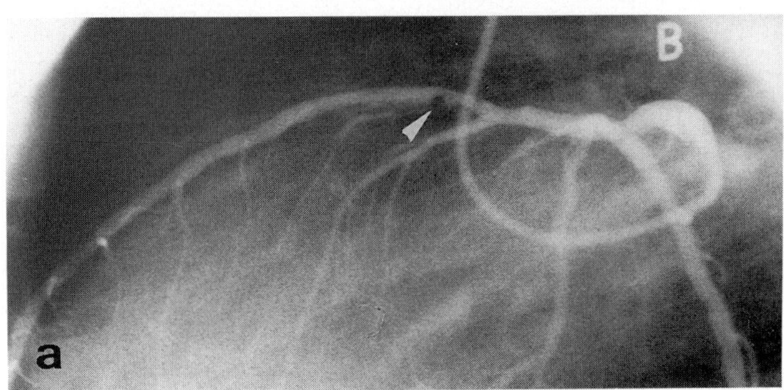

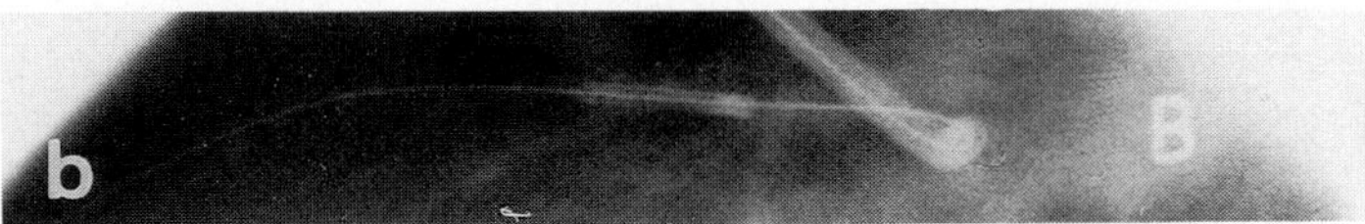

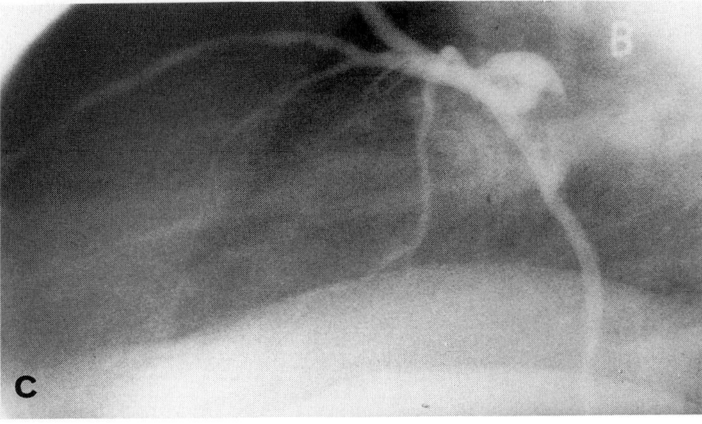

Figure 96

and long-term results. This is demonstrated in a 69-year-old man who underwent angioplasty for serial stenoses of the LCx (Fig 95a) with a Magnum–Magnarail system (Fig. 95b). The procedural result was excellent (Fig. 95c). However, a 3-month follow-up evaluation revealed an occluded LCx (Fig. 95d). Such lesions should always be looked upon with suspicion in view of their poor long-term results.

3.3 ECCENTRIC STENOSES

An eccentric stenosis may be associated with a higher risk of dissection. While crossing such stenoses, it is imperative to avoid a subintimal passage, since there is a high probability of entering with the wire below a plaque in such cases. Occasionally, an eccentric membrane-like or wedge-shaped lesion may be seen which persists unchanged after angioplasty. Such a stenosis is well handled by stenting, using half a Palmaz-Schatz stent, for example. For eccentric lesions situated in the proximal segment of a large coronary artery (Fig. 96a), directional atherectomy (Fig. 96b) may be an alternative technique. This allows the plaque to be excised and removed (Fig. 96c). However, a large contribution to the result is due to the Dotter effect of the atherectome and the angioplasty effect of the balloon used to impinge the device on the plaque. Additionally, the procedure is cumbersome, requiring large guiding catheters, and since it has been shown to have no procedural or long-term advantages over conventional balloon angioplasty, its routine use is not advocated. An approach using balloon angioplasty with stenting in case of need appears to be the better alternative.

3.4 RELAPSING STENOSES

A 65-year-old man with stenosis of the LAD (Fig. 97a) underwent angioplasty with a 3.5-mm balloon. However, the stenosis persisted despite prolonged inflations of the balloon (Fig. 97b). The balloon could be inflated fully each time, without a waist (in contrast to a tough stenosis with a persisting waist), but the stenosis recurred immediately following deflation of the balloon, indicating a relapsing lesion,

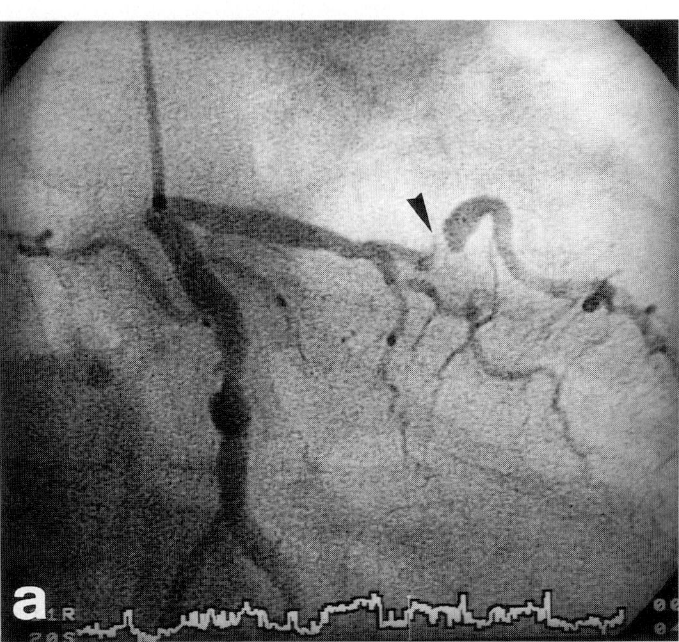

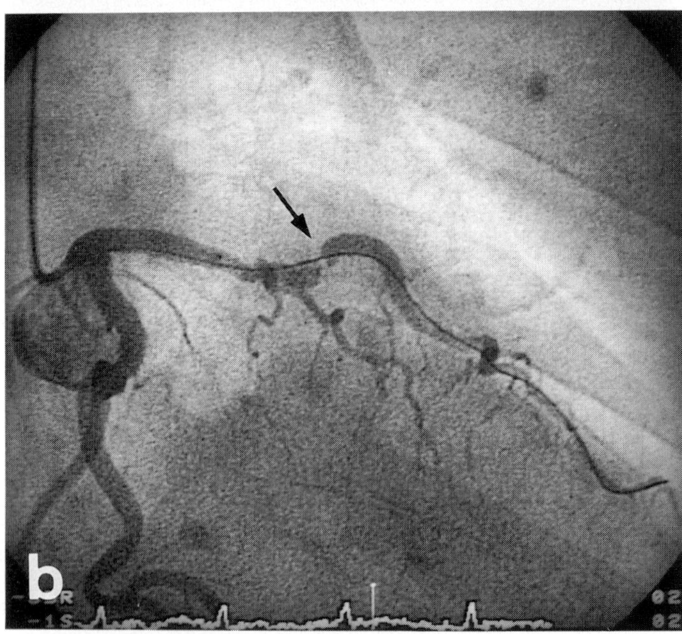

Figure 97

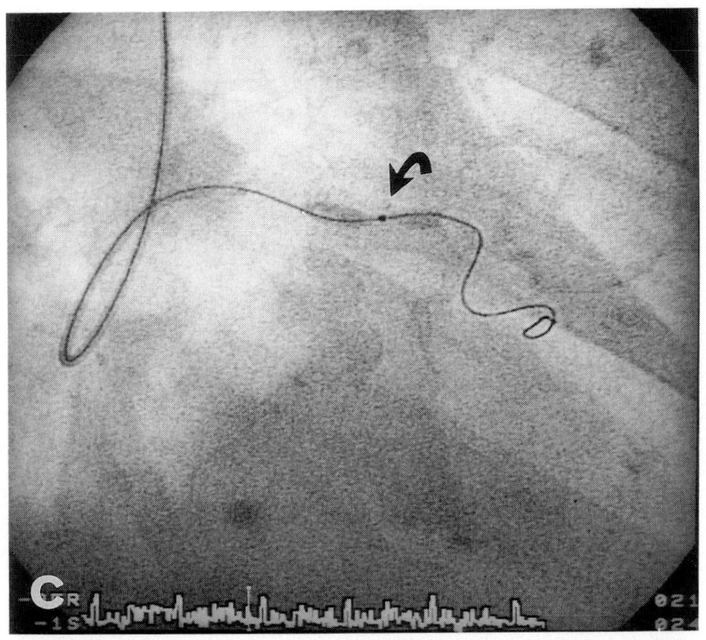

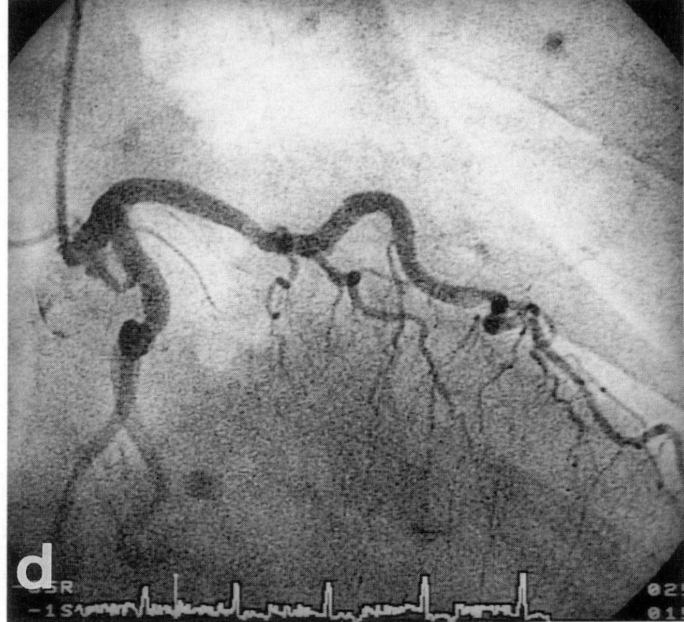

which in most cases represents a dissection flap falling back into the lumen with each deflation. Half a Palmaz-Schatz stent was implanted (Fig. 97c), with a good result (Fig. 97d). Such an approach is eminently suitable for such stenoses. Patients with a half stent in a sufficiently large vessel with good peripheral runoff, as well as selected patients with a full stent, may be managed with aspirin alone.

3.5 STENOSIS WITH THROMBUS

A thrombus at the site of a plaque (thrombotic plaque) indicates a complex lesion for PTCA. A fresh thrombus, as in unstable angina or acute myocardial infarction, is a harbinger of acute occlusion following angioplasty. However, when a thrombus is seen distal to a lesion (Fig. 98a) (related to sluggish flow and thrombosis in the downstream "sink"), it is not associated with increased risks, although it may be dislodged during the procedure and transiently block a peripheral vessel. Good immediate and long-term angioplasty results can be expected in this setting (Fig. 98b).

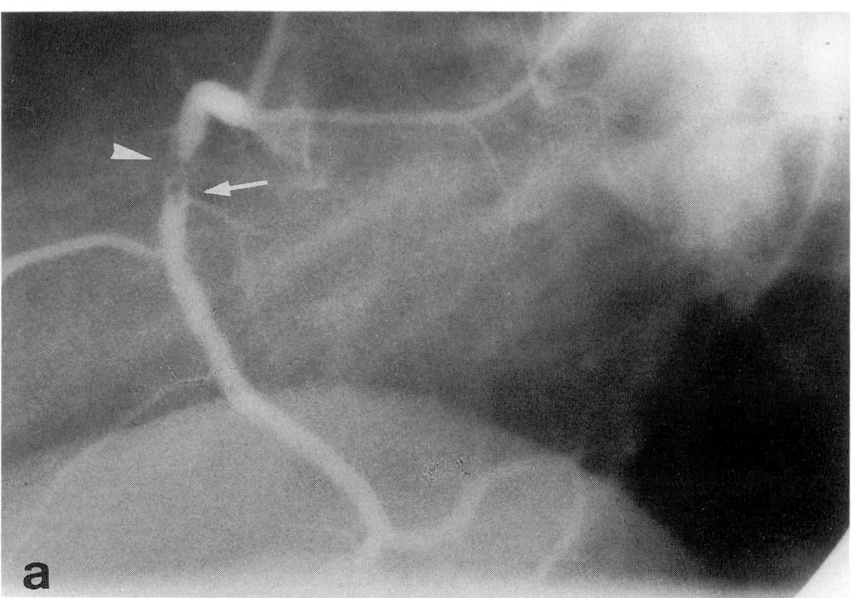

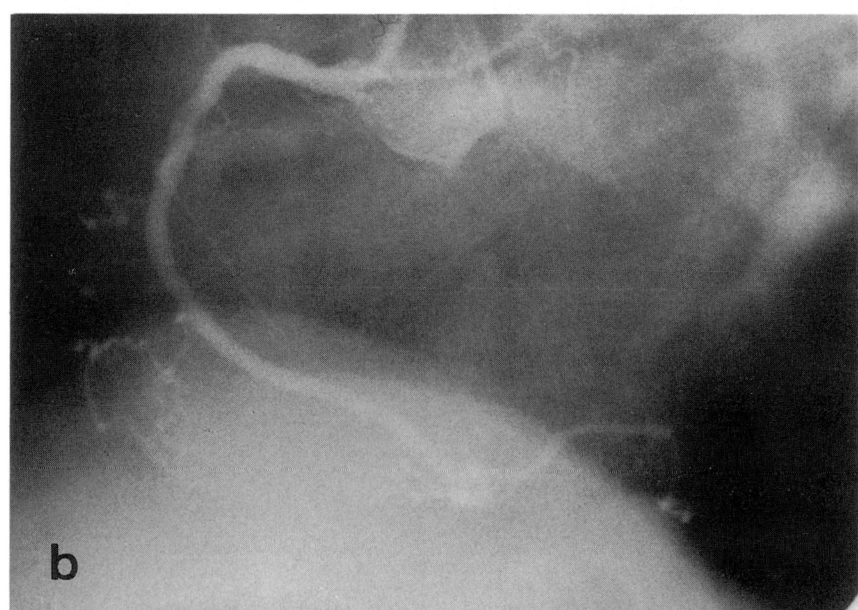

Figure 98

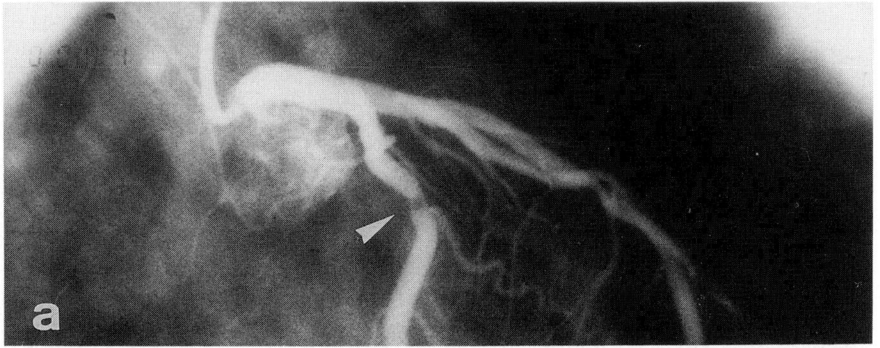

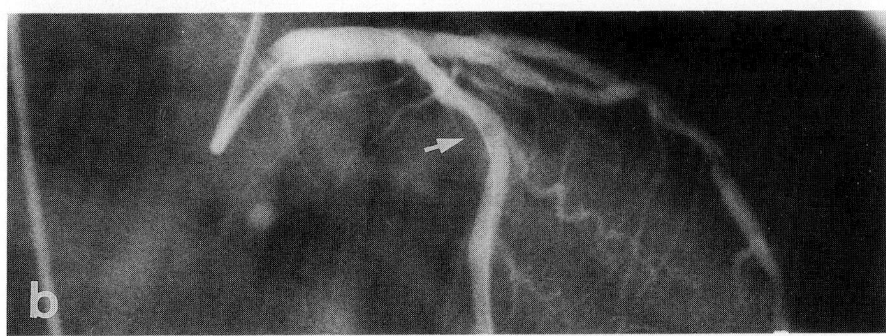

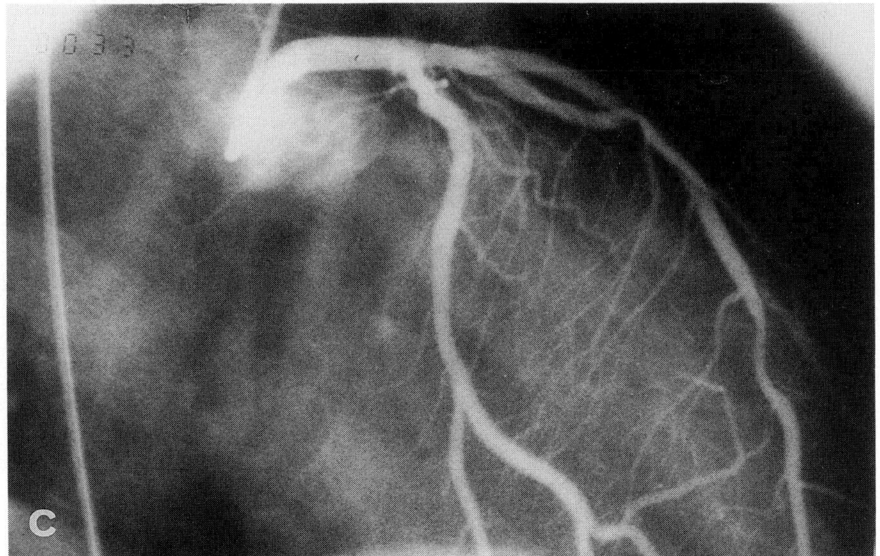

Figure 99

A lesion with a thrombus, as in a patient with unstable angina (Fig. 99a), may show an insufficient result after balloon angioplasty (Fig. 99b). This problem can often be overcome by stenting. In a small lesion, half a Palmaz-Schatz stent can be used with good results (Fig. 99c). The chances of stent thrombosis are probably somewhat higher when dealing with thrombotic lesions, but this can be reduced to some extent by using half a stent (which is less thrombogenic, owing to its reduced metal content).

It is advisable, in patients in whom thrombus is suspected (e.g., unstable angina, following myocardial infarction, etc.), to perform angioplasty after a few days of pretreatment with heparin (if clinically possible). Additionally, patients with a visible thrombus should receive generous (additional) heparin during the intervention and prolonged intravenous heparin after the intervention. Intravenous administration of 1 to 2 million units of urokinase may also advisable during angioplasty, although its benefit has not been documented. A 49-year-old man presented with crescendo angina. A previous coronary angiogram 3 years earlier had revealed insignificant stenoses of the LAD (Fig. 100a). The current angiogram showed the LAD lesions unchanged but there was a thrombotic lesion of the LCx (Fig. 100b). The thrombotic nature of this lesion is evident from its eccentric droplike appearance. The risk of angioplasty of such a lesion is high. Hence PTCA was not performed; instead, the patient received 2 million units of urokinase intravenously. A control angiogram performed the next day revealed some thrombolysis with an improvement in flow and lysis of the distal clot fragments (Fig. 100c). The patient was treated medically with intravenous heparin and subsequently coumadin, and symptoms abated. However, 1 week later, angina at rest recurred. Angiography revealed recrudescence of the thrombotic lesion (Fig. 100d). Angioplasty was performed, the

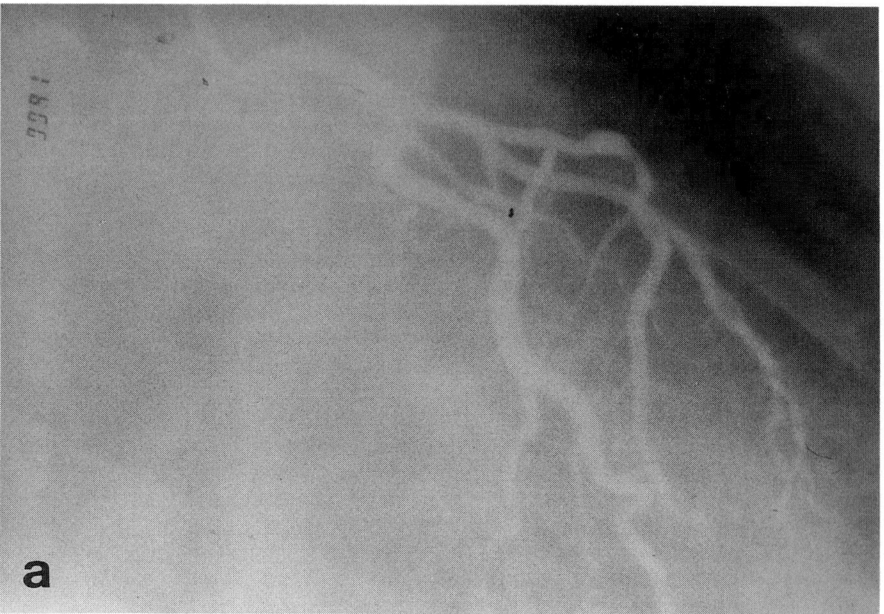

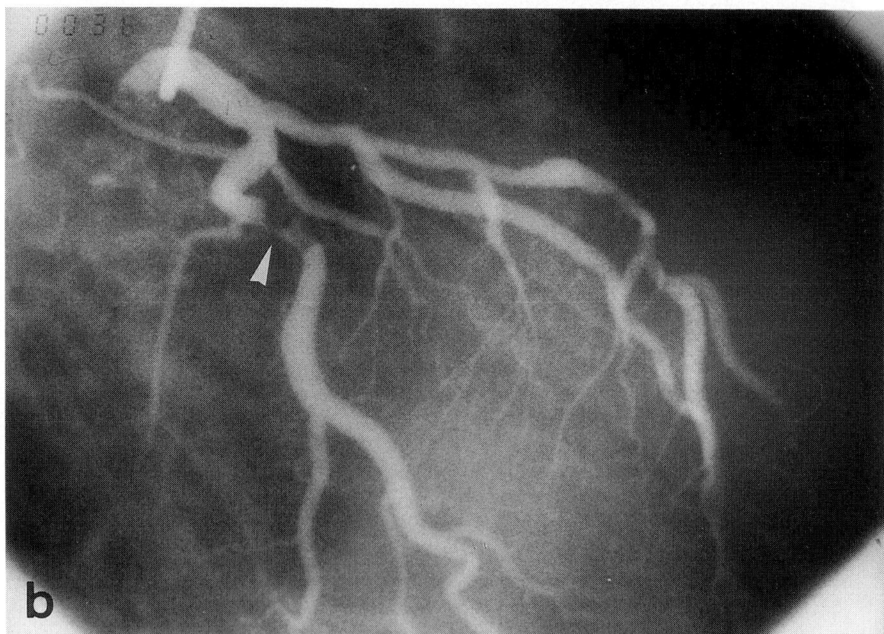

Figure 100

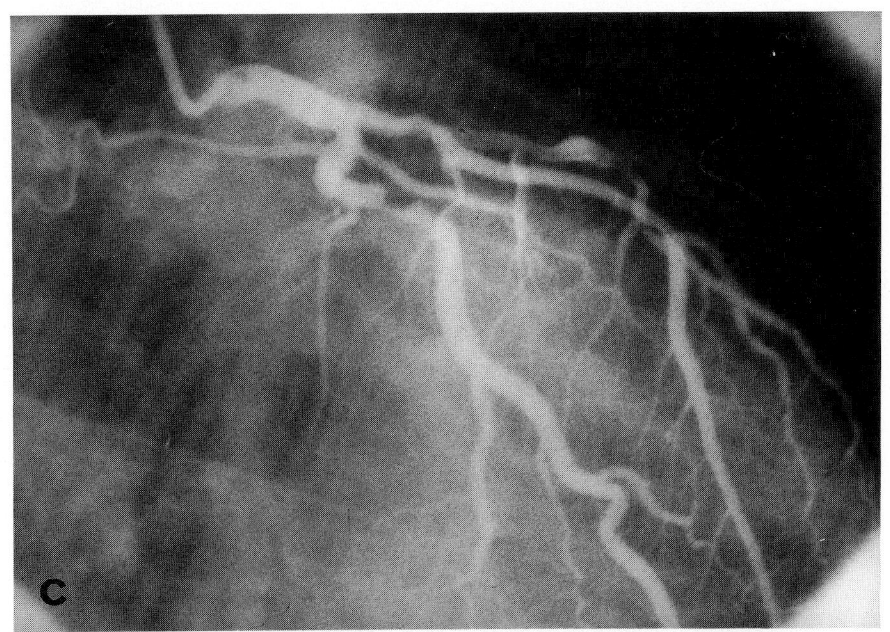
c

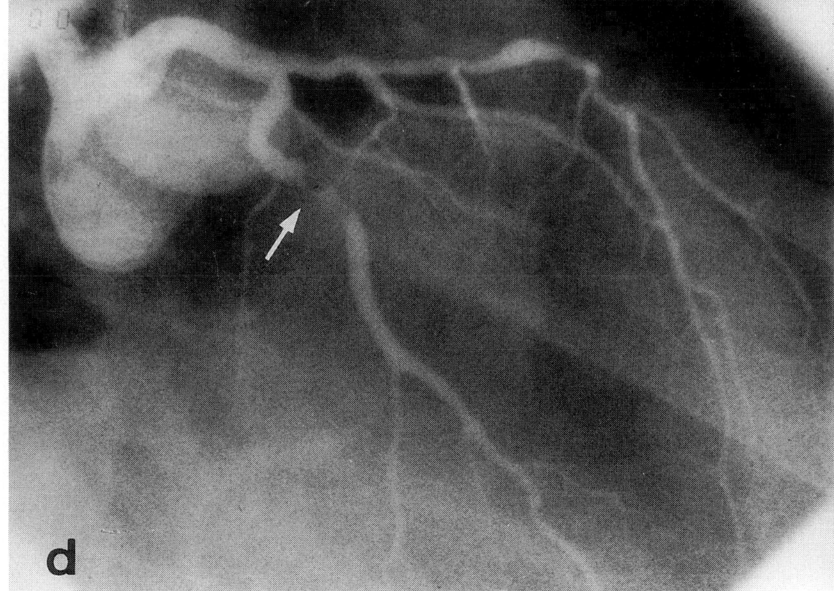
d

result being satisfactory at first, leaving only a slight irregularity at the dilated site (Fig. 100e). Yet, the next day, symptoms recurred with ST segment elevation in the ECG. Angiography revealed progression of the thrombus at the dilated site with sluggish flow (Fig. 100f). Reangioplasty with a larger balloon resulted in a long spiral dissection (Fig. 100g). The lesion was stented, with a good result (Fig. 100h). The following day, symptoms recurred again. Angiography revealed good patency of the stented site but a distal occlusion of the LCx (nonstented distal end of the spiral dissection) (Fig. 100i). No further intervention was performed, and a "controlled infarction" was accepted as a final result in this case.

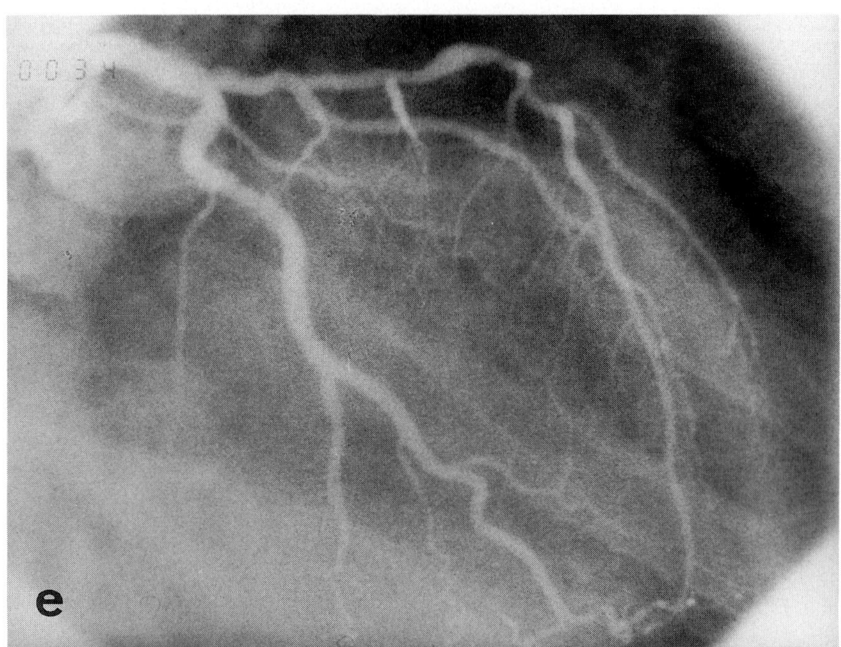

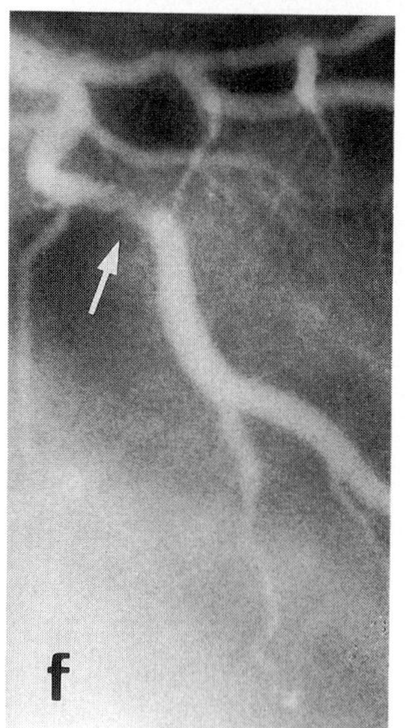

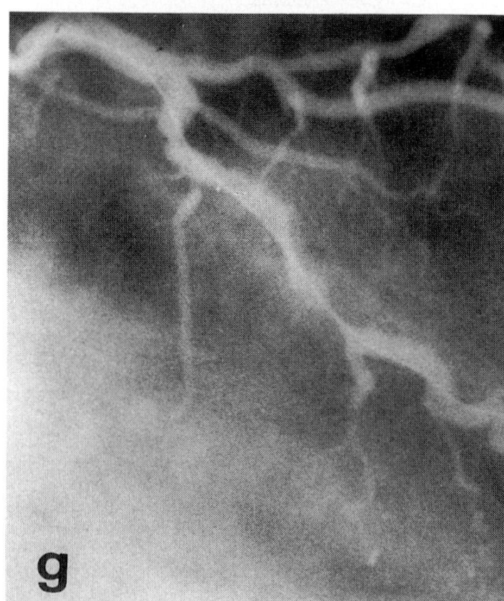

Figure 100 (Continued)

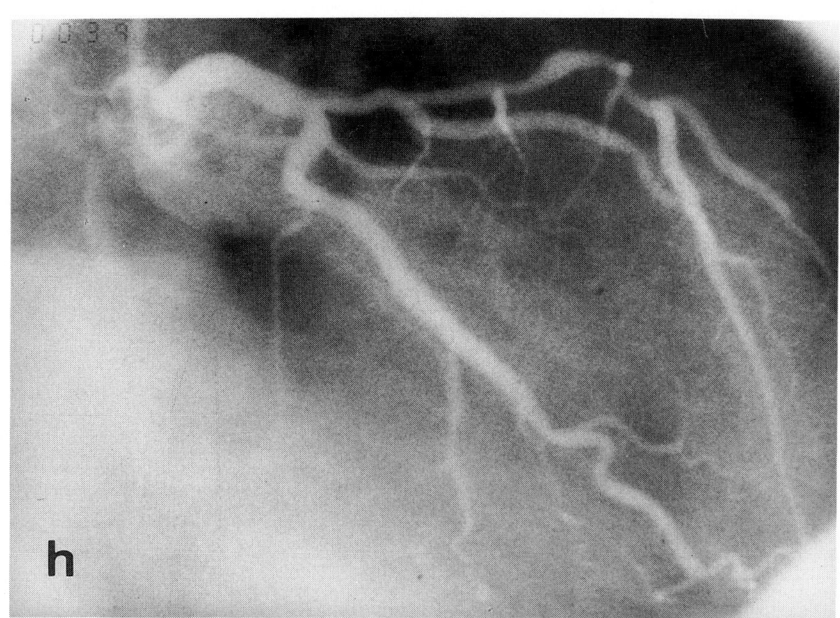
h

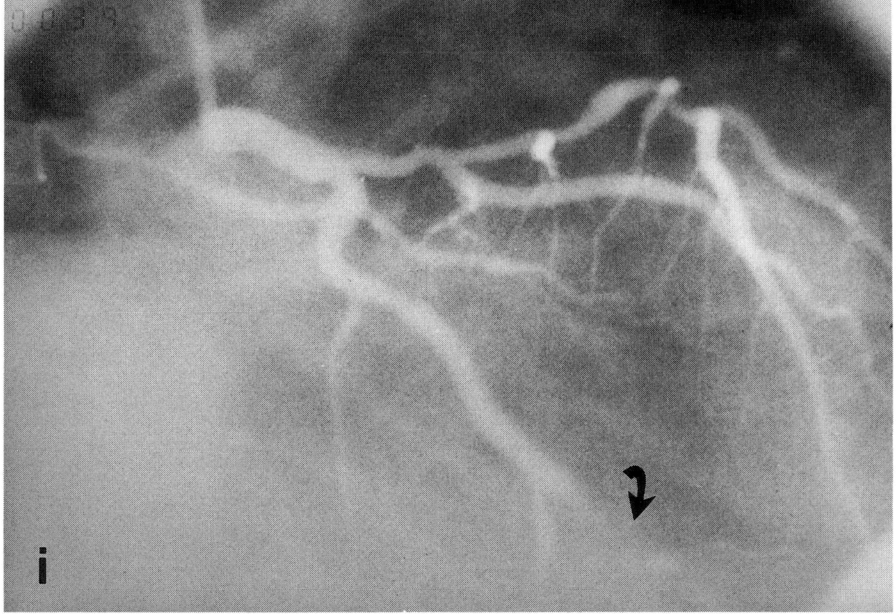
i

It may sometimes be possible to aspirate a fresh thrombus from coronary arteries and grafts to relieve an obstruction. A 53-year-old male presented with an acute anterior myocardial infarction. Coronary angiography revealed a fresh thrombus (arrow) in the proximal segment of the vein graft to the LAD (Fig. 101a). The clot was aspirated with a 7F guiding catheter and a 60-mL syringe (Fig. 101b). The lesion distal to the thrombus was dilated, with a good result (Fig. 101c), and a 3-week follow-up angiogram revealed a patent graft and distal vessel (Fig. 101d). Figure 101e shows the 3.5-cm-long aspirated thrombus.

3.6 CORONARY ARTERY ECTASIA OR ANEURYSM WITH STENOSIS

Coronary artery ectasia or aneurysms may arise spontaneously or consequent to angioplasty. Stenoses in ectatic or aneurysmal coronary arteries can pose problems for PTCA. These include difficulties in adequately judging the correct balloon size, since a residual relative stenosis will persist

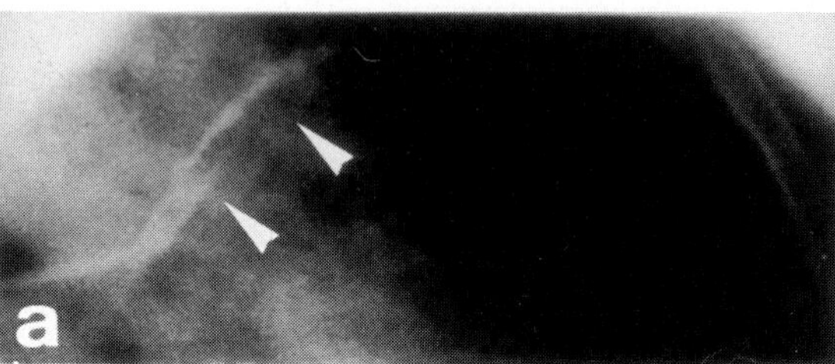

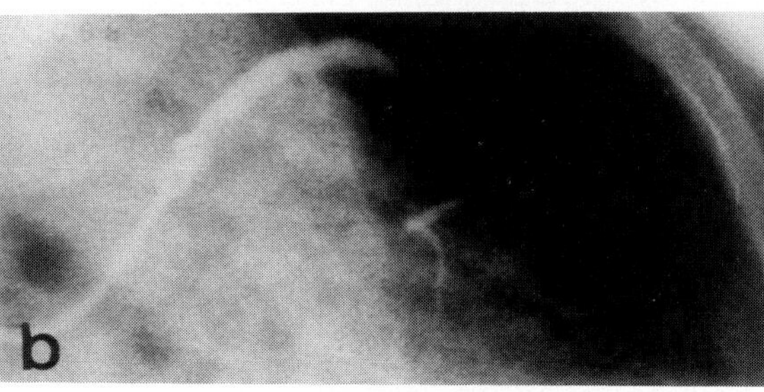

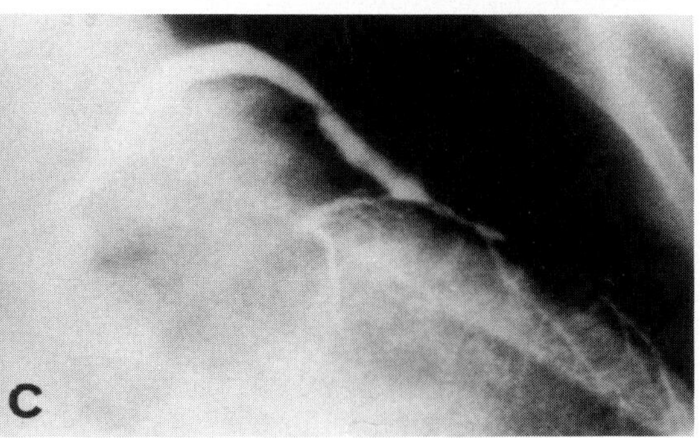

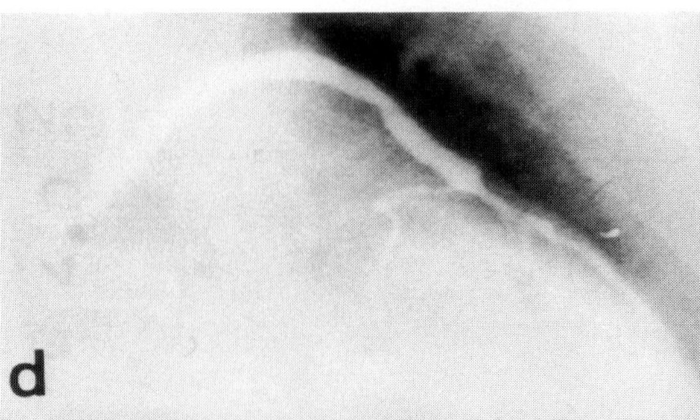

Figure 101

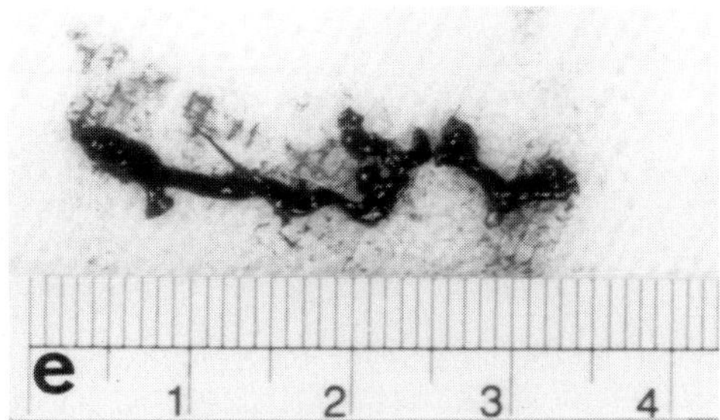

Figure 101 (Continued)

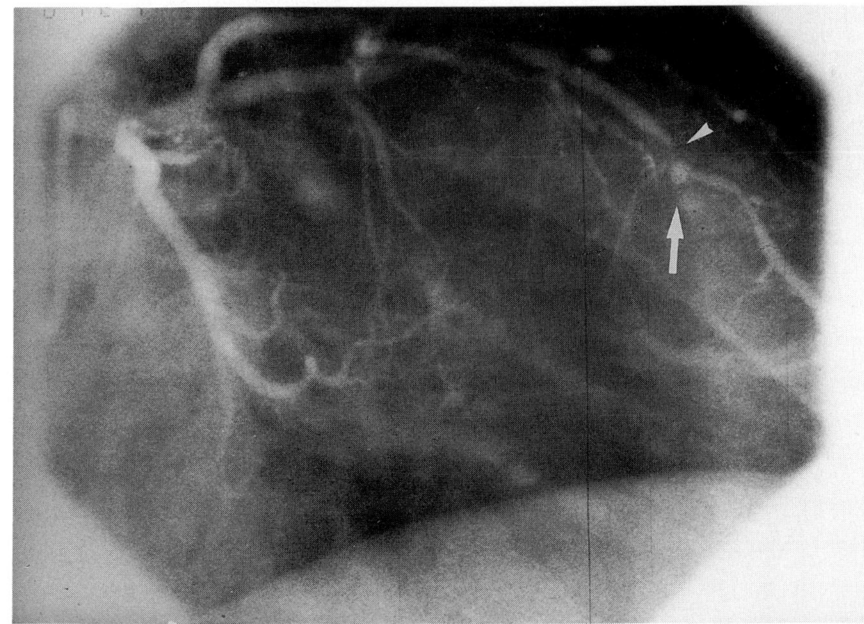

Figure 102

even with an optimal result. Lesions in ectatic segments may look severe in relation to the neighboring vessel but may not necessarily be associated with the hemodynamic consequences of similar degrees of stenoses in normal vessels. Using large balloons may result in overdilation and damage to the normal segments of the vessel. In case stenting becomes necessary, it is associated with the same problem. Underdilation will result in a poorly seated stent, overdilation in damage to the adjacent normal vessel. Moreover, devices such as the directional atherectome harbor the risk of overly deep cuts and vessel leakage.

Anticoagulation for a couple of weeks after angioplasty may be advisable to reduce thrombus formation in a dissected plaque situated in a vessel with sluggish flow. A stenosis situated near such an aneurysm can pose procedural difficulties during PTCA. It is difficult to negotiate the aneurysmal segment with a guidewire that is impeded in its steerability by a stenosis proximal to the aneurysm. In this example shown in Figure 102, it proved impossible to take the left turn out of the ectatic segment (arrowhead) because the tip of the guidewire was straightened by the tight stenosis at the entrance. In another such patient with a large aneurysm situated distal to an LAD stenosis (Fig. 103a), angioplasty was ultimately successful (Fig. 103b), but not before over an hour had been spent in attempts to cross the aneurysm with the guidewire.

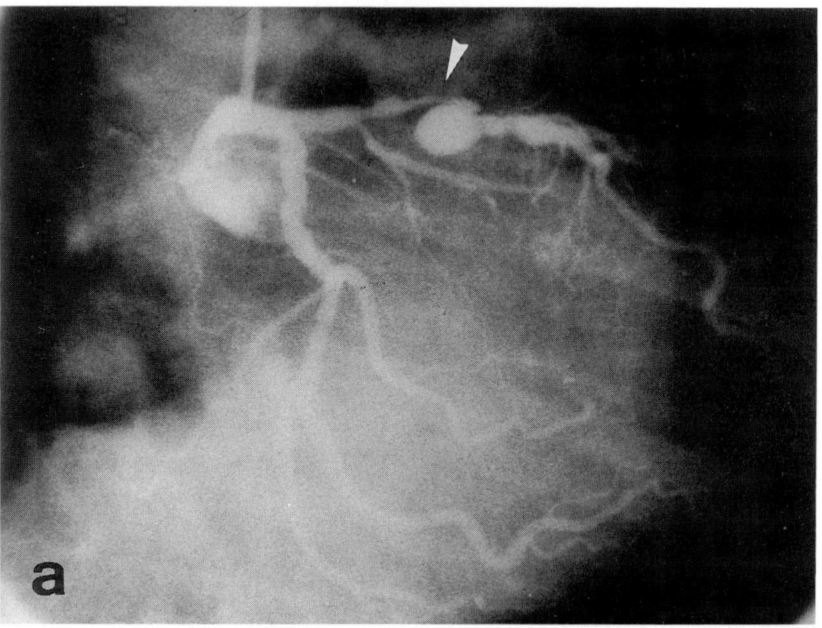

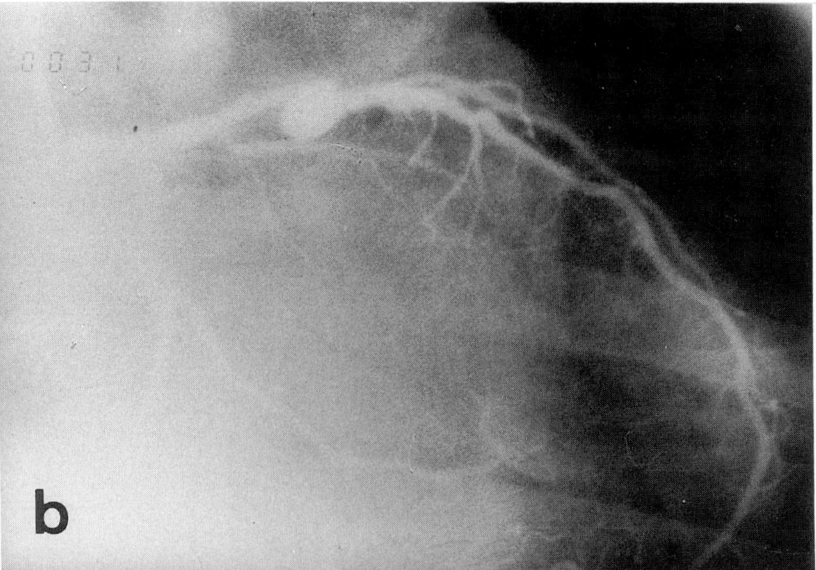

Figure 103

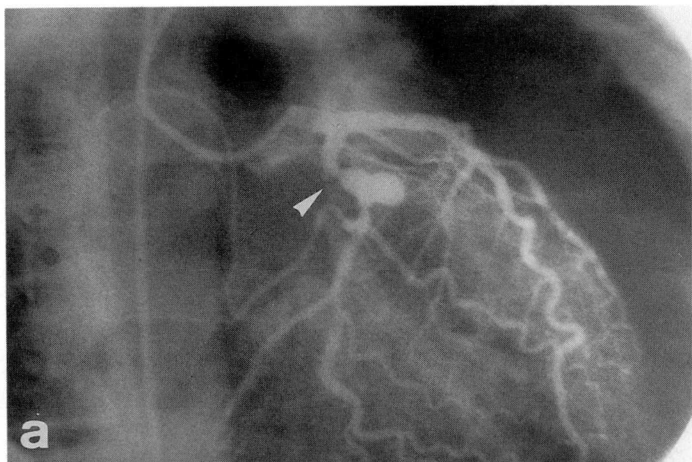

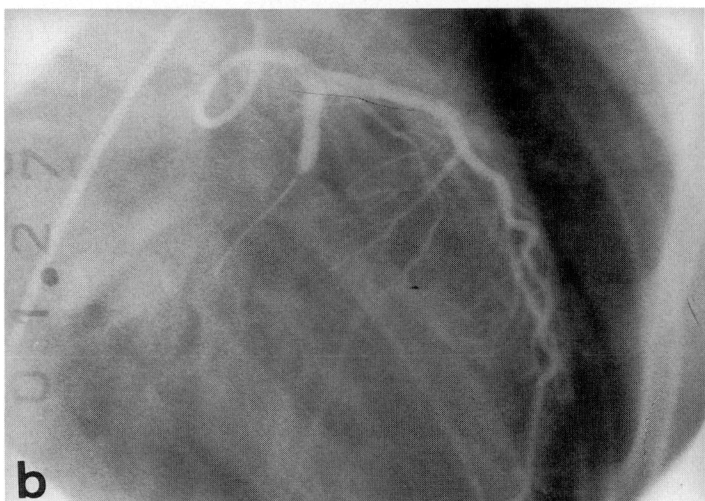

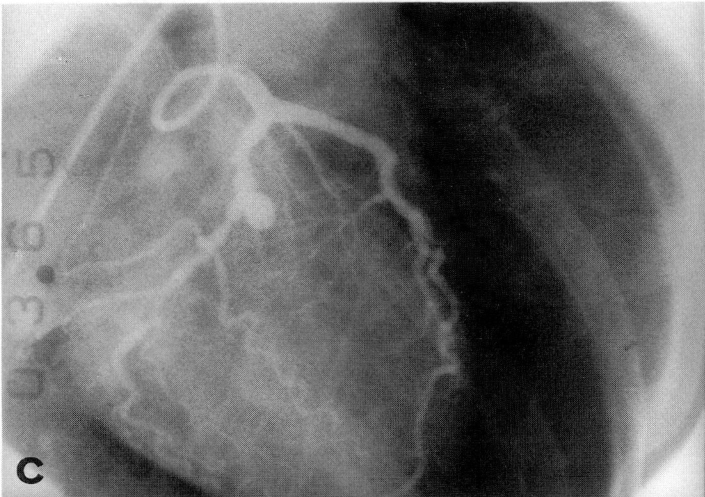

Figure 104

An aneurysm need not always increase procedural difficulties. A 54-year-old male with angina had a stenosis of the proximal LCx. Again, there was an aneurysm just distal to it (Fig. 104a). However, in this case the aneurysm had a large exit in the direction the guidewire of the fixed-wire balloon took spontaneously (Fig. 104b). The angioplasty could be performed with ease and a good result (Fig. 104c).

A Magnum wire, with its ball tip and its relative stiffness, may be helpful to negotiate an aneurysm and avoid the cul de sac. Such an approach was useful in a 57-year-old man (Fig. 105a), in which a 0.014-in. guidewire could not be passed into a stenosed diagonal branch of the LAD (arrowhead), owing to a small stump of the occluded LAD forming a sort of aneurysmal cul de sac (arrow). The problem was overcome by a Magnum wire (Fig. 105b) and angioplasty could be performed successfully (Fig. 105c).

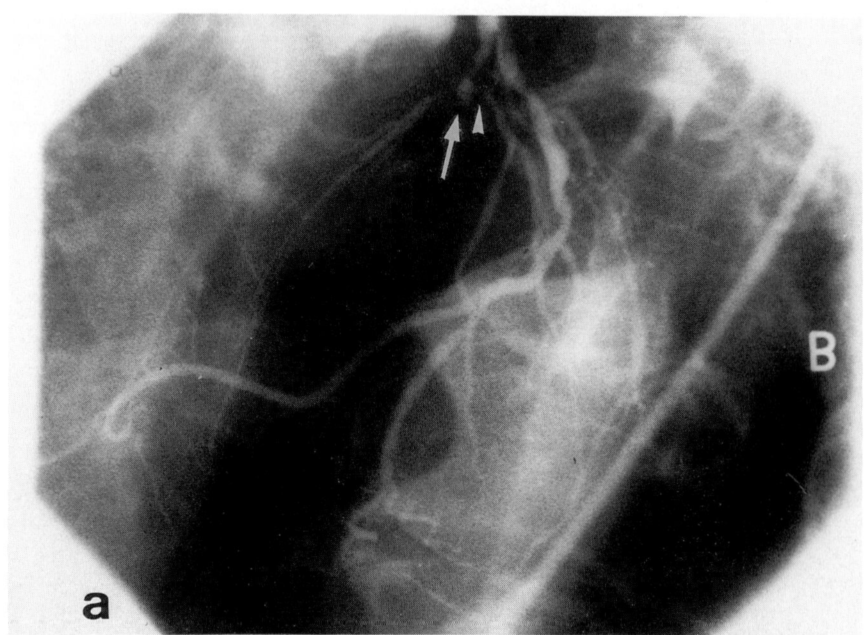

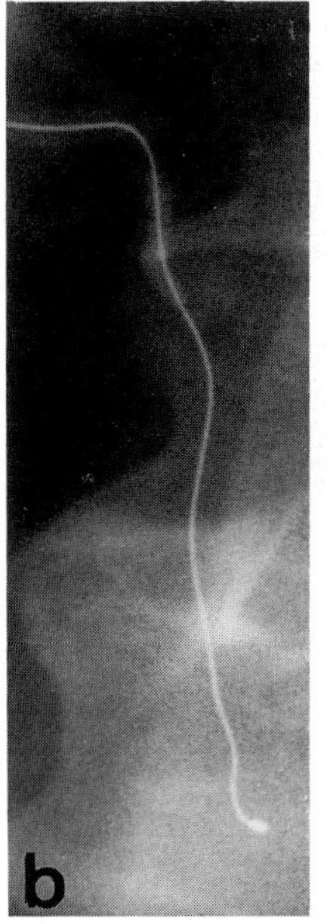

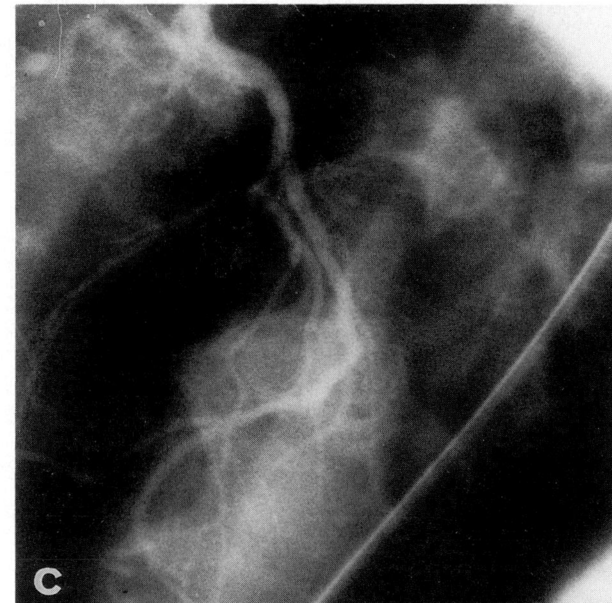

Figure 105

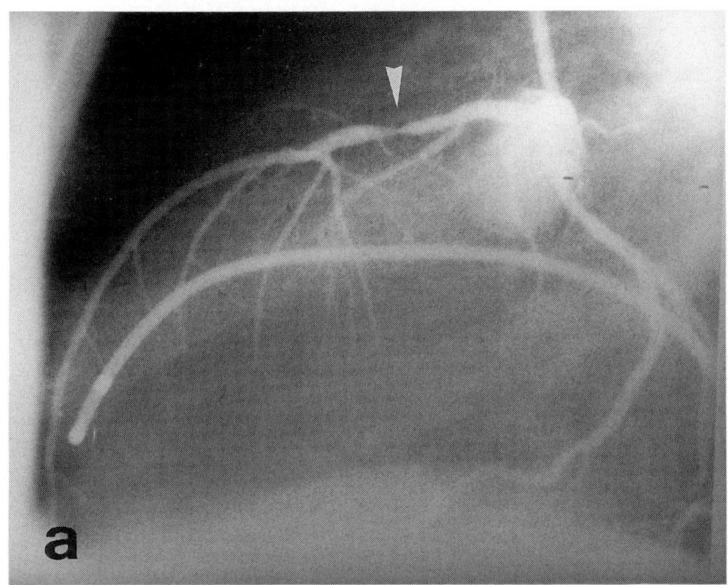

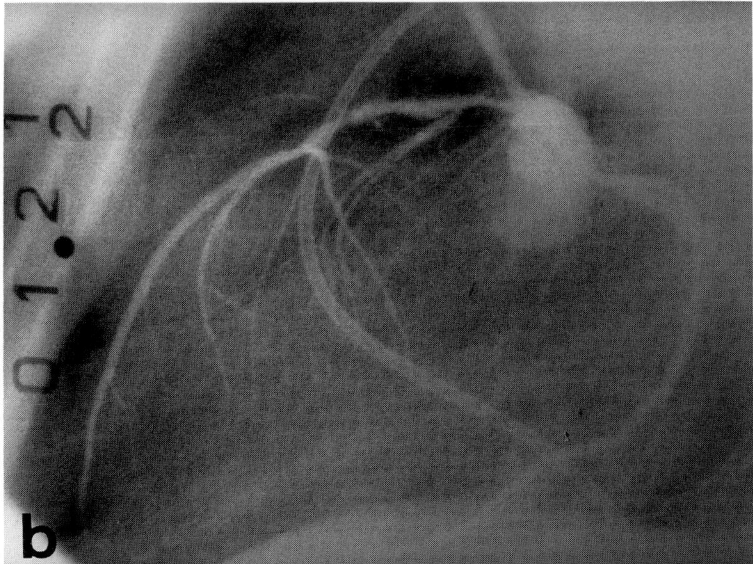

Figure 106

Aneurysms appearing following angioplasty are usually benign. A 34-year-old man underwent angioplasty for an LAD stenosis (Fig. 106a), with a good result and a local dissection (Fig. 106b). A 2-year follow-up revealed healing of the dissection with appearance of an aneurysm at the dilated site (Fig. 106c). The picture persisted on an angiogram performed 6 years later (Fig. 106d). Some of these aneurysms may even regress spontaneously over time.

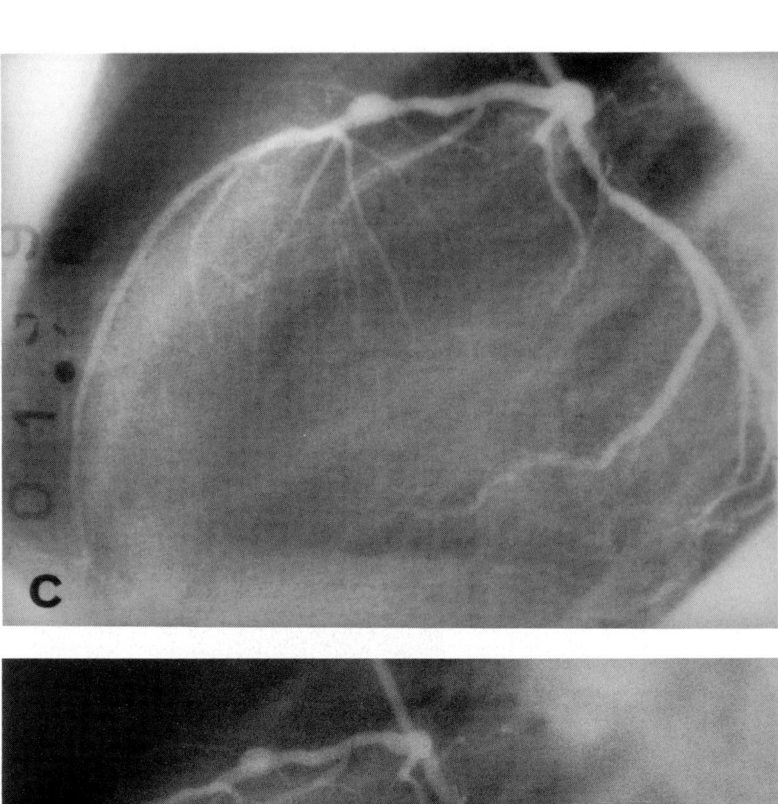

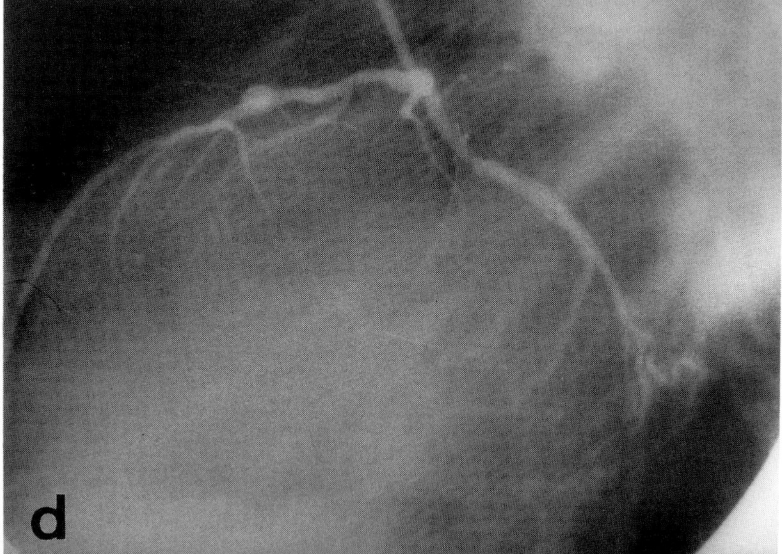

Figure 106 (Continued)

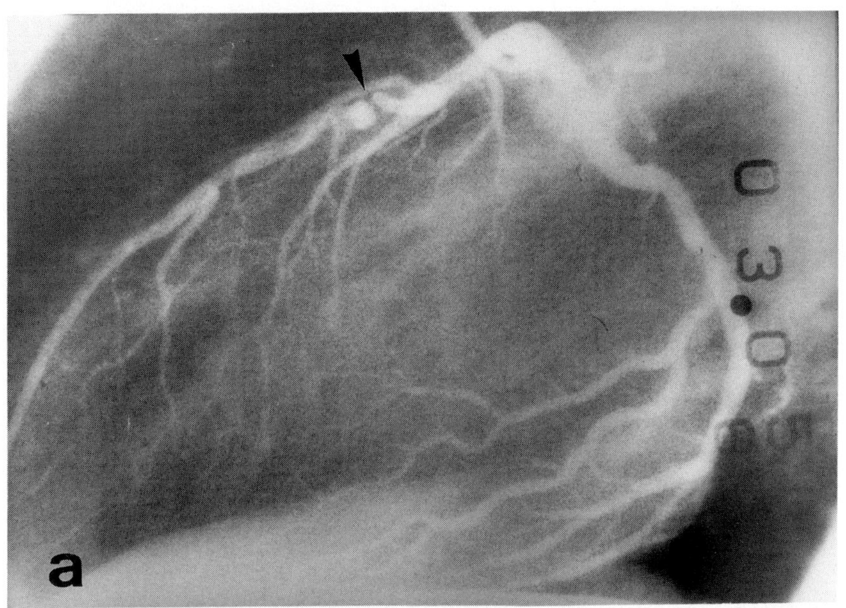

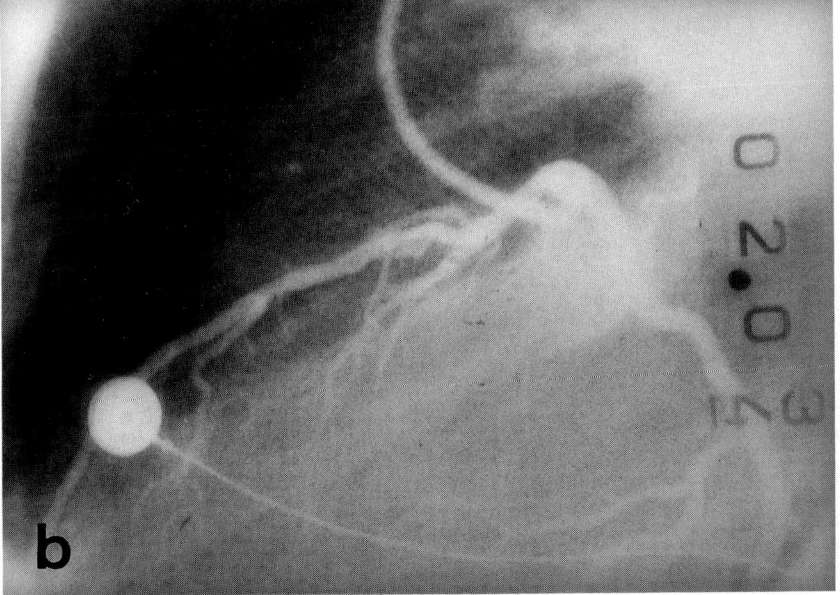

Figure 107

Occasionally, aneurysms may diminish in size or disappear immediately following angioplasty. This is demonstrated in an angioplasty operator who underwent angioplasty himself. He had an aneurysm distal to a mid LAD stenosis (Fig. 107a). Following successful angioplasty, the aneurysm was less apparent (Fig. 107b), probably related to the altered flow pattern. A stress test performed the next morning was normal, and the patient performed an angioplasty that afternoon as he had done the morning before his own procedure ("do one, have one done the same day, do one the next day"). This case nicely demonstrates the early discharge and return-to-job potential of angioplasty, one of its major advantages.

3.7 TOUGH STENOSES

Occasionally, a tough stenosis resists even high inflation pressures. In such situations, a noncompliant balloon is preferable, since a compliant balloon grows in size at high pressures and may damage the neighboring normal vessel. However, some lesions may resist all attempts at dilatation. This occurred in a 70-year-old male with a tandem stenosis of the RCA, with the tighter lesion distal (Fig. 108a). Despite inflation with a 3.5-mm PET balloon up to 23 bar, a waist remained from the distal lesion (Fig. 108b), which persisted almost unchanged while the proximal lesion was clearly improved (Fig. 108c).

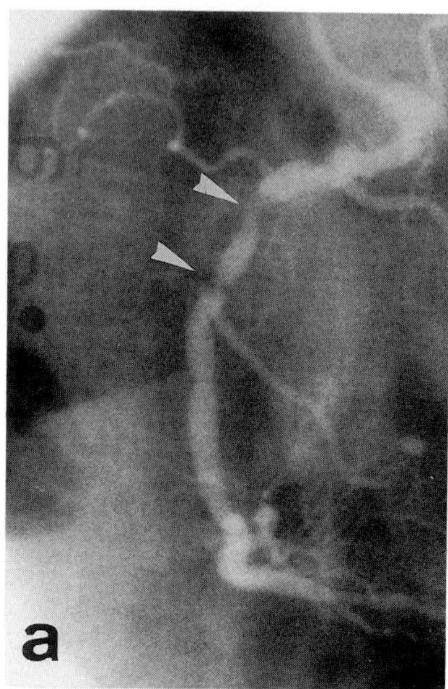

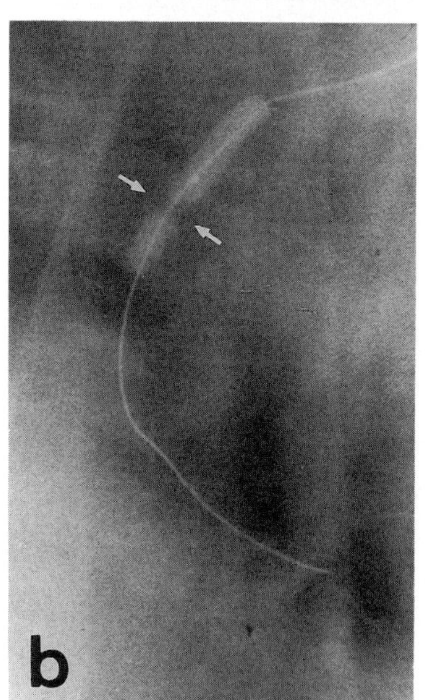

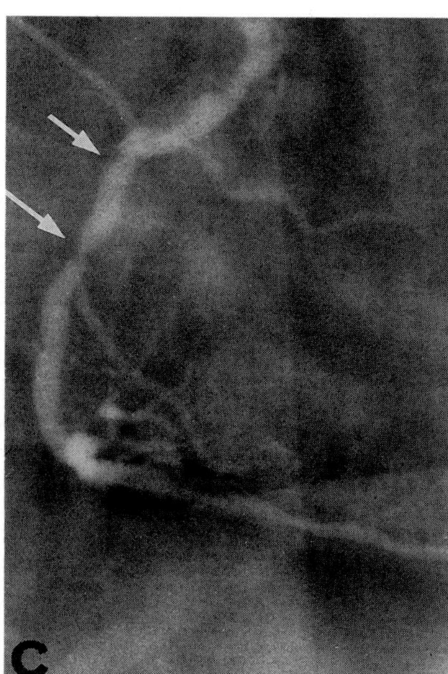

Figure 108

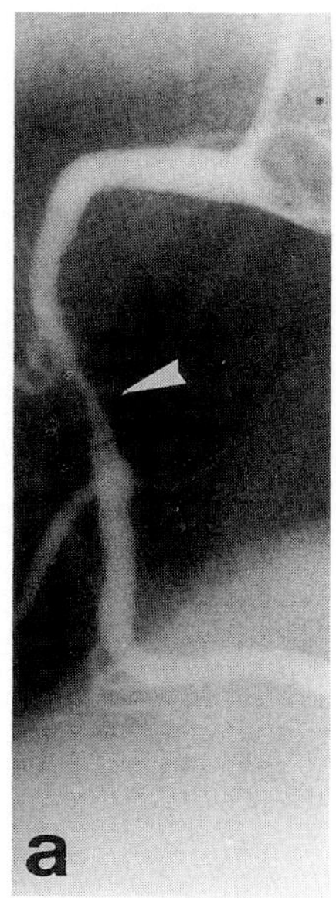

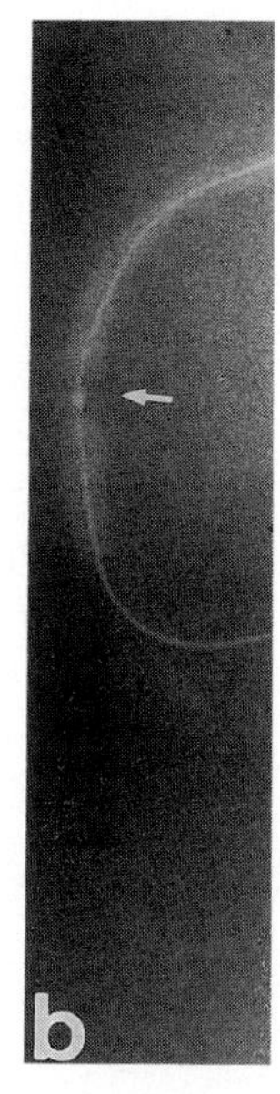

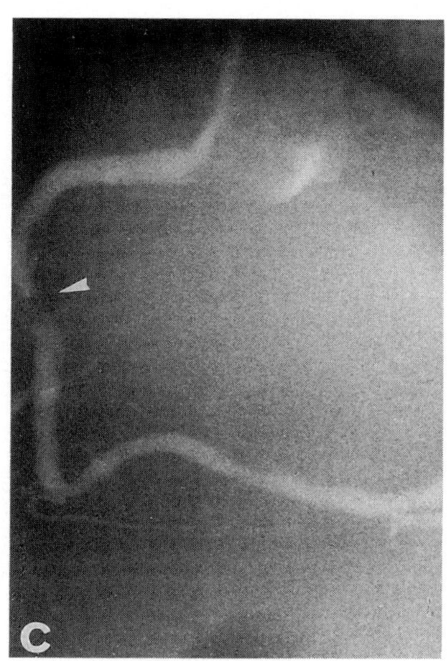

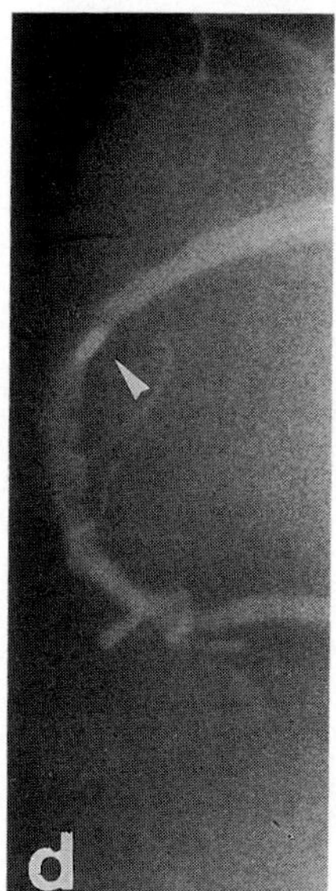

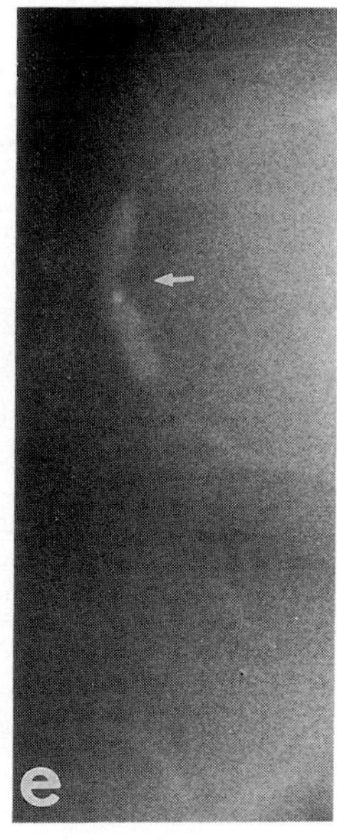

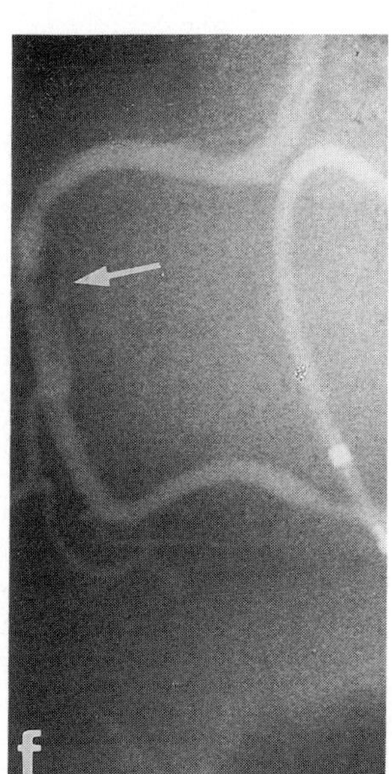

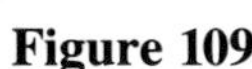
Figure 109

Some of these problems can be overcome by the use of a Rotablator initially to crack the usually circumferential and calcified lesion. Rotablation can so enable balloon angioplasty, which on its own failed. Figure 109a reveals a tight stenosis of the LAD which despite 25 bar pressure with a 3.0-mm balloon (note the unyielding balloon waist in Fig. 109b, arrow) persisted in its midportion (Fig. 109c). Rotablation with a 1.75-mm burr (arrow) was performed (Fig. 109d). This was followed by balloon angioplasty with the 3.0-mm balloon inflated up to 22 bar, the resultant waist being much reduced (Fig. 109e). The final result was acceptable, albeit not optimal (Fig. 109f). This is one of the niches where Rotablation shows a unique potential, the other being a failure to cross the lesion with the balloon, as explained in the following section.

3.8
TIGHT STENOSES

Tight stenoses may be difficult to cross and may require a stiffer wire. The left coronary angiogram in a patient with angina showed collateral supply to the right coronary artery (Fig. 110a), indicative of the tight stenosis of the RCA (Fig. 110b). The RCA lesion could not be crossed with a fixed-wire balloon, despite its very small profile (Fig. 110c). The system was changed for a Magnarail system, which permits significantly more force and succeeded in crossing the lesion (Fig. 110d). Angioplasty was performed with a satisfactory result (Fig. 110e).

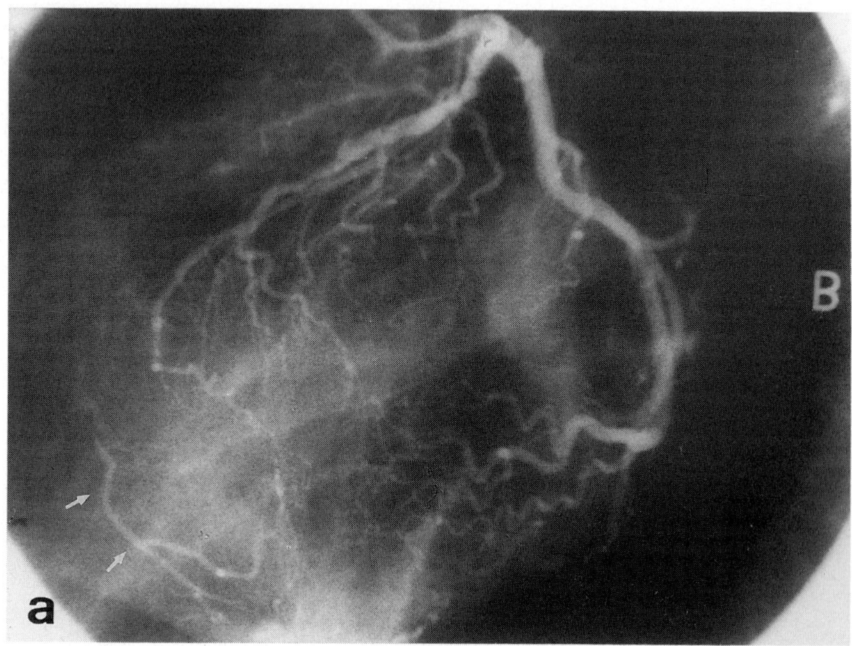

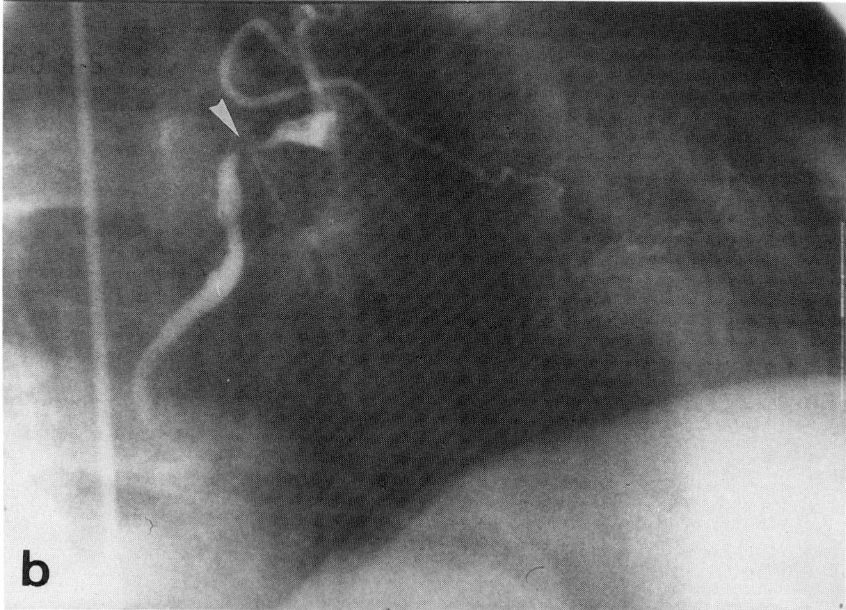

Figure 110

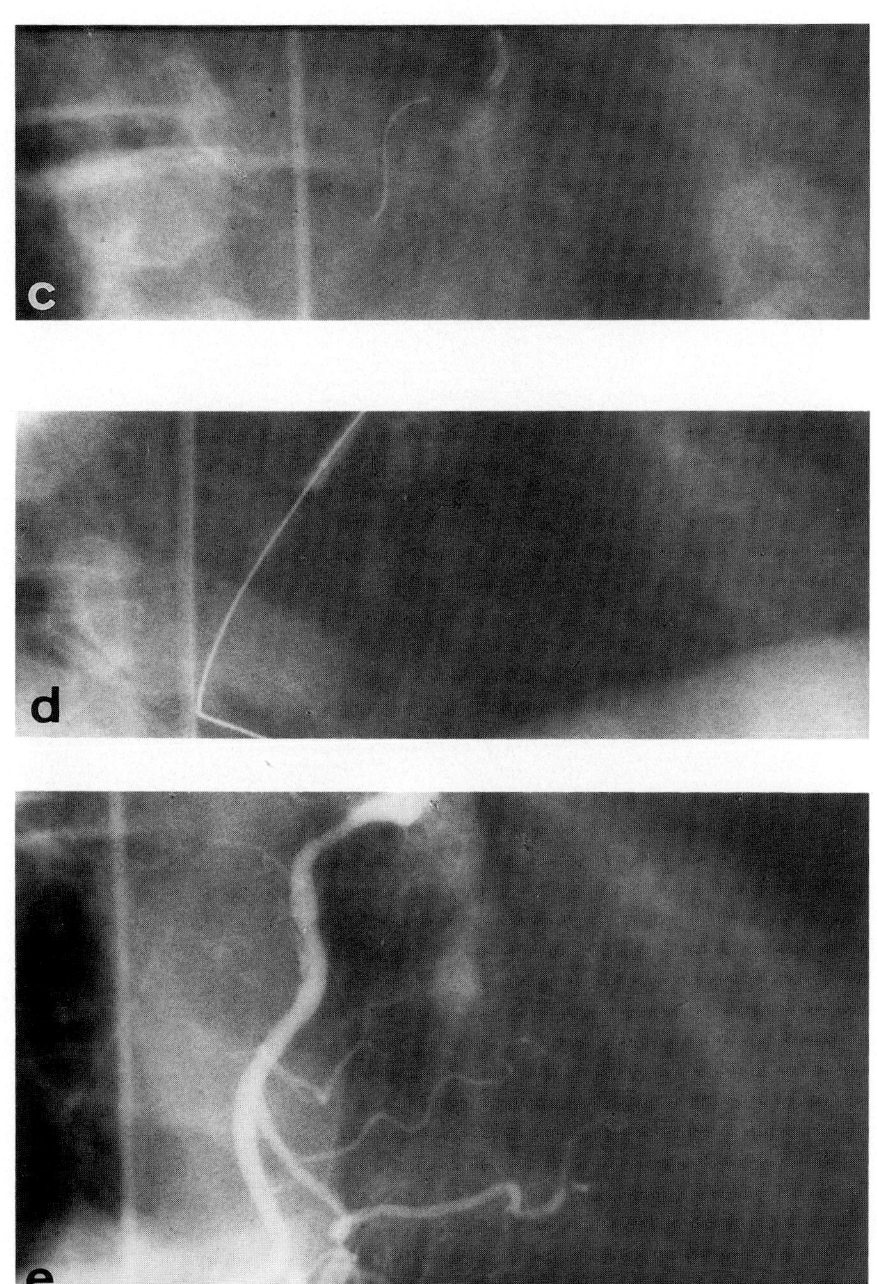
c
d
e

It may sometimes be necessary to exert considerable force to cross a tight stenosis. This is facilitated by deep intubation with the guiding catheter for increased backup. This technique succeeded in an old patient with a tight stenosis of the distal LCx (Fig. 111a) using a stiff wire (Magnum) with additional support of the deeply intubated 7F guiding catheter (the arrow indicates its tip) (Fig. 111b), after failed attempts with other techniques.

Tight stenoses can be tackled with various techniques, including use of a smaller balloon with its smaller crossing profile, changeover to a fixed-wire system from an over-the-wire system, or use of a stiffer wire, as the Magnum system used in this case. Rotablation is an option for an occasional lesion that cannot be crossed with even the smallest balloons (mentioned in the preceding section as one of the two niches for the Rotablator). This is subject to being able to cross the lesion with the Rotablator wire. Adjunctive balloon dilatation is almost always necessary.

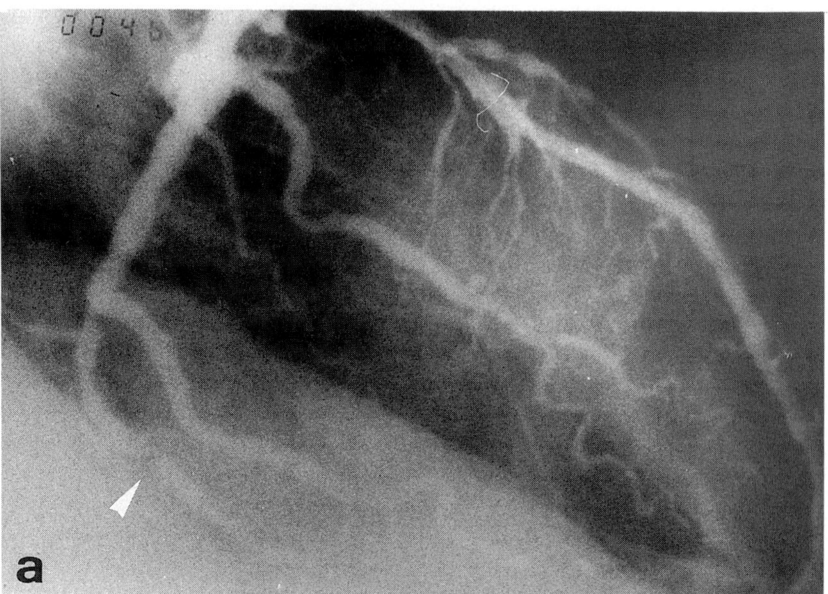

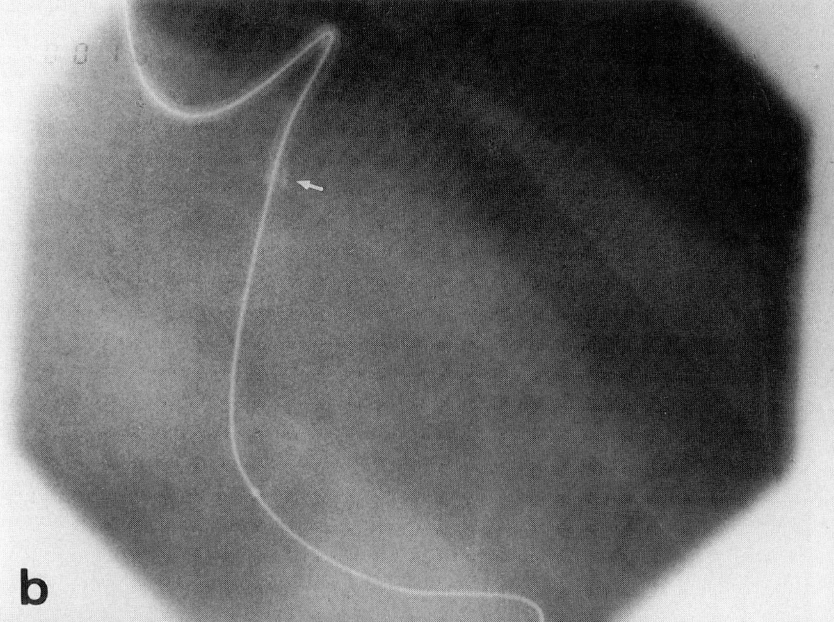

Figure 111

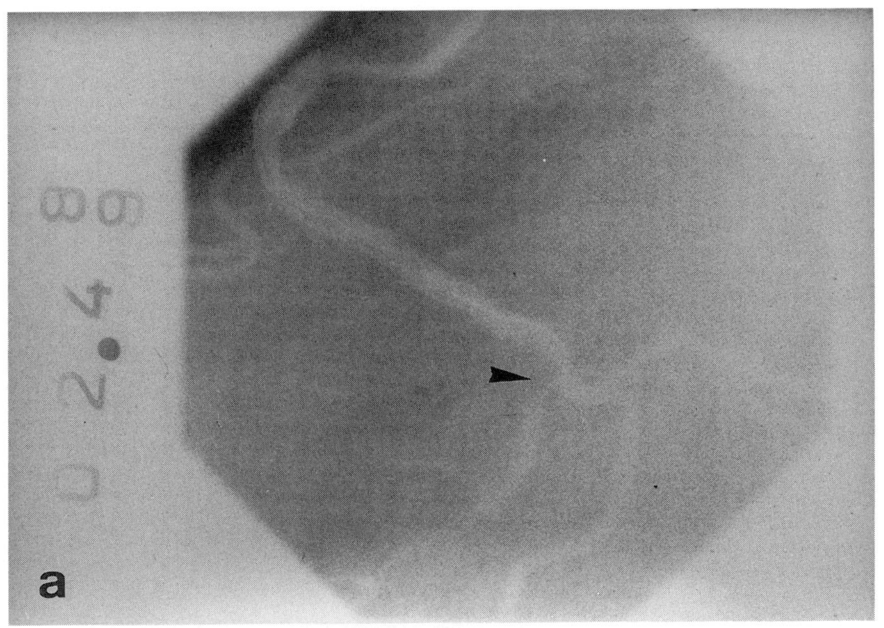

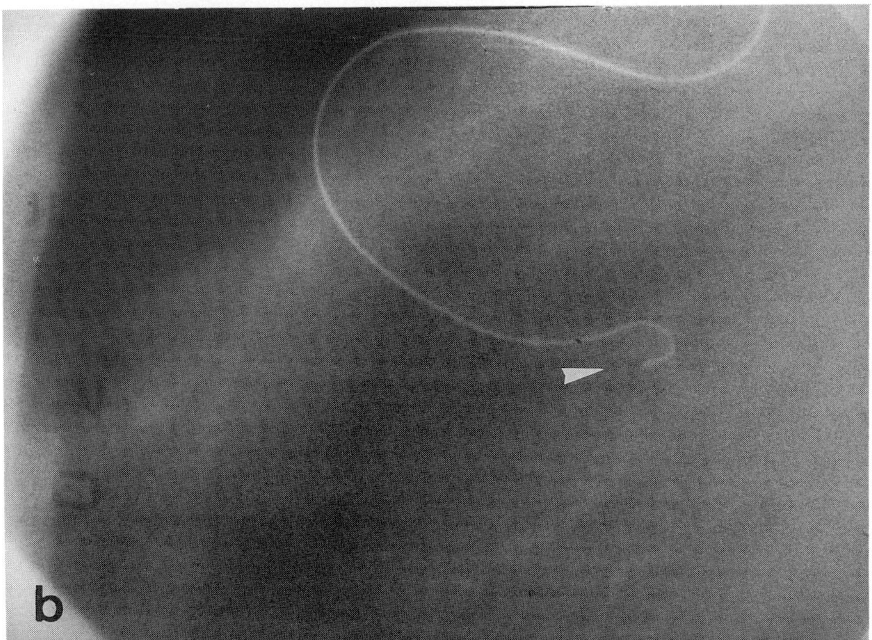

Figure 112

Sometimes a lesion cannot be crossed despite all attempts. A typical example of such a situation is a tight ostial lesion just beyond an acute angle or takeoff. Such a tight lesion in the posterior descending coronary artery could not be crossed with an ACS intermediate wire due to buckling (Fig. 112a). A Magnum wire braced with a Magnarail balloon met with the same fate (Fig. 112b).

3.9 OSTIAL STENOSES

Ostial stenoses pose a different set of problems, ranging from difficulty in seating the guiding catheter and positioning the balloon, to the elastic nature of these lesions with a higher restenosis rate. A 75-year-old man presented with a stenosis of the RCA ostium (Fig. 113a). Angioplasty was performed using a Monorail system (Fig. 113b) (note the position of the balloon straddling the ostium and the guiding catheter situated far away from the coronary artery). The initial result was good (Fig. 113c). An 8-month follow-up showed a good long-term result (Fig. 113d).

The problems when dealing with ostial stenoses are well demonstrated in the example of this 67-year-old woman with an ostial (Fig. 114a, arrowhead) and a proximal stenosis of the RCA (Fig. 114a, arrow). Balloon angioplasty of the two lesions was performed with a 3.0-mm balloon (Fig. 114b,c). The result (Fig. 114d) was acceptable. The patient's symptoms abated transiently but she returned 3 months later with recurrent symptoms.

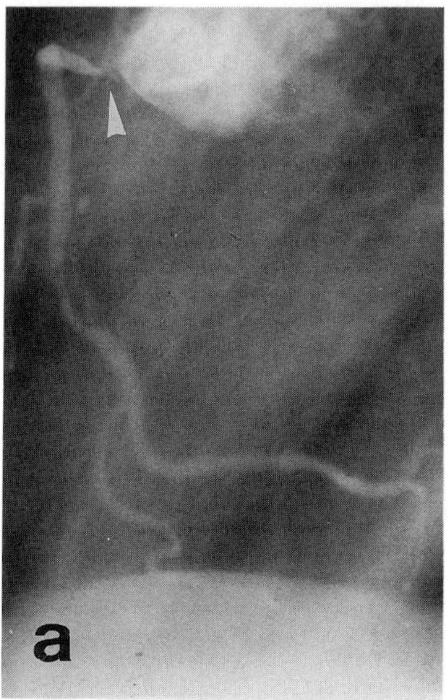

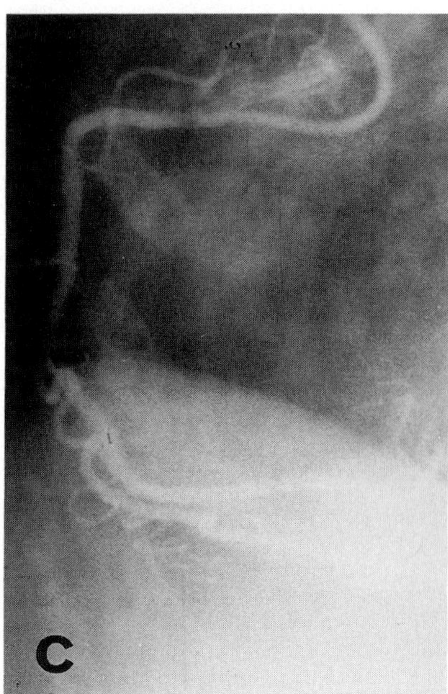

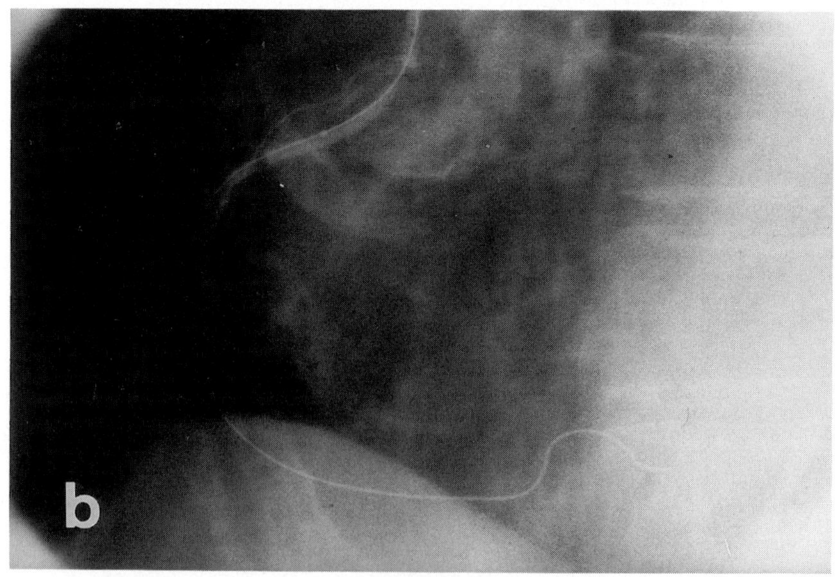

Figure 113

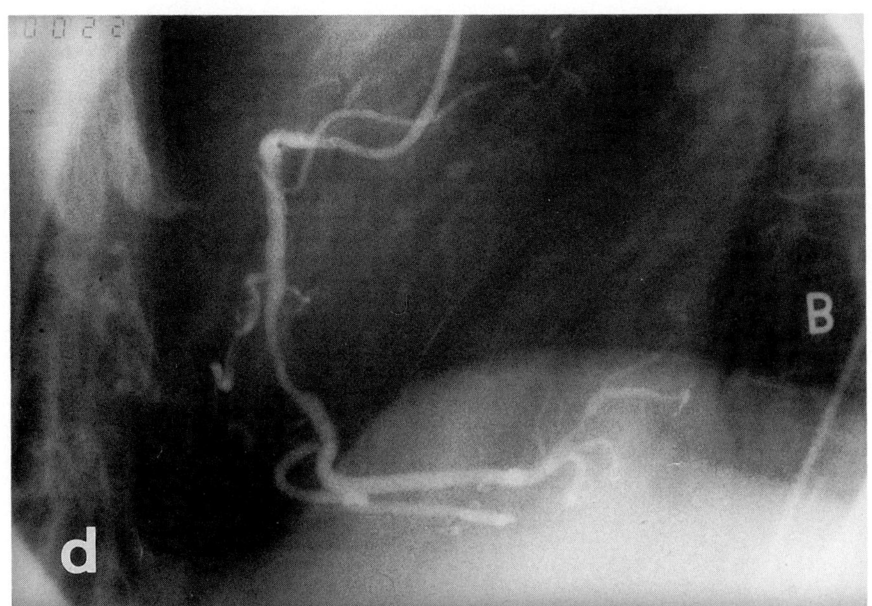

Figure 113 (Continued)

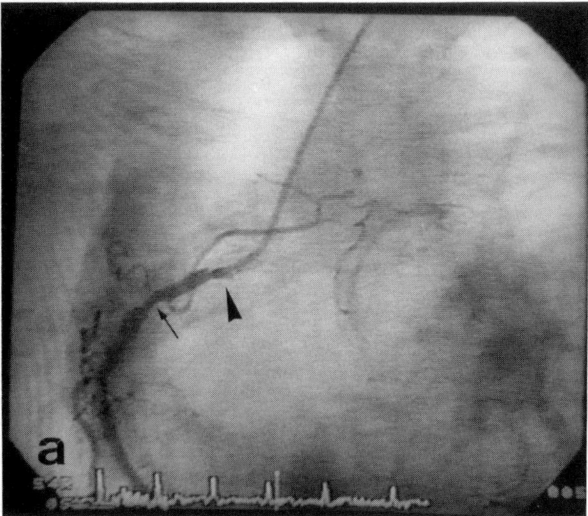

Figure 114

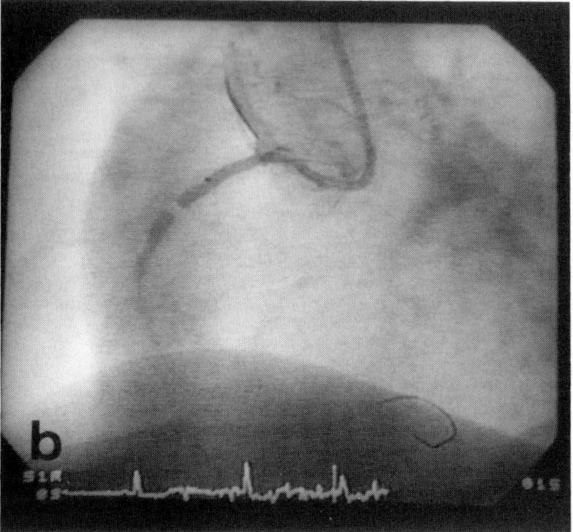

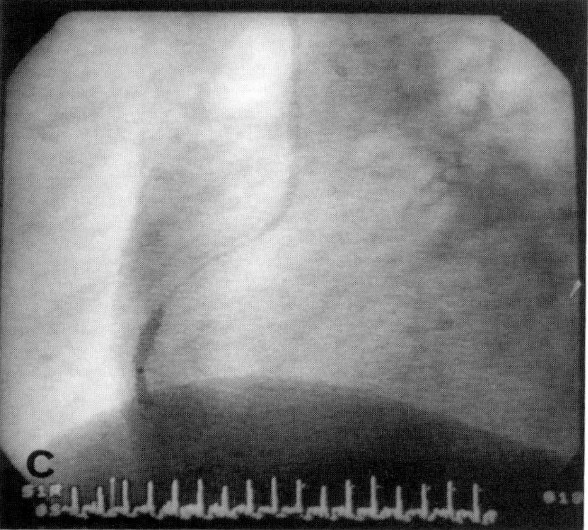

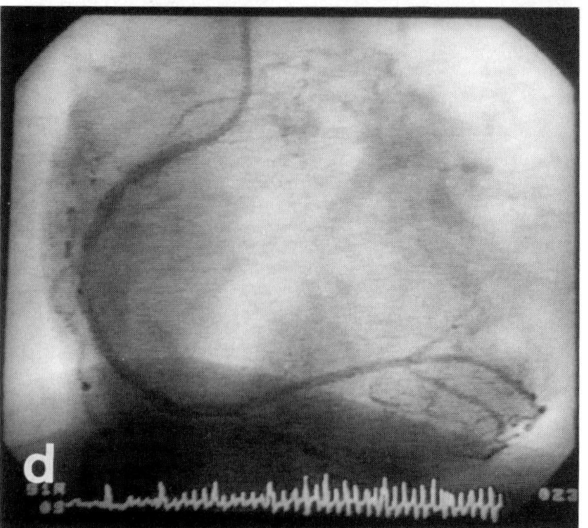

Figure 114 (Continued)

Angiography revealed an isolated restenosis of the ostial lesion (Fig. 114e). Balloon angioplasty was again performed, this time with a 3.5-mm balloon (Fig. 114f). The angiographic result was good (Fig. 114g). However, the patient returned 7 months later with chest pain and a positive stress test. A tight restenosis of the RCA ostium and a significant restenosis of the proximal RCA site were seen (Fig. 114h). This time an alternative approach was tried. Rotablation with a 1.75-mm burr was performed (Fig. 114i), followed by adjunctive balloon angioplasty (Fig. 114j). The result was unsatisfactory (Fig. 114k). Hence a directional atherectomy was performed with a 6F device (Fig. 114l). The final result (Fig. 114m), although not perfect, was accepted. The patient had chest pain with ECG changes the next morning after stopping the heparin. Angiography revealed a severe narrowing of the ostium (Fig. 114n, arrowhead). At this time it was decided to stent the vessel. A half (disarticulated) Palmaz-Schatz stent was implanted into the proximal RCA lesion with a 3.5-mm balloon (Fig. 114n, arrow). The other half Palmaz-Schatz stent was implanted at the ostium (Fig.

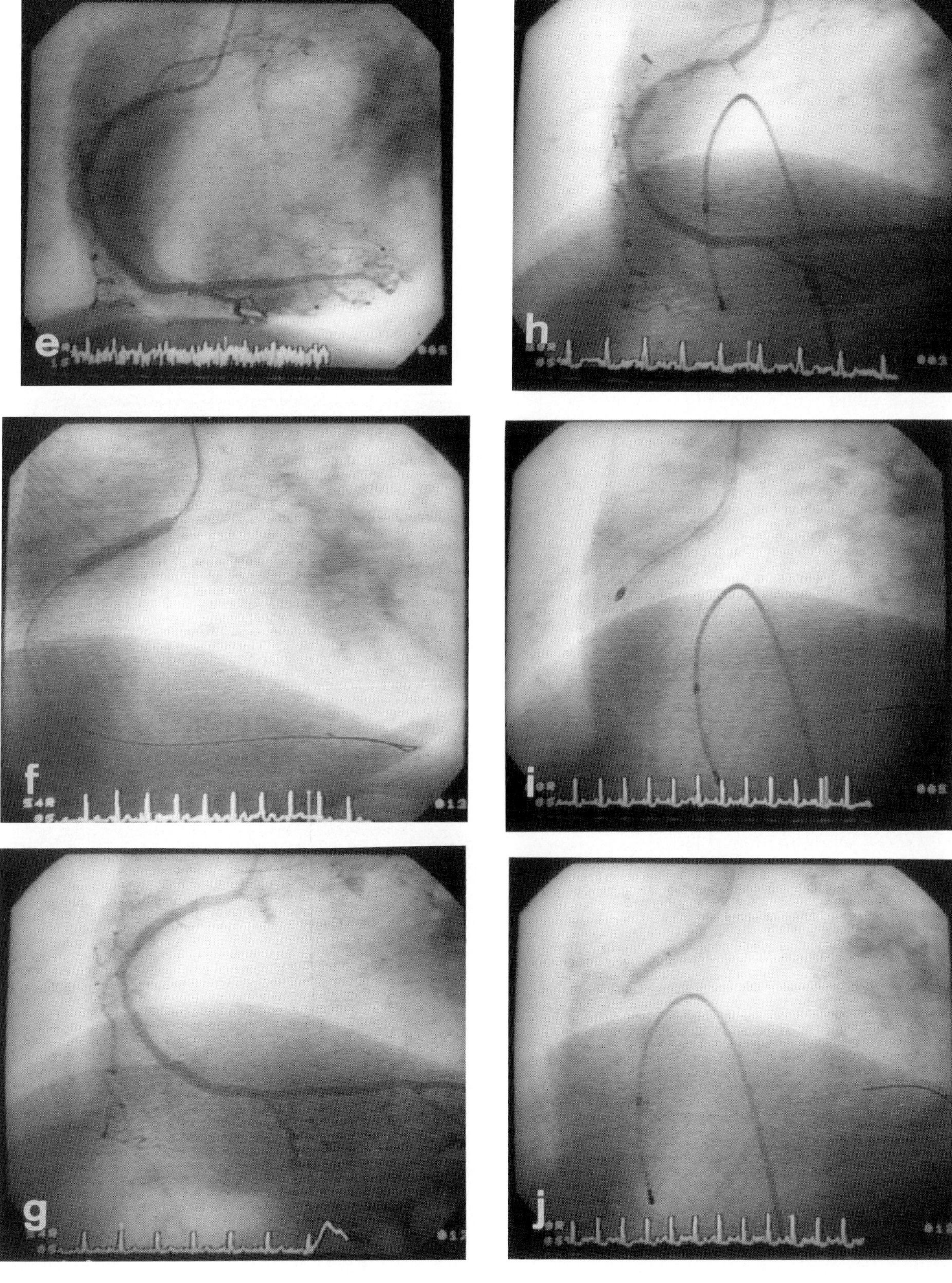
e
h
f
i
g
j

114o). The final result was good (Fig. 114p). The patient remained asymptomatic for 5 months when she had a relapse of symptoms. A tight restenosis of the stented ostial stenosis was seen (Fig. 114q, arrowhead) with a mild restenosis of the more distal stented lesion (Fig. 114q, arrow). It was assumed that some endothelial proliferation had occurred in both sites but that the ostial stent had been squeezed by the elastic aortic wall in addition. This was confirmed by the result following a 16-bar inflation with a 3.5-mm balloon in both lesions. The distal lesion showed a wide patency (Fig. 114r, arrow), while the ostial lesion immediately recoiled markedly (Fig. 114r, arrowhead). Therefore, a second half (disarticulated) Palmaz-Schatz stent was implanted within the first one to reduce the compressibility of the ostial segment. This yielded a perfect angiographic result (Fig. 114s). The patient was discharged the following day on aspirin alone. This case highlights the poor angioplasty results of ostial lesions. It also demonstrates that of the new devices, the stent fares best but may need a stronger design to withstand the compressing force of the highly elastic aortic wall.

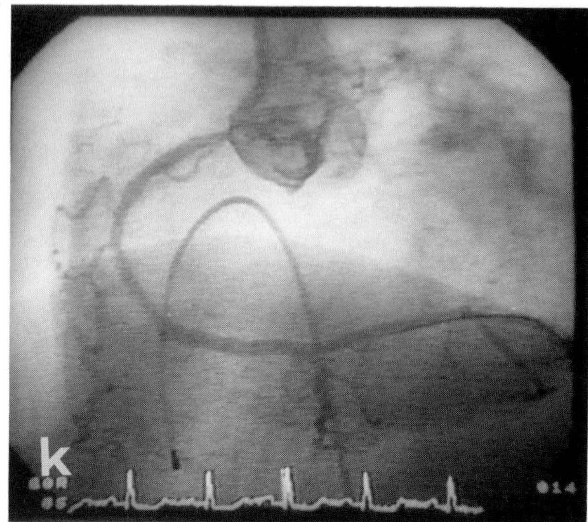

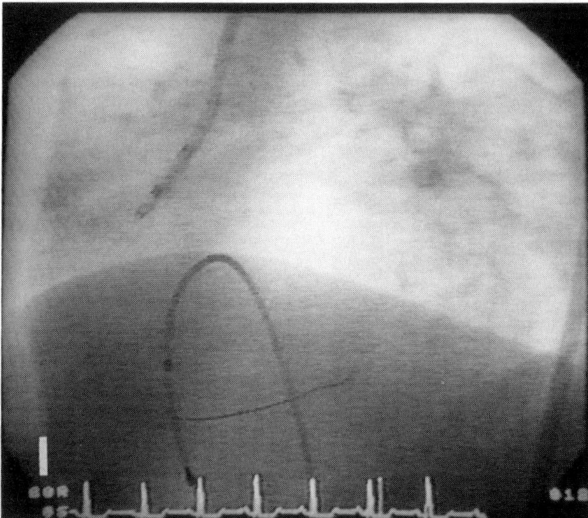

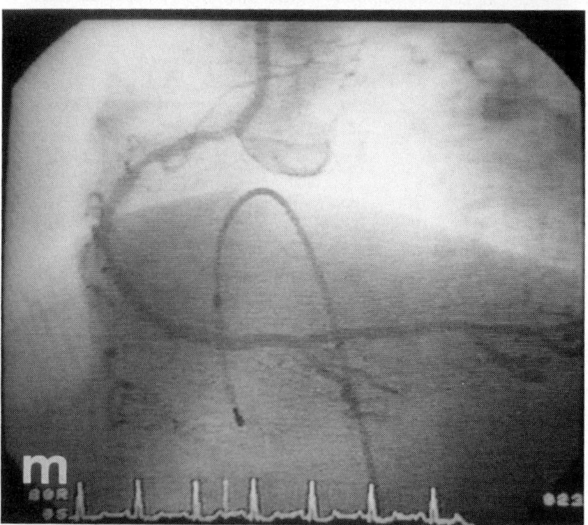

Figure 114 (Continued)

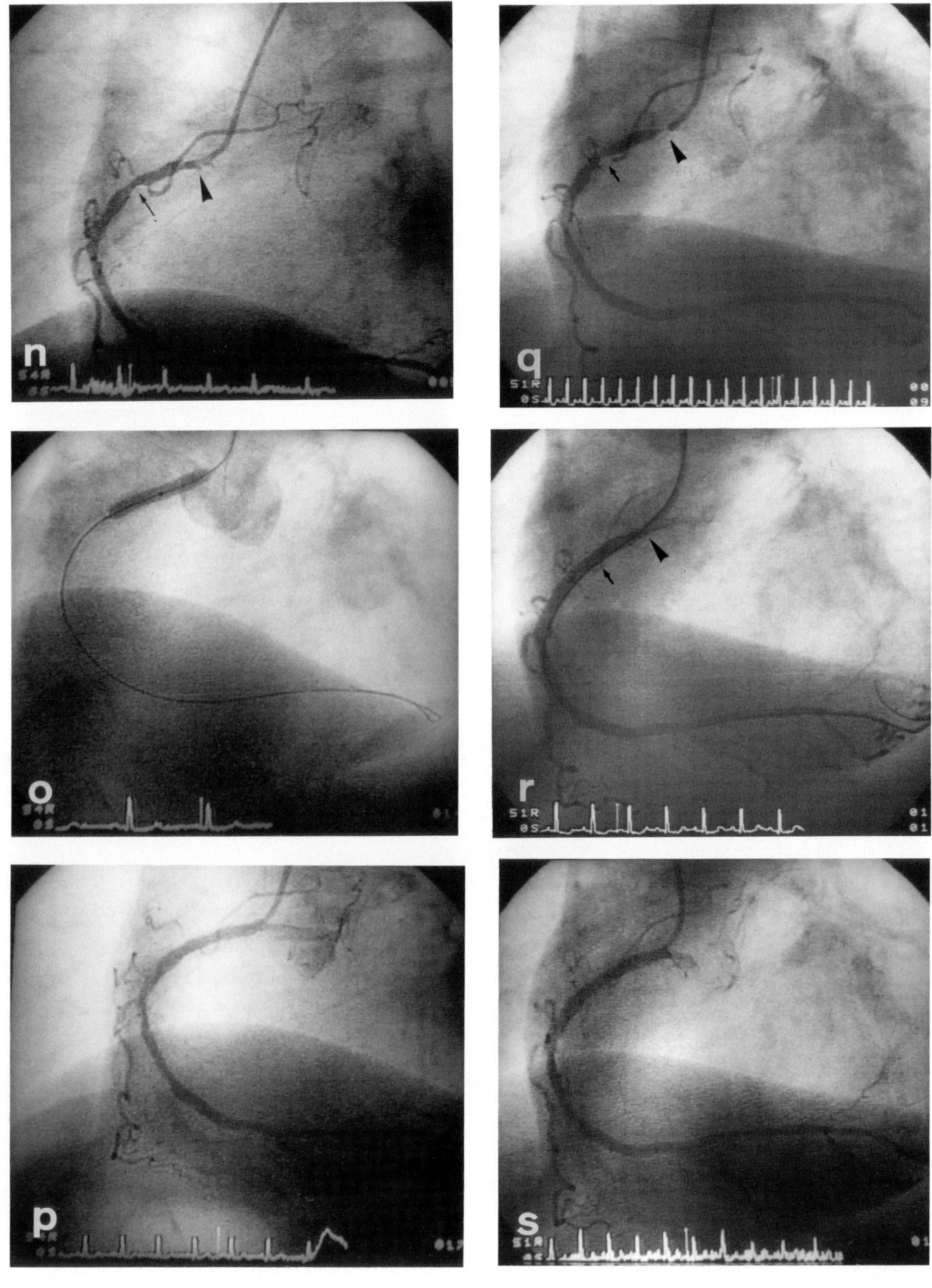
n
q
o
r
p
s

3.10 TORTUOUS VESSELS

Extremely tortuous vessels may make a lesion unreachable. A 61-year-old woman with a stenosis of a LIMA graft anastomosis with an occluded LAD presented with angina. However, the extreme curve of the LIMA, which was in addition fixed by a suture, rendered it impossible to reach the stenosis despite the use of several wires, including a Magnum wire (with a radiolucent ball tip) (Fig. 115, arrow). It is possible to reach and dilate lesions situated in seemingly impossible locations, such as in the patient with a stenosis of the distal anastomotic site of a right internal mammary artery graft to the LAD shown in Figure 116. The balloon marker is indicated by an arrow. In such situations, a balloon catheter or some other soft catheter [e.g., a Tracker catheter (Target Therapeutics)] can be advanced over the guidewire to support it for access through the vessel.

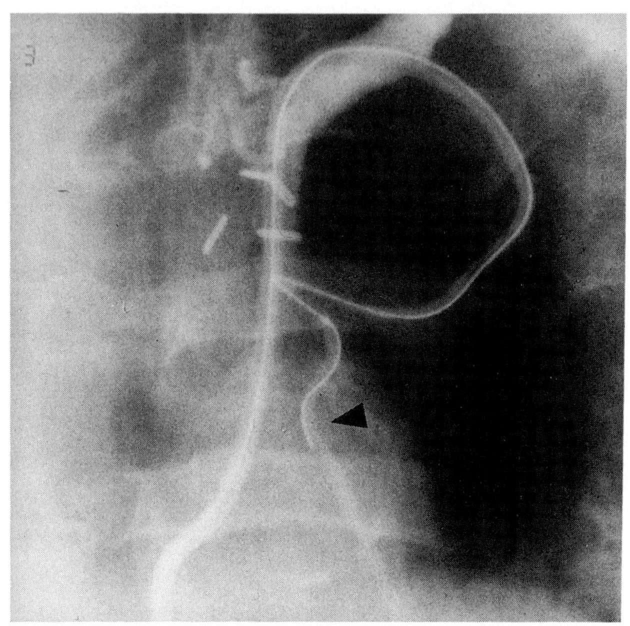

Figure 115

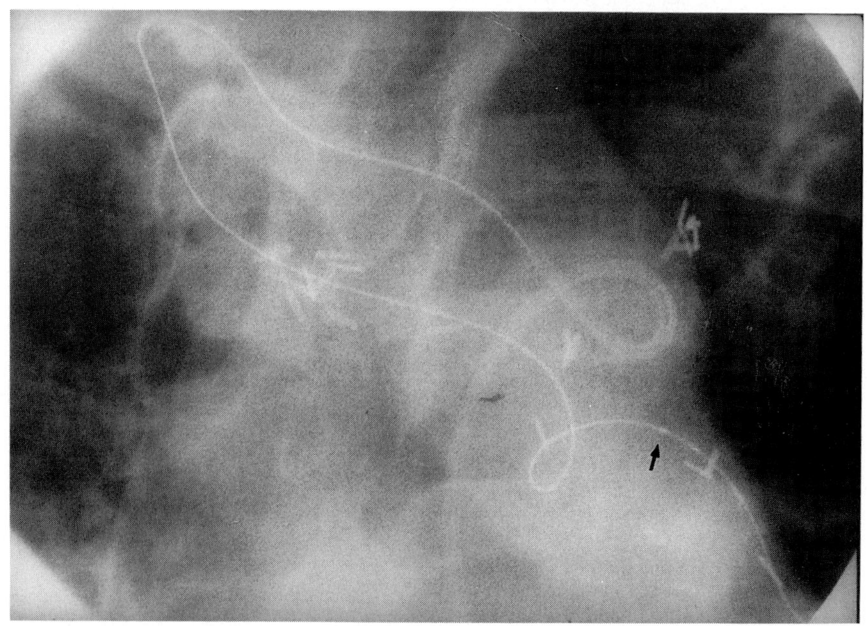

Figure 116

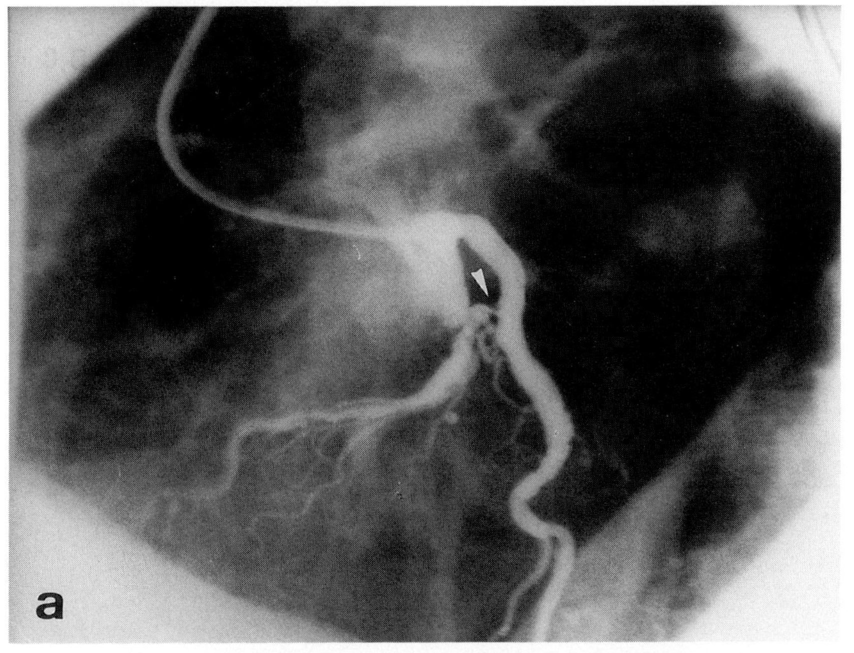

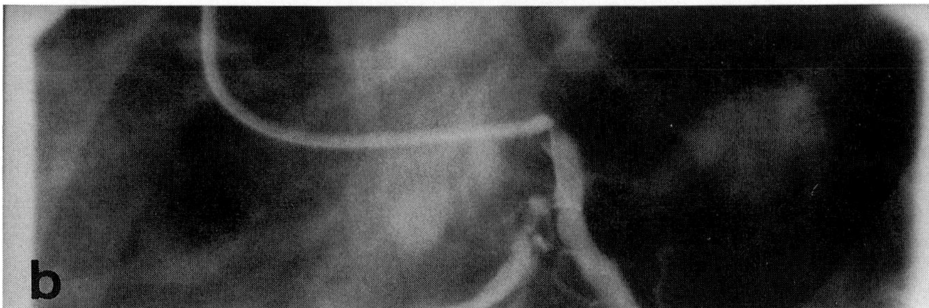

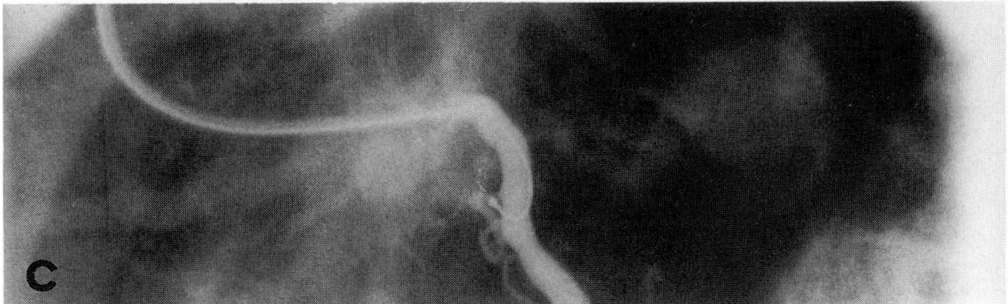

Figure 117

A Magnum wire with its enhanced stiffness can often help to negotiate difficult lesions. This is demonstrated by the case of a 70-year-old man with a tight stenosis of the origin of the LAD (Fig. 117a). The lesion, located in an acute angle, could not be crossed with a 0.012-in. wire (Fig. 117b). Success was obtained by a Magnum wire (Fig. 117c,d), which in contrast to the thinner wire did not buckle into the LCx and could be negotiated across the lesion. The final angioplasty result was satisfactory (Fig. 117e). However, at

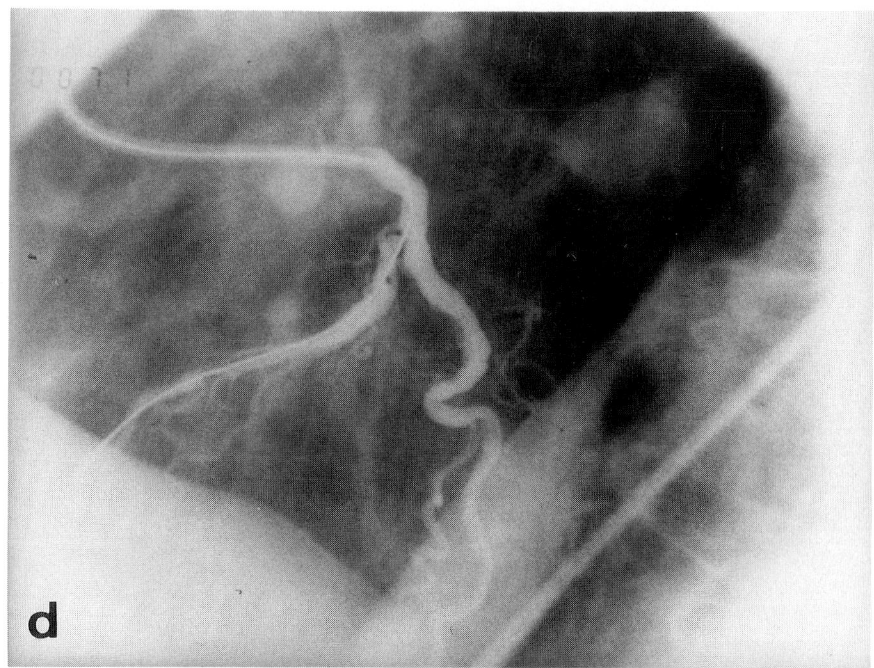

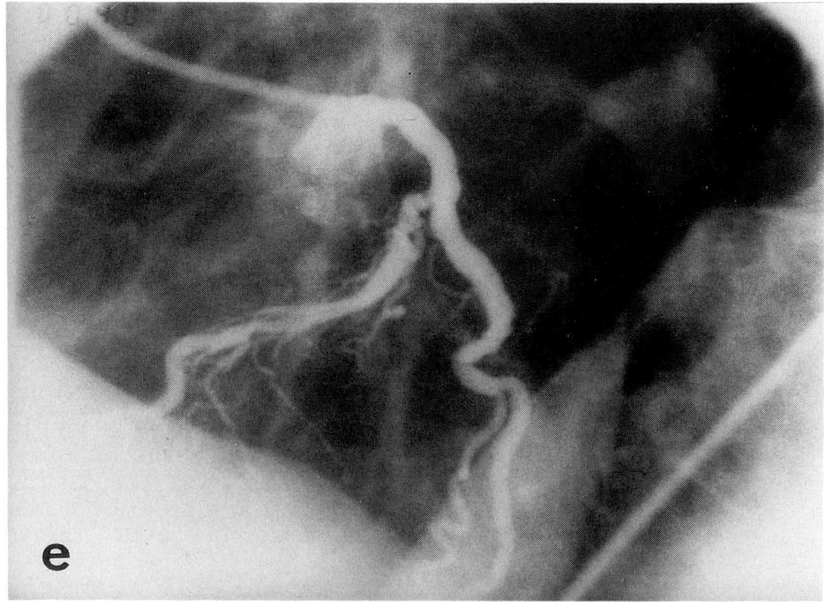

Figure 117 (Continued)

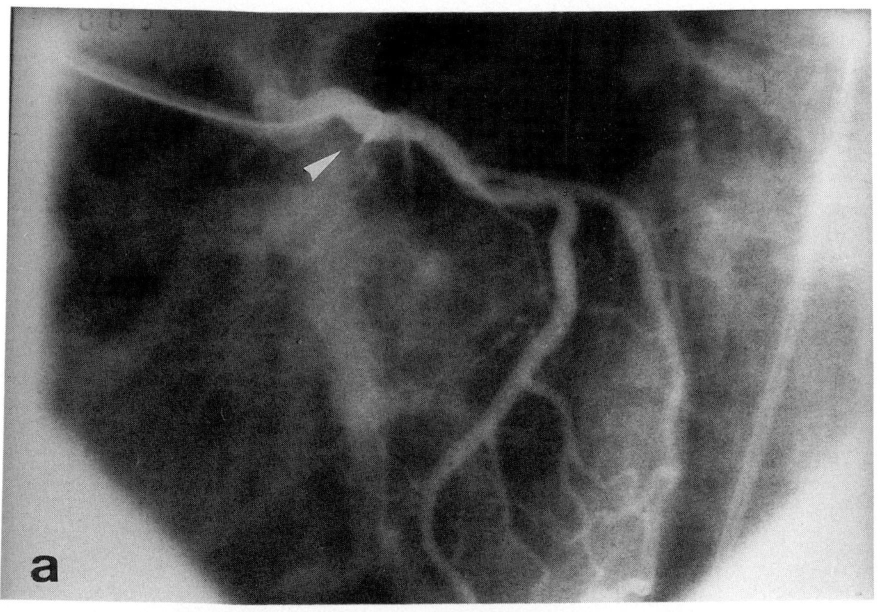

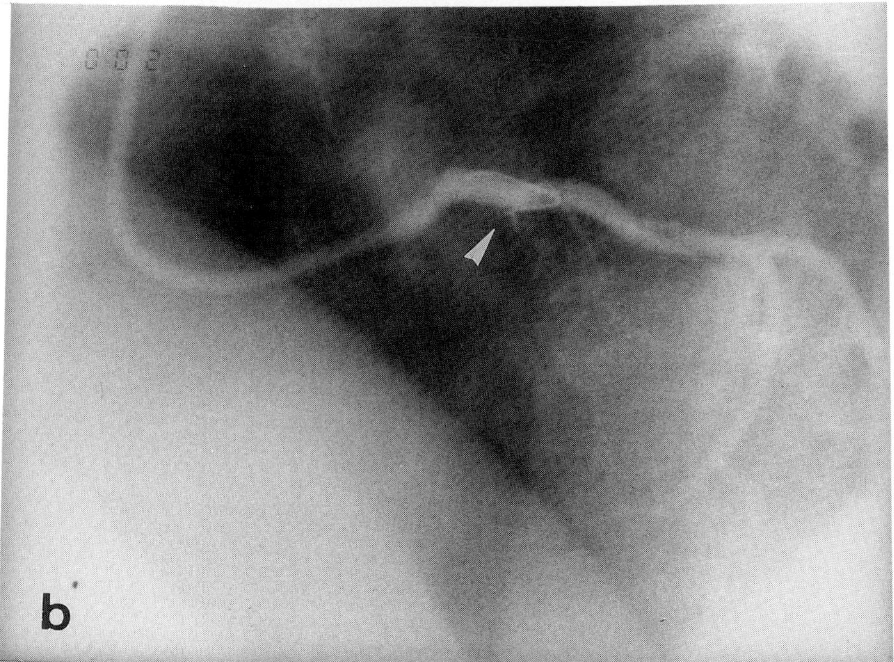

Figure 118

times it may be impossible even for a Magnum wire to enter a lesion situated at a sharp takeoff, as in this case with an occluded LAD. Attempts with a Magnum wire failed (Fig. 118a), the wire prolapsing into the LCx. An ACS standard wire was then tried with the same result (Fig. 118b). The case had to be abandoned. Lesions of this kind are occasionally met and represent some of the few remaining technical shortcomings of PTCA.

3.11 BIFURCATION LESIONS

Lesions at vessel bifurcations may be divided into three major subgroups for angioplasty purposes:

1. The plaque does not involve the ostium of the side branch. This may be thought of as a pseudo-bifurcation lesion. Although the balloon will obstruct this branch during inflation, it is unlikely to damage it. Such a lesion does not need special protection during angioplasty.

2. The plaque involves the ostium of the side branch but does not extend into it. Dilatation of such a bifurcation lesion may lead to the plaque being displaced into the side branch during angioplasty. This has been called the "ping-pong effect." The "ping" part of the ping-pong effect is demonstrated by an example where a plaque in the LAD (Fig. 119a) is pushed into the diagonal branch following PTCA of the LAD (Fig. 119b). If the diagonal lesion had now been dilated, the plaque may be shifted back into the LAD (the "pong" part). This could go on and on. The displaced plaque can on occasions significantly impair blood flow into the side branch. In such a situa-

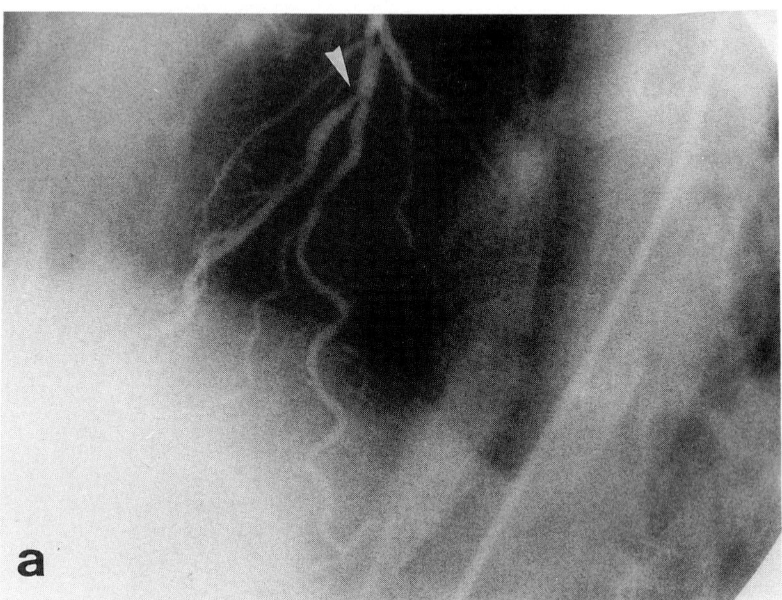

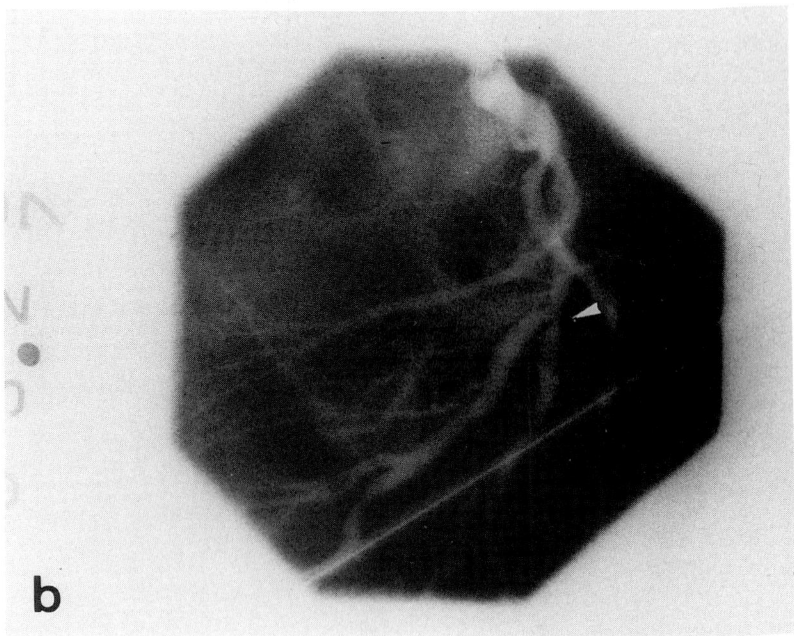

Figure 119

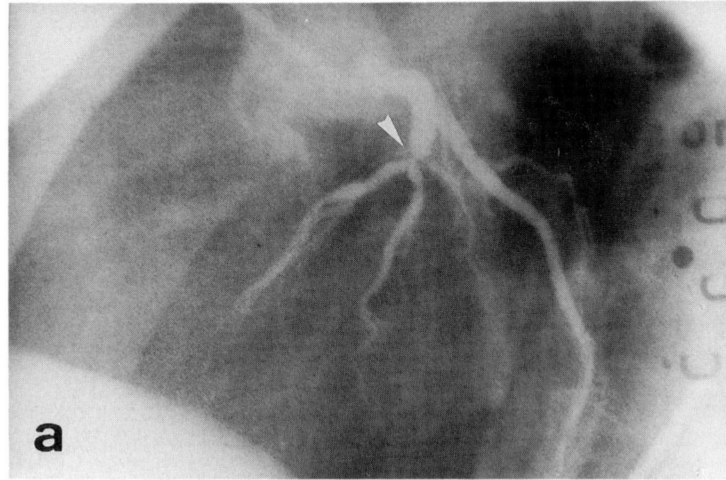

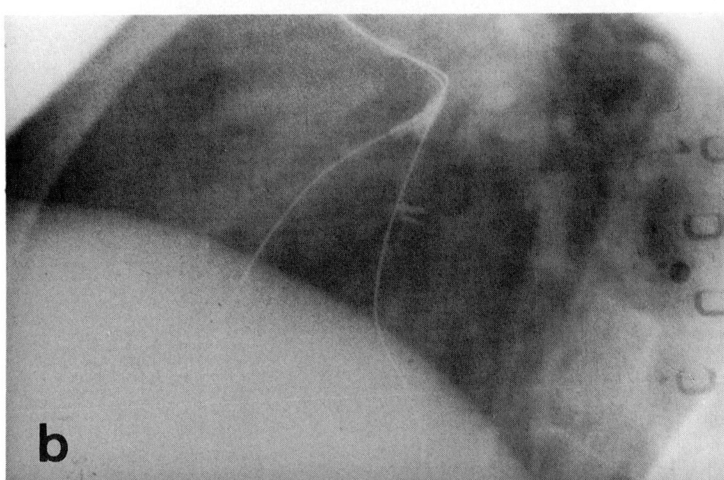

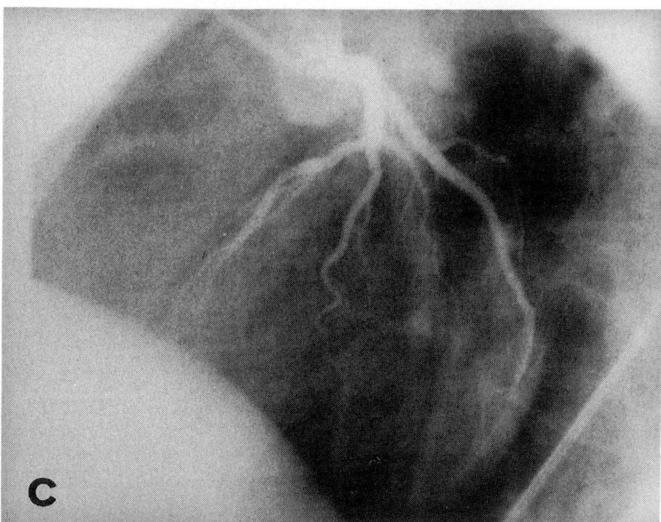

Figure 120

tion, a double (kissing) wire is recommended, especially if the branch is large. This facilitates rapid dilatation of the branch in the event of closure. However, a small or medium-sized side branch of this type need not be protected. Angioplasty of the main lesion results in splitting of the plaque, and this may even improve flow into the side branch. If such a branch gets occluded following the inflation, it can frequently be accessed using the same wire. Such an approach is more economical and time efficient than using a kissing wire for all such lesions.

3. The plaque extends into both branches. This can be considered as a true bifurcation stenosis. Such a lesion is best approached by a double (kissing) wire or a double (kissing) balloon technique. The kissing balloon technique prevents the ping-pong effect and achieves adequate dilatation of both branches simultaneously. This is shown in an example with a bifurcation stenosis of the LAD and the first diagonal branch, which are of comparable size (Fig. 120a). A kissing balloon technique using two 2.5-mm Monorail balloons inserted through a single 8F guiding catheter was used (Fig. 120b). The result was good (Fig. 120c).

A kissing wire technique suffices in most cases, since it is rare that an adequate result cannot be achieved by serial dilatations of the two branches. The smaller branch should be dilated before the major vessel. This ensures that the plaque displacement (if any) at the end of the procedure is into the less important branch. A 52-year-old male presented with a bifurcation stenosis of the LAD and its first diagonal branch (Fig. 121a). A kissing wire was employed, with dilatation of the diagonal branch being performed first (Fig. 121b). A subsequent angiogram showed the plaque to be shifted into the LAD, as expected (Fig. 121c). The LAD lesion was dilated next (Fig. 121d). A test angiogram with the wire in place revealed an adequate result (Fig. 121e), which was confirmed after wire removal (Fig. 121f). Note that the result is better in the LAD, which corroborates the initial strategy.

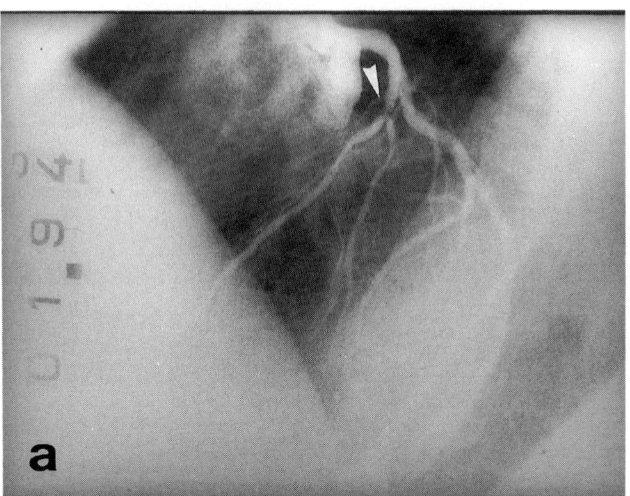

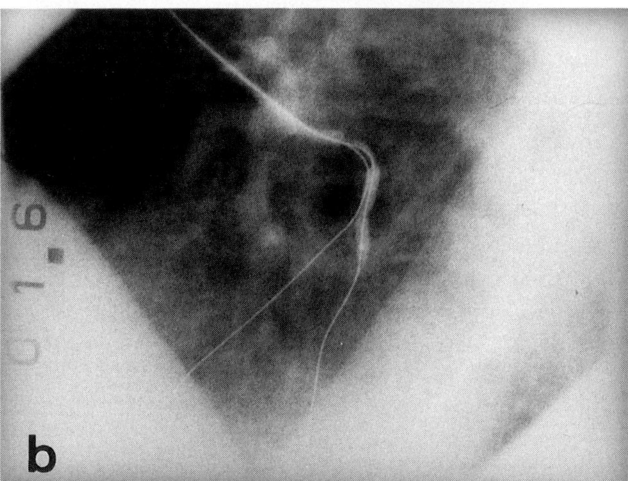

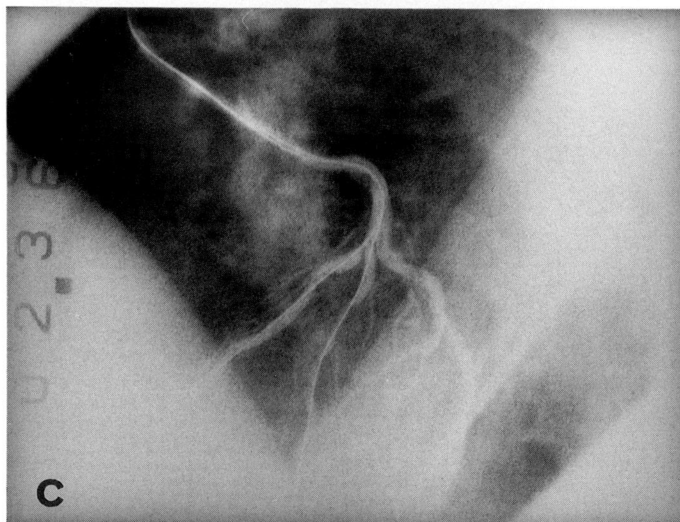

Figure 121

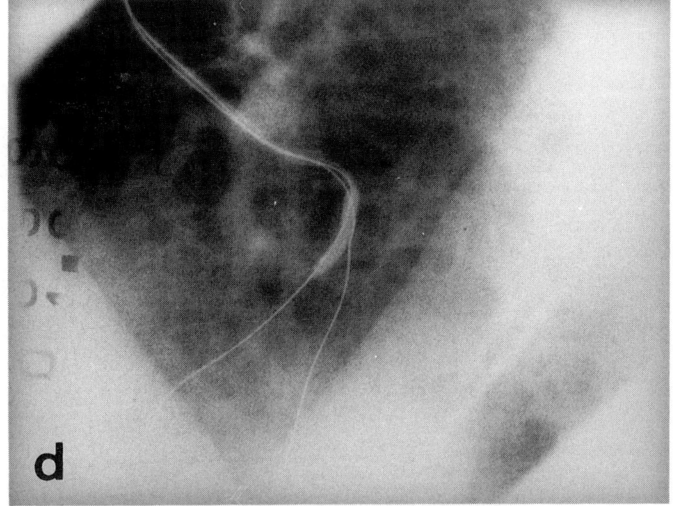
d

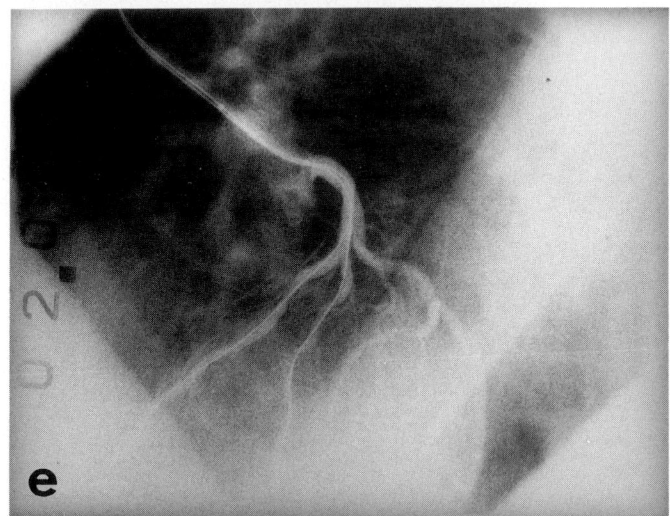
e

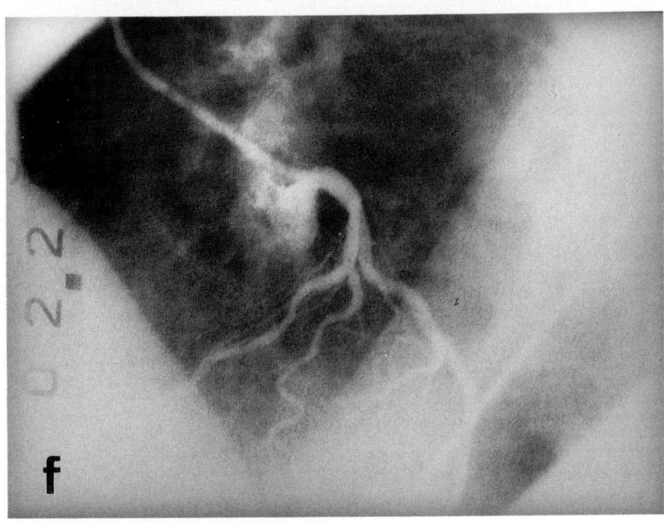
f

A precaution to be taken with the kissing wire technique is to prevent the two wires from getting twisted. A 45-year-old man had significant stenoses of the LAD and the second diagonal branch (Fig. 122a). The lesions were crossed with two kissing wires (Fig. 122b) and the diagonal branch dilated first according to the established rule. However, after withdrawing the balloon the two wires were seen to be twisted (Fig. 122c). This prevented balloon advancement into the LAD. The problem was overcome simply by withdrawing the wire of the diagonal branch. The final result was acceptable, again showing a better result in the vessel dilated second because of the ping-pong effect (Fig. 122d). Although the problem of twisted wires is petty, it is unavoidable in cases that require extensive torquing with the second wire. Thus it is recommended to wire the more difficult vessel first.

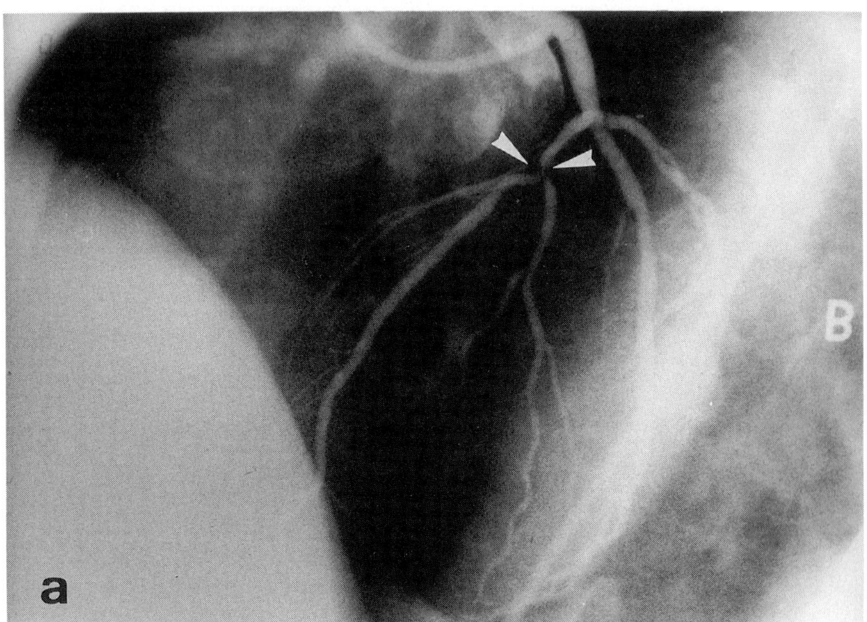

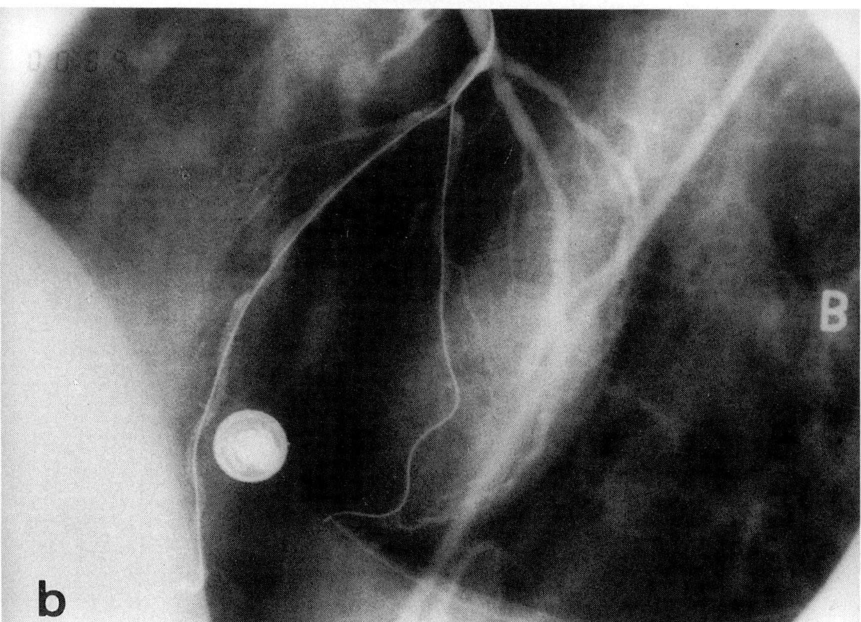

Figure 122

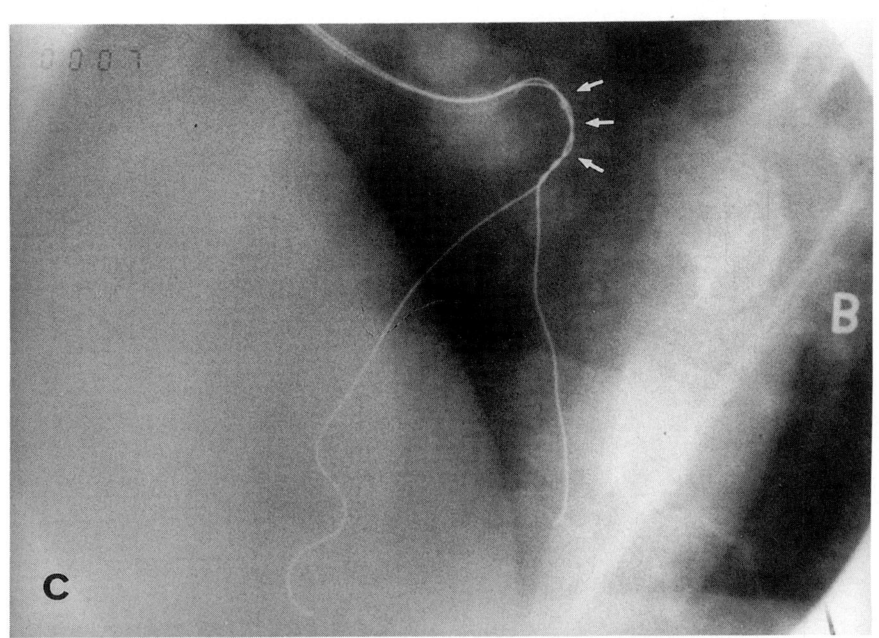
c
B

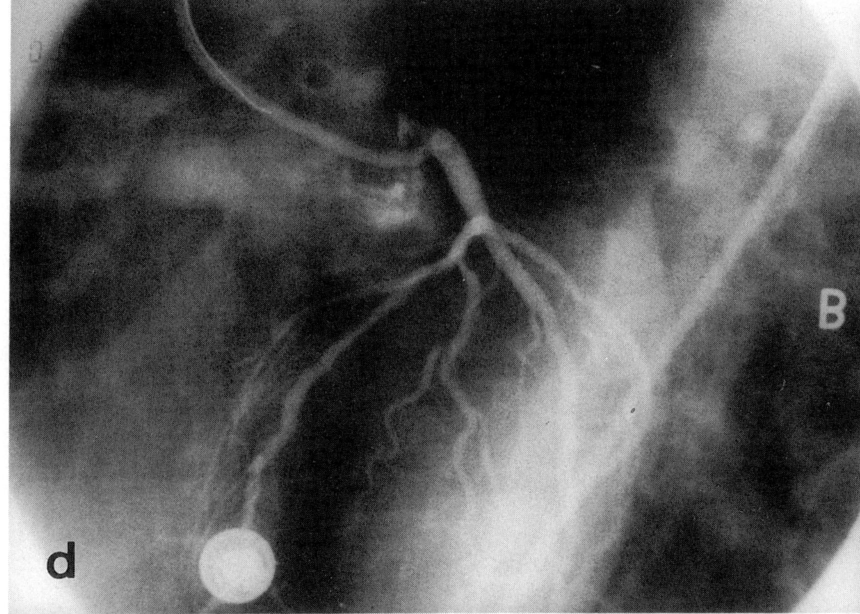
d
B

4
Ancillary Techniques

4.1
INTRACORONARY PRESSURE MEASUREMENTS

A diameter stenosis of less than 50% typically creates no significant pressure gradient. Increasing stenoses generate growing gradients which are also dependent on coronary flow. The gradient across a coronary stenosis can be measured with over-the-wire balloons by subtracting the mean pressure at the tip of the balloon placed beyond the lesion from the mean pressure measured through the guiding catheter in the coronary ostium. Alternatively, pressures distal to the lesion may be assessed using coronary wires with a fluid channel or a tip manometer. Stenoses with a resting gradient of less than 20 mmHg are insignificant and may not warrant angioplasty. In a typical example of intracoronary pressure measurements (Fig. 123) the surface ECG (leads I, II, III) and the intracoronary ECG (ic) are shown along with the pressure recordings from the guiding catheter and the tip of the balloon catheter. The first column depicts the lack of gradient while the balloon is proximal to the stenosis. The next col-

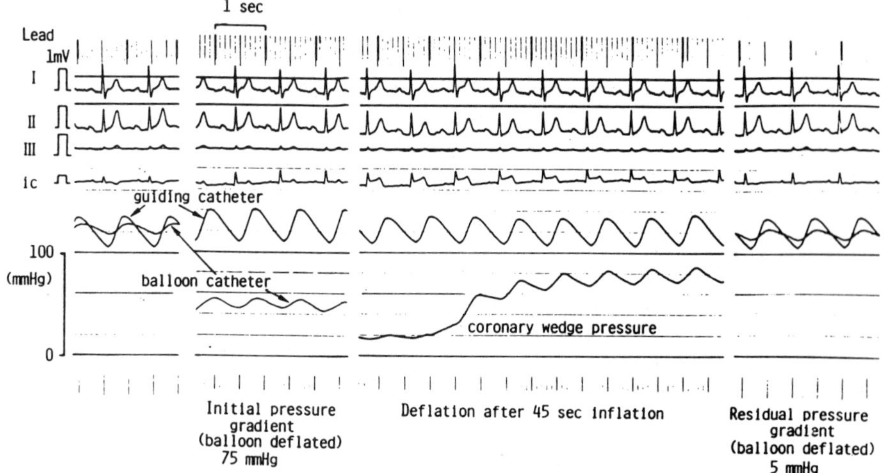

Figure 123

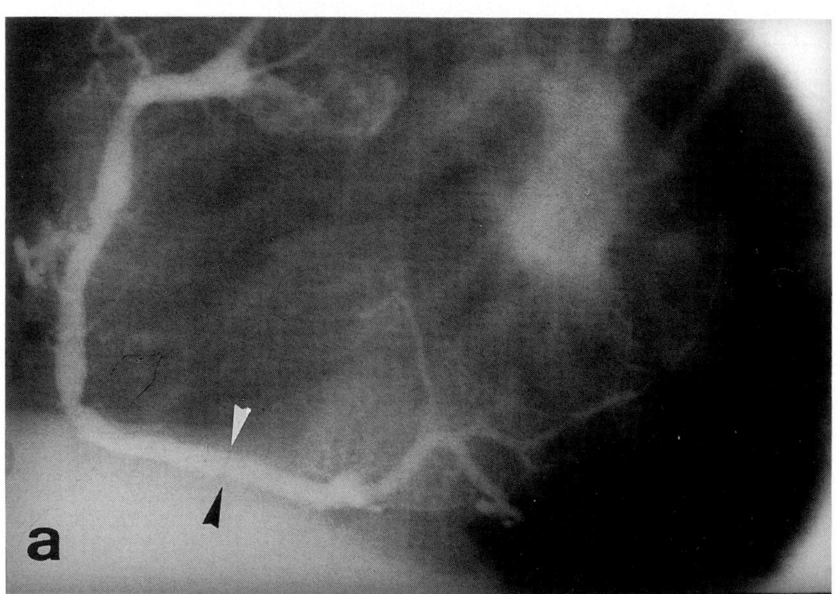

Figure 124

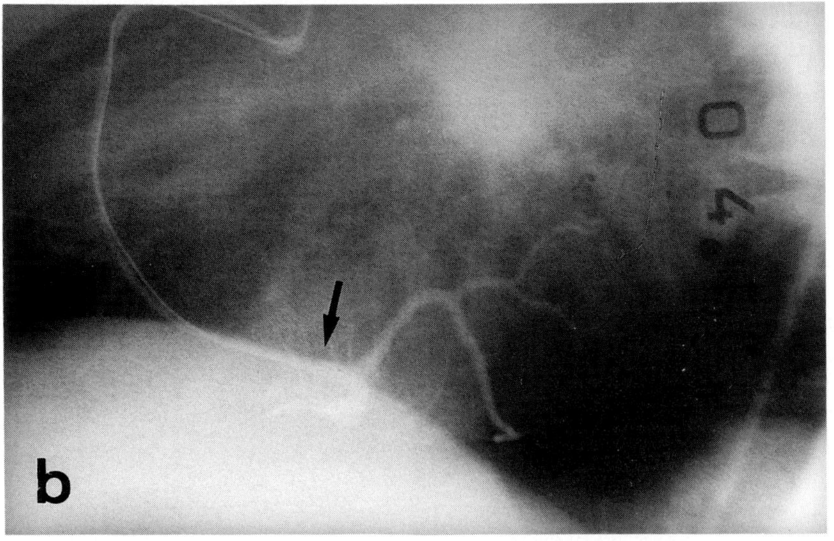

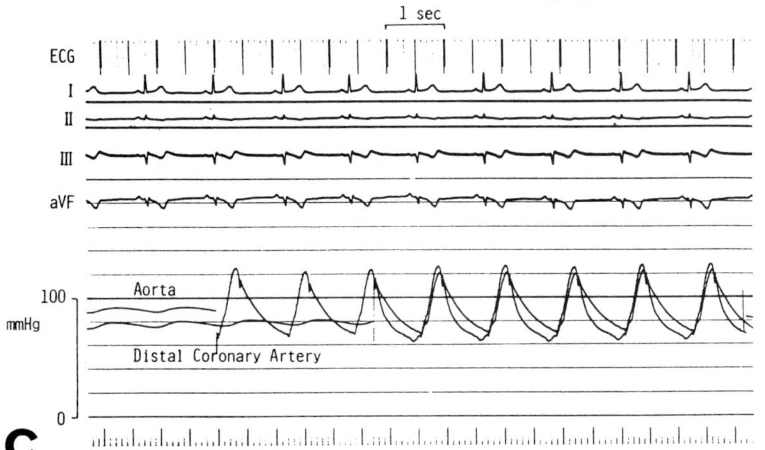

Figure 124 (Continued)

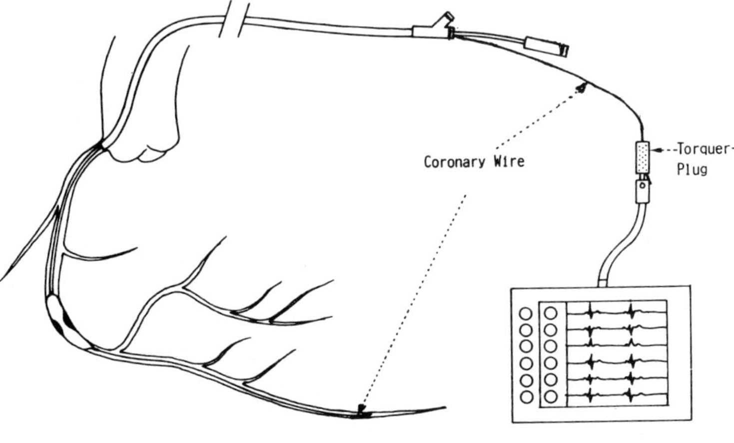

Figure 125

umn shows a mean gradient of 75 mmHg across the stenosis. In the third column, the tracing denotes the events occurring during balloon deflation. Note that the intracoronary ECG rapidly normalizes as the peripheral coronary pressure rises reflecting the resumption of flow. Also note that although the intracoronary ECG showed dramatic changes, the surface ECG had hardly changed. The intracoronary pressure at the beginning of the curve is below 20 mmHg, reflecting a low coronary wedge pressure and testifying to the absence of collaterals. This pressure rapidly rises after balloon deflation. The final result (column 4) shows a minimal residual pressure gradient across the stenosis, indicating a good functional result of the dilatation.

The measurement of gradients can also be used to assess the functional significance of the stenosis in order to determine the indication for angioplasty. A 53-year-old man presented with angina. A RCA angiogram revealed a membrane-like lesion of the distal RCA (Fig. 124a). The functional significance of this lesion could not be estimated by angiography, hence pressure gradients were measured. A 4F Monorail perfusion catheter was ad

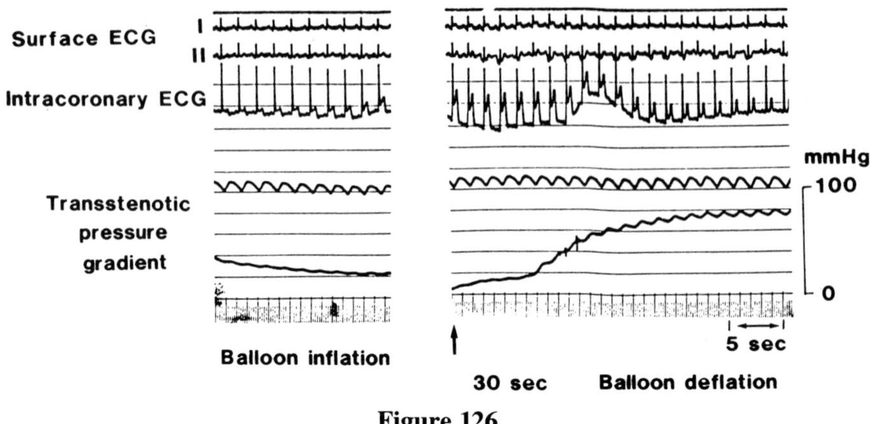

Figure 126

vanced over a coronary guide wire distal to the stenosis (Fig. 124b) (tip position distal to the lesion demonstrated by dye injection). Simultaneous pressure recordings from the aorta and the distal RCA failed to reveal a significant pressure gradient (Fig. 124c), indicating a non-significant stenosis. Angioplasty was not performed.

Intracoronary pressure measurements constituted an important part of the angioplasty procedures in the past. They have contributed significantly to the understanding of the pathophysiology of coronary stenoses. However, with improved imaging techniques, and the increasing use of Monorail catheters which do not allow the measuring of pressure gradients, this functional assessment has been abandoned.

4.2 INTRACORONARY ECG

The intracoronary ECG is a helpful feature during angioplasty. It can be obtained by connecting the guidewire to the chest lead terminal of the ECG. The setup involved in obtaining the intracoronary ECG is shown in Fig. 125. It is important to ensure good contact between the wire and the ECG plug, which can be ensured by pinching the wire between the plug and the hollow torquer (see also Fig. 8).

The intracoronary ECG is overall more sensitive than the surface ECG in detecting ischemia. It reveals ischemic changes in the myocardium supplied by the target vessel oftener, sooner, and more conspicuously than the surface ECG since it yields larger signals and always reflects the territory of interest by definition. The advantage of the intracoronary ECG over a surface ECG is more pronounced when dealing with vessels subtending the lateral wall, which is poorly represented by standard leads (e.g., PTCA of obtuse marginal or diagonal branches). The intracoronary ECG rapidly normalizes following balloon deflation. The presence of intracoronary ECG changes after balloon deflation should lead to the suspicion of an insufficient angioplasty result, or impending acute occlusion. Figure 126 shows leads I and II of the surface ECG and the intracoronary ECG during PTCA of an LAD. Note the prompt and prominent changes in the intracoronary ECG which rapidly normalize after balloon deflation, while the surface ECG hardly changes. The intracoronary ECG recording is thus a highly sensitive index of ischemia that can be obtained with minimal effort and at no additional cost.

4.3 CORONARY AND LEFT VENTRICULAR PACING

The setup utilized for recording of the intracoronary ECG can be used for pacing. It is important to place the guidewire tip as distally as possible, preferably in an intramyocardial branch and in a noninfarcted area of myocardium. The guidewire is connected to the negative terminal of the temporary pacemaker, the positive terminal being a large plate electrode attached, for instance, to the leg of the patient. Pacing should be begun at maximal

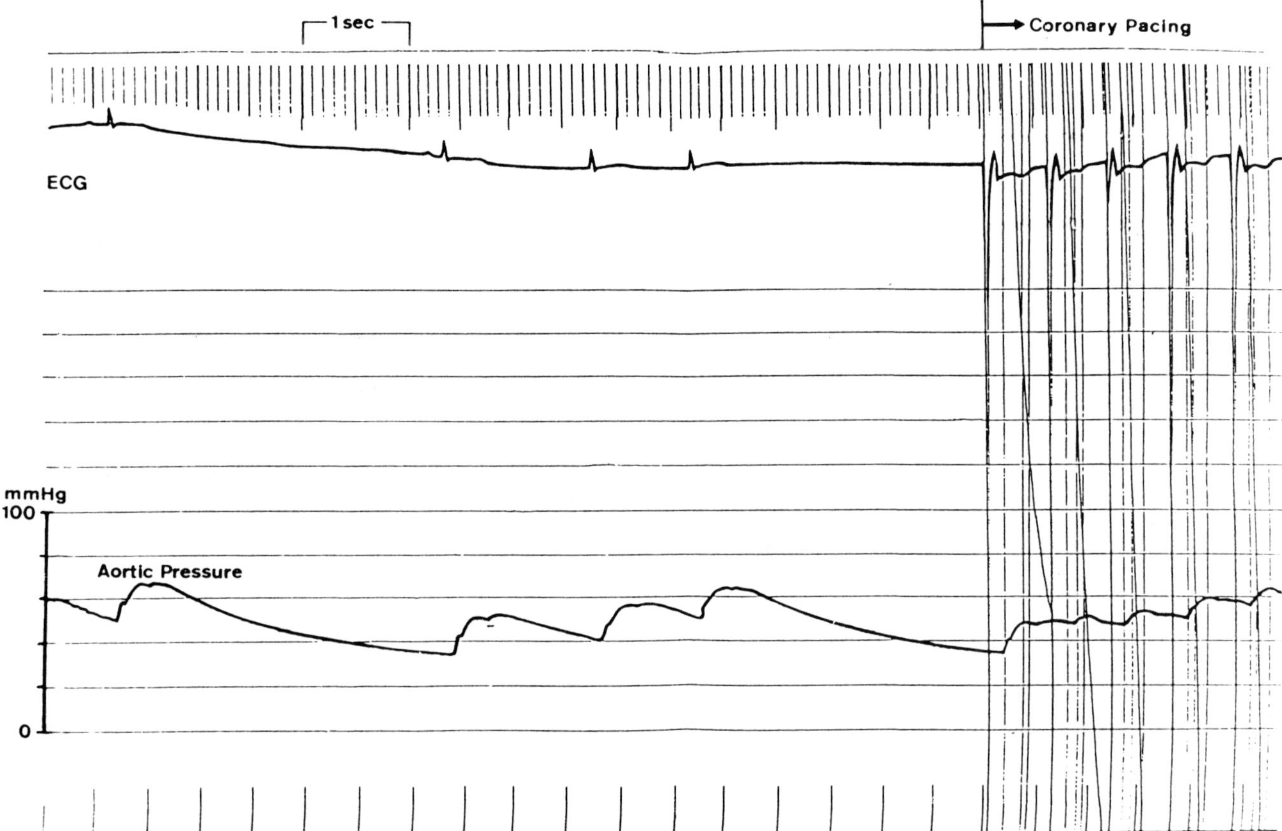

Figure 127

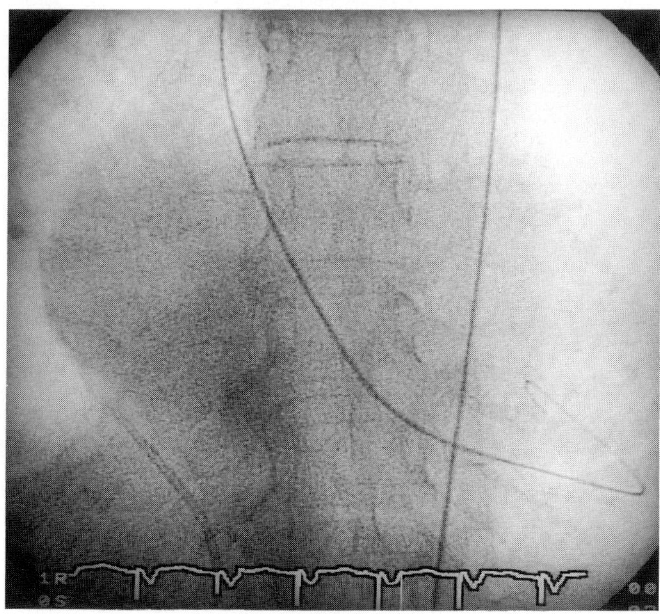

Figure 128

output, although a threshold of below 5 mA is frequent. Coronary spasm sometimes occurs after prolonged coronary pacing, but it can be reversed promptly by intracoronary nitrates or calcium antagonists. This technique rapidly allows pacing during angioplasty in the event of bradycardia without the need for a venous pacing wire. Figure 127 shows an example of coronary pacing. The patient had developed sinus node dysfunction during PTCA. Coronary pacing was required for a few minutes until the sinus node recovered.

Similarly, during diagnostic studies or during PTCA phases without a wire in the coronary artery, the 0.035-in.

wire used for catheter insertion can be advanced deeply into the left ventricle, positioned as depicted, and pacing performed with the method described above. If prolonged pacing becomes necessary, a right ventricular pacemaker lead can be inserted under the protection of coronary or left ventricular pacing.

4.4 CORONARY ANGIOPLASTY THROUGH SMALL CATHETERS

Coronary angioplasty through small catheters is of interest if performed immediately following a 4F or 5F diagnostic study. The same diagnostic catheter is used as a "guiding" catheter. Use of a smaller catheter is associated with several advantages, including a small arterial access, with reduced risk for bleeding, arteriovenous fistulae, and pseudoaneurysms. Moreover, a smaller catheter has less tendency to wedge in the coronary artery and can be deeply intubated for increased backup support if required. Advancement beyond the lesion permits the assessment of translesional pressure gradi-

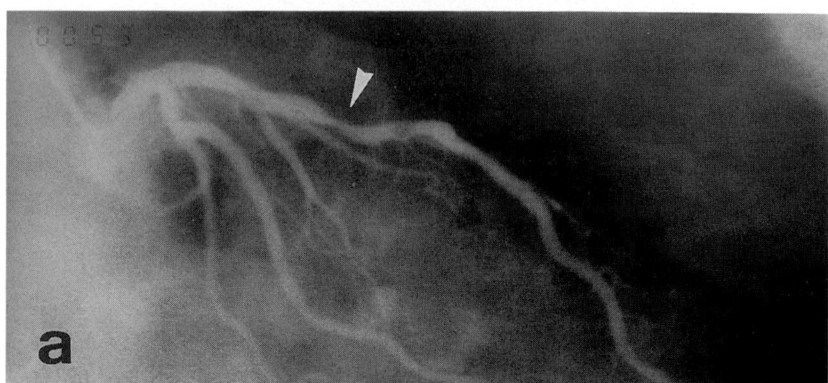

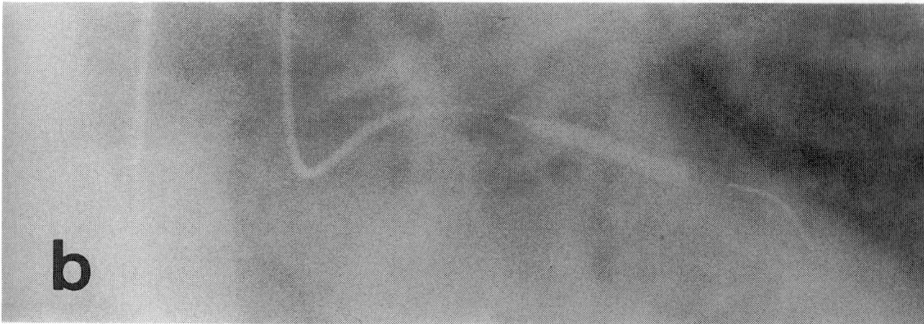

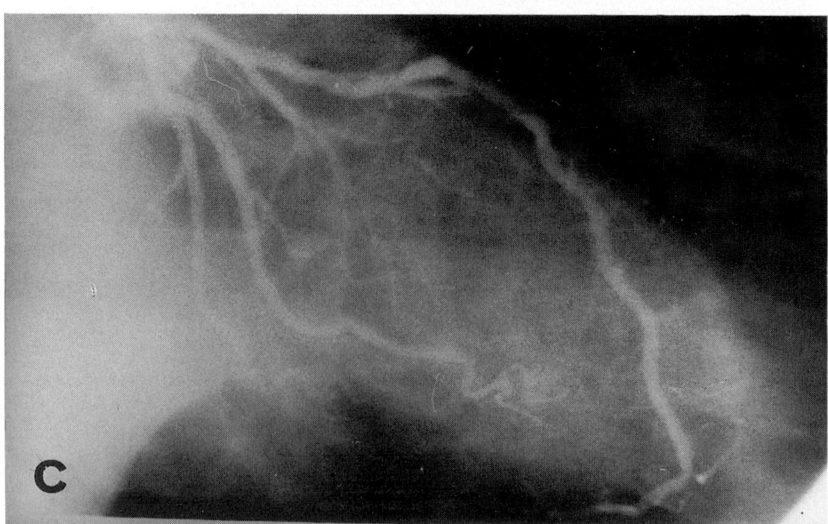

Figure 129

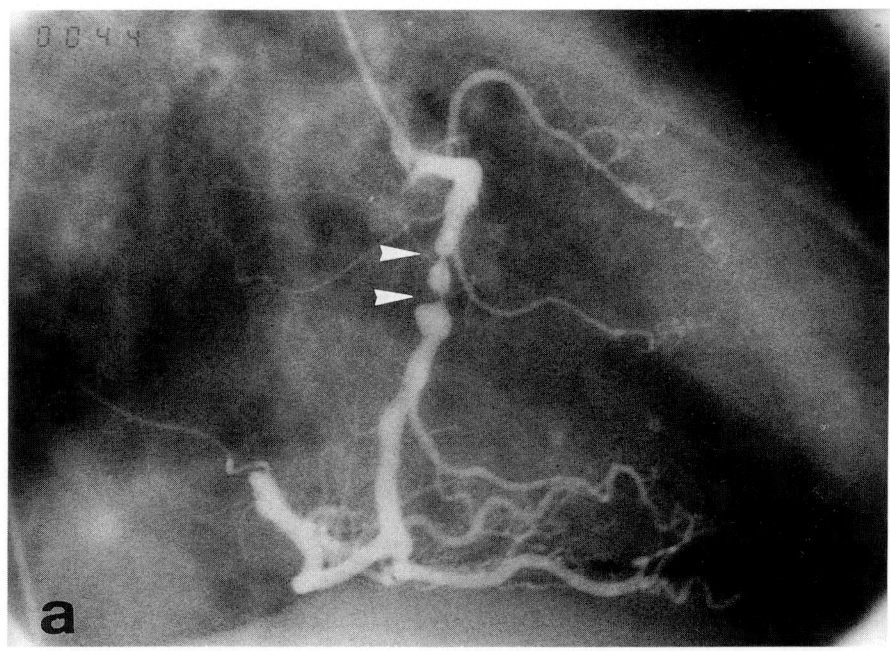

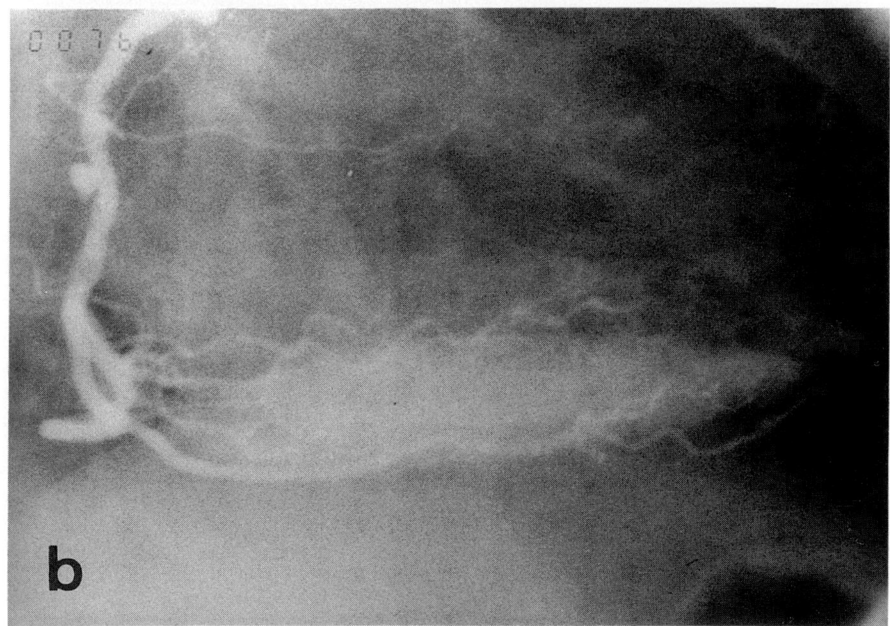

Figure 130

ents. However, only fixed-wire balloons can be used through 4F or 5F catheter [e.g., Lightning (Cordis), Ace (Scimed) etc.]. This entails all the disadvantages of fixed-wire systems, including the need to renegotiate the lesion in case of an insufficient result. An additional drawback of the 4F or 5F system is the poor coronary opacification while the balloon resides within the catheter. This can be largely overcome by forceful injections using a 2-ml glass syringe.

A 56-year-old man presented with unstable angina. Angiography with 4F catheters revealed a presumably partially thrombotic lesion of the mid LAD (Fig. 129a). Angioplasty was performed immediately following the diagnostic study with a 3.0-mm Ace (Scimed) balloon (Fig. 129b). Note the deeply intubated 4F "guiding" catheter for increased backup support. The result was good (Fig. 129c), although a slight local haziness remained due to the thrombotic nature of the lesion. One million units of urokinase were administered intravenously following the procedure, which might be beneficial in such cases.

The 4F "guiding" catheter can also be used for measuring translesional gradients. A 68-year-old woman with a tandem RCA stenosis (Fig. 130a) underwent successful angioplasty with a 4F system (Fig. 130b). To measure the postprocedure translesional gradient, the "guiding" catheter was advanced over the balloon distal to the lesion (Fig. 130c), and a pull-back pressure gradient obtained by withdrawing the catheter proximal to the stenosis (Fig. 130d). Figure 130e shows the pressure recording with a residual gradient of 10 mmHg across the lesion. Also note the difference in the intracoronary (IC) ECG recording (increase in p waves and decreased QRS amplitude in the proximal tracing), related to the shift in the position of the wire tip of the balloon, bringing it closer to the atrioventricular groove.

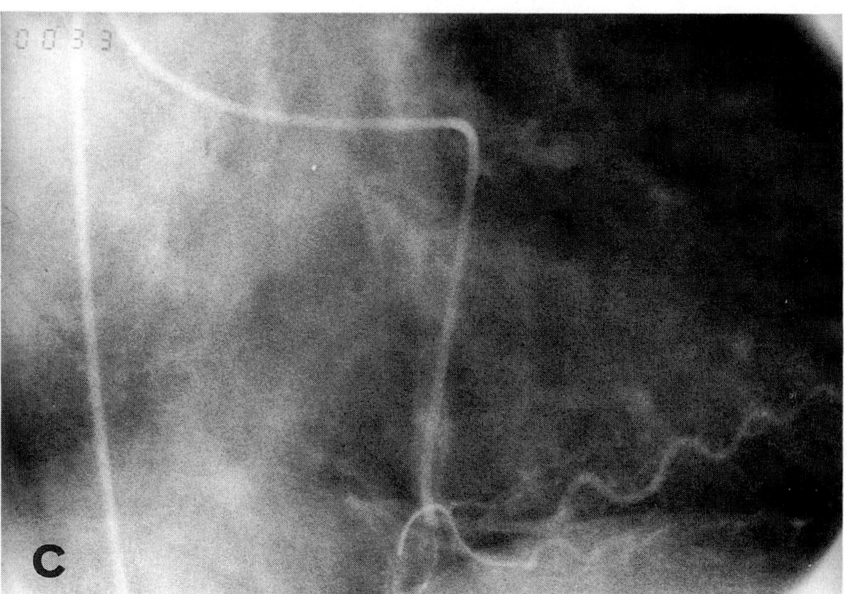

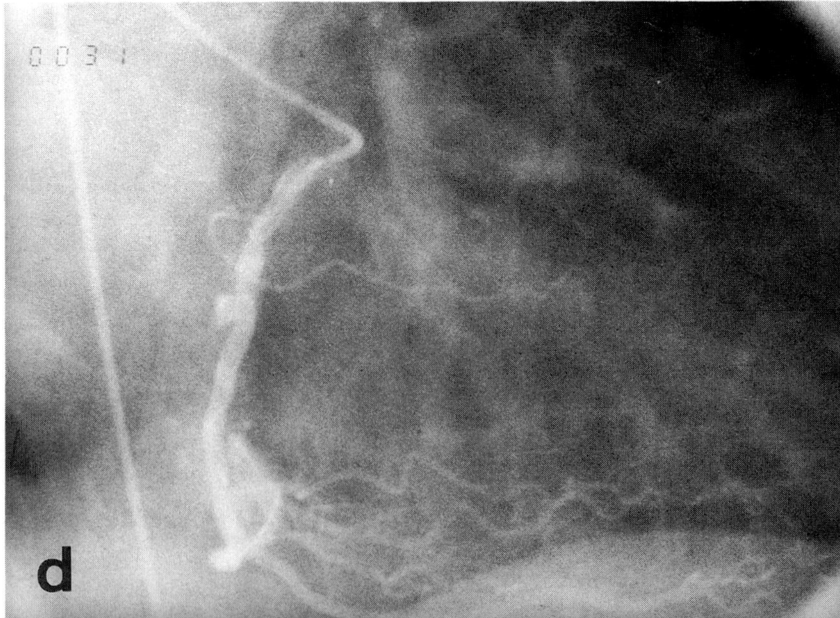

Figure 130 (Continued)

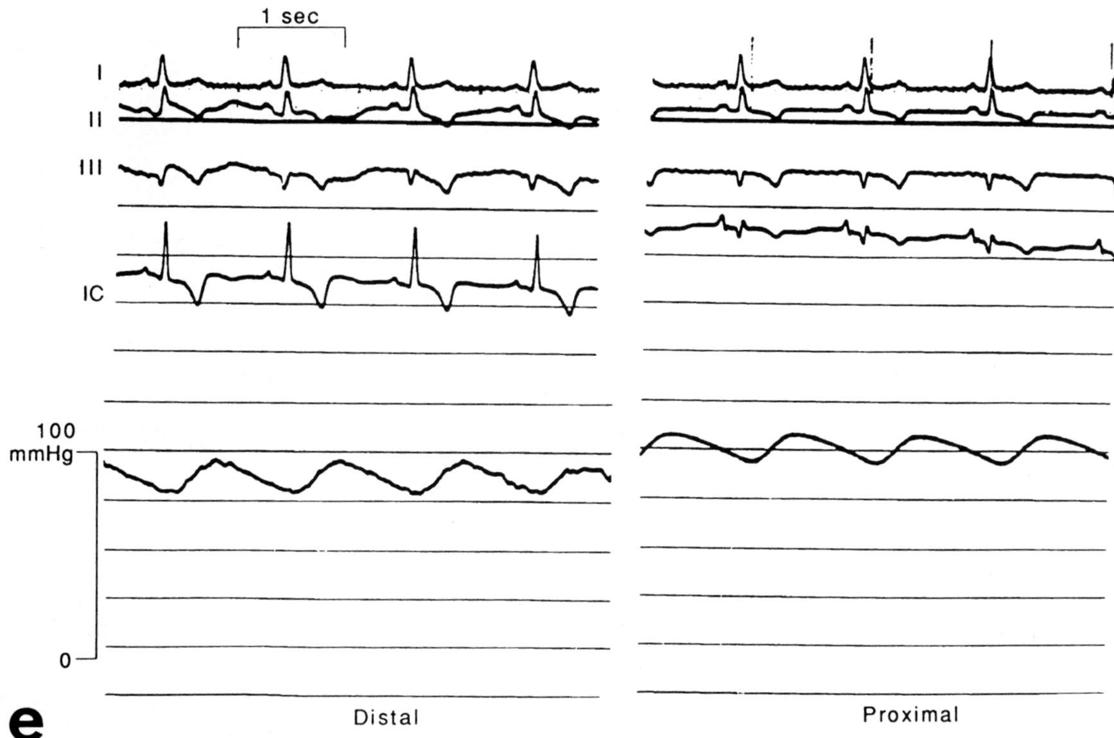
1 sec
I
II
III
IC
100
mmHg
0
e
Distal
Proximal

5
Complications

5.1 DISSECTION

Dissections can occur from the guiding catheter, guidewire, or balloon. A guidewire may be advanced subintimally under a plaque. This event can be recognized by the resistance encountered in advancing the wire, by a buckling of the wire, and occasionally by a dye staining and an occlusion of the coronary artery. The problem can usually be overcome by withdrawing the wire and searching for the true lumen. However, in some cases it may be necessary to change the wire and use a softer wire or a Magnum wire. A wire dissection occurred in a 44-year-old man with an LCx stenosis (Fig. 131a) while attempting to cross the lesion through the 4F diagnostic catheter with a 3.0-mm Ace balloon (Scimed), resulting in occlusion of the artery (Fig. 131b). The system was changed and a 7F guiding catheter and a Magnum wire were utilized to cross the occlusion (Fig. 131c). The Magnum wire with its ball tip often finds the true lumen in such cases. Angioplasty was subsequently performed with a 3.0-

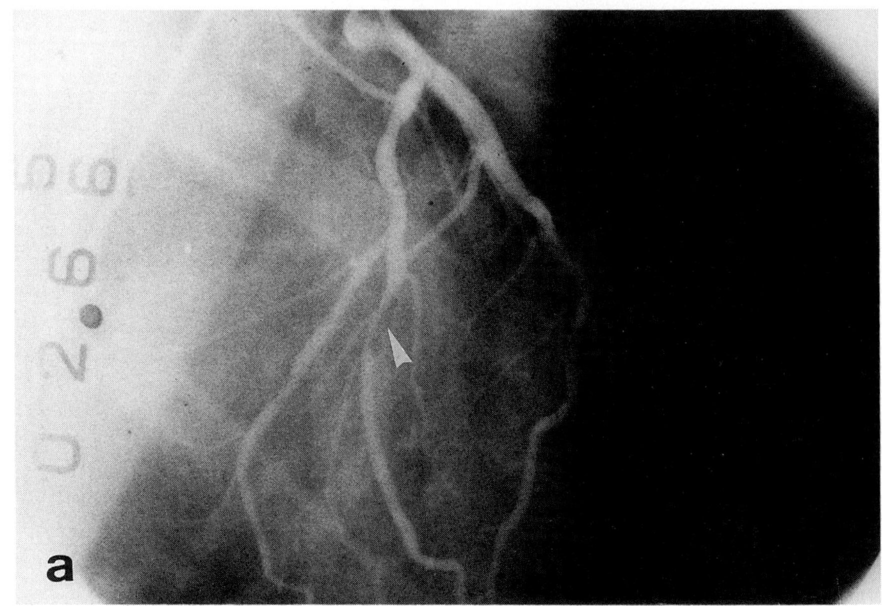

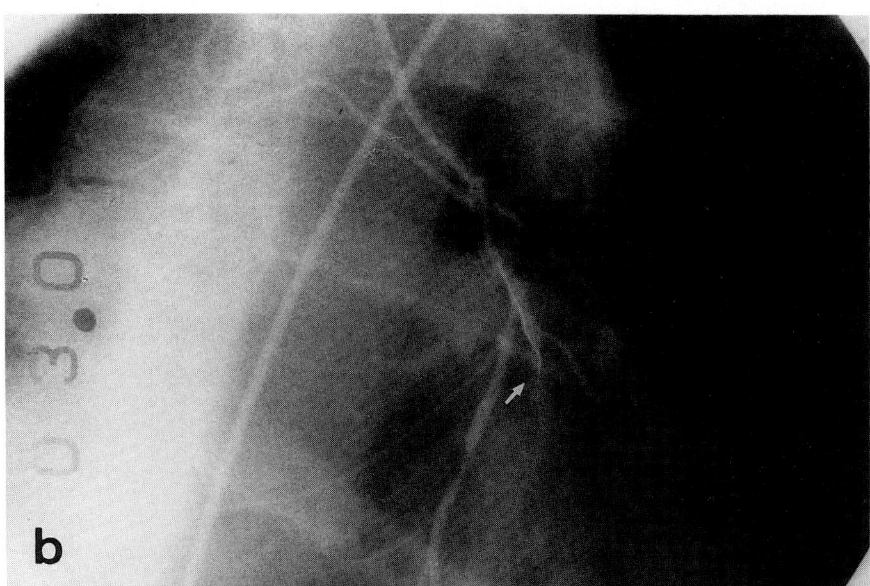

Figure 131

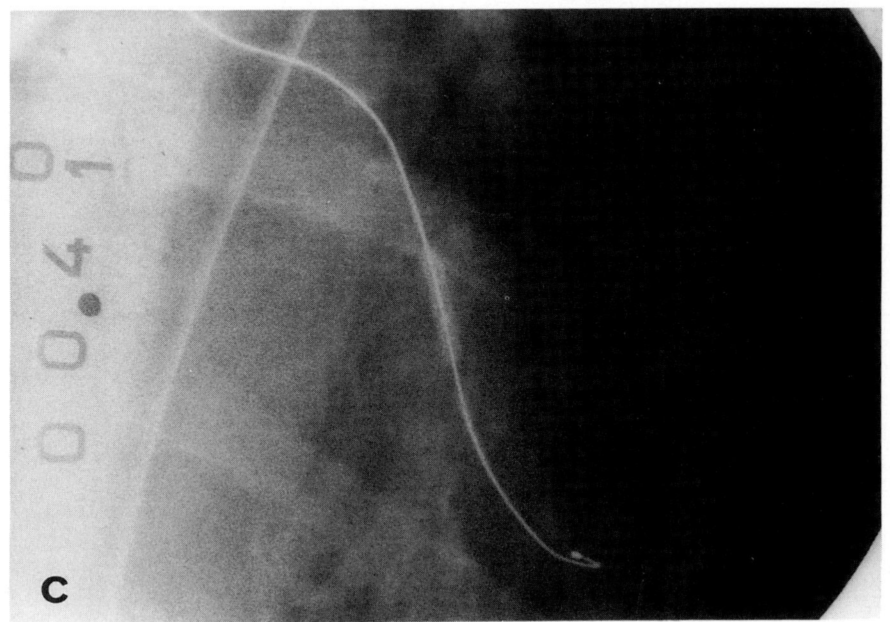
c

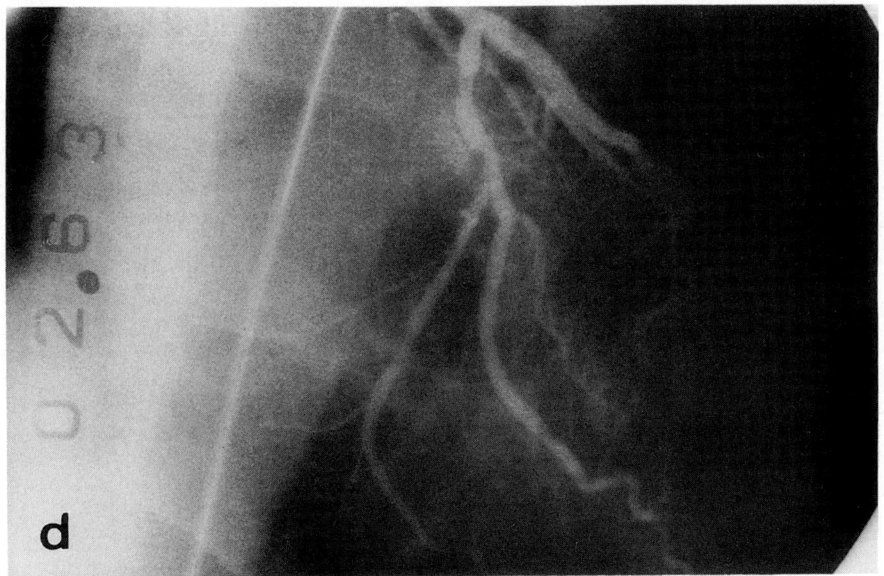
d

mm Magnarail balloon and yielded a good result (Fig. 131d).

A local dissection after balloon inflation is a normal consequence of angioplasty. Smaller dissections should be left alone, since they tend to heal spontaneously. A 44-year-old man underwent angioplasty for an occluded LCx (Fig. 132a), with a resultant local dissection (Fig. 132b). The patient remained asymptomatic after the procedure with negative stress tests. A follow-up examination 19 months later revealed healing of the dissection (Fig. 132c).

Dissections need to be evaluated for their risk of acute closure. A dissection in which the flap faces upstream, or one associated with a sluggish flow or dye retention, is associated with a high risk of acute occlusion. Such a lesion needs to be stabilized. Occasionally, a repeat dilatation of the segment with a higher balloon pressure (associated with a larger balloon diameter in the case of a compliant balloon), a larger balloon, and/or a prolonged inflation period may result in the tacking up of the dissection. The larger balloon diameter may sometimes succeed in changing the configuration of the dissection (e.g., splitting of a cul-de-sac-

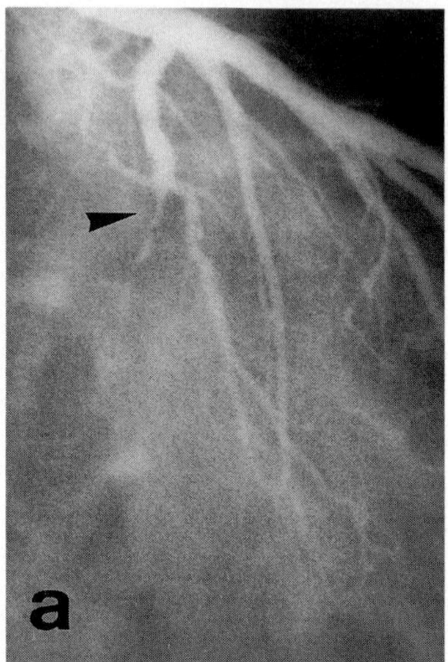

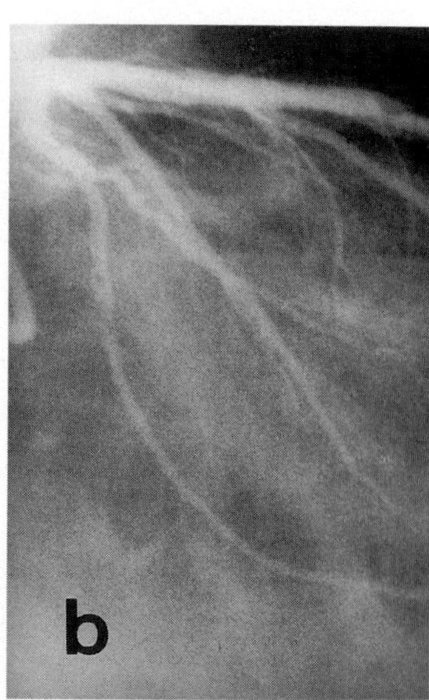

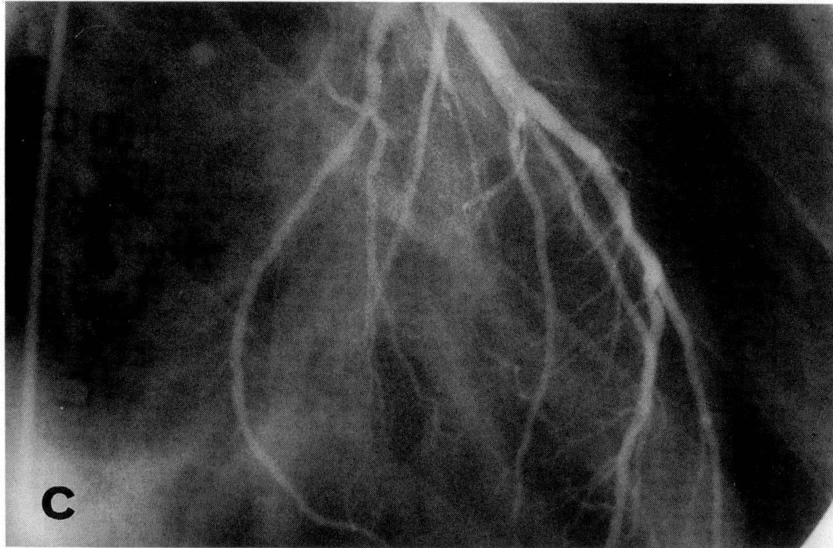

Figure 132

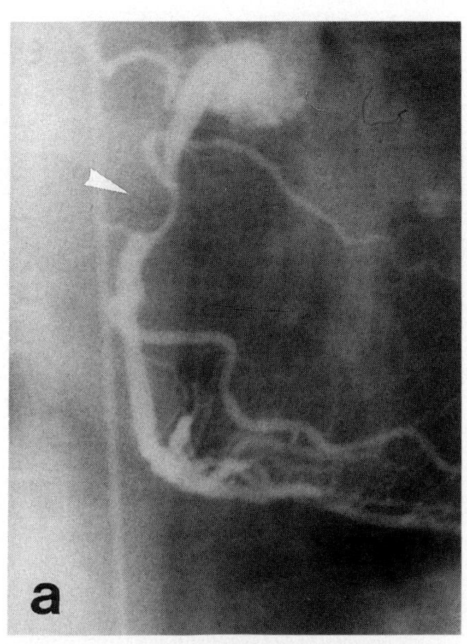

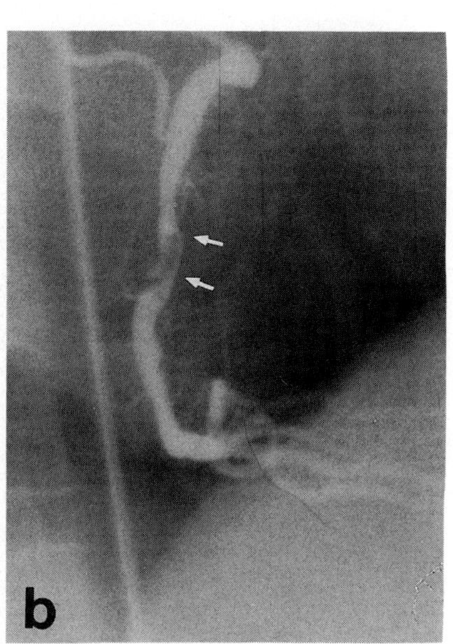

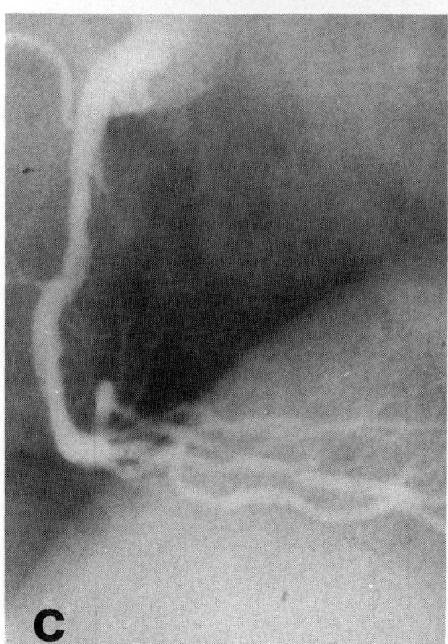

Figure 133

type distal end of the dissection), thereby normalizing flow. A 45-year-old man underwent angioplasty of an eccentric midsegment RCA lesion (Fig. 133a), with a 3.5-mm balloon. This resulted in a local dissection, which remained unchanged after a prolonged inflation with the same balloon (Fig. 133b). At this stage a 4.0-mm balloon was utilized. After a prolonged (3-minute) inflation, the result was good (Fig. 133c). The larger balloon may have helped to plaster the flap against the wall, in addition to reducing the elastic recoil of the artery. Such a technique may be tried before the implantation of a stent. If the patient does not tolerate ischemia, a prolonged inflation may require a perfusion balloon. Immediate results after prolonged balloon inflations may look good at first but have a tendency to deteriorate over the ensuing minutes. Therefore, the result should be observed over a period of time, and stent implantation may become necessary after all. Our policy is to try as long an inflation as tolerated with the standard balloon and spare the expense of a perfusion balloon by proceeding directly with stent implantation if the result is not satisfactory.

In case of long spiral dissections with a distal cul-de-sac phenomenon, it may be necessary to extend the dissection down the artery intentionally until the distal end of the dissection is unobstructive. A 60-year-old woman underwent angioplasty of a mid RCA stenosis (Fig. 134a) with a 3.0-mm balloon, with an acceptable result and a local dissection (Fig. 134b). The next day she experienced chest pain. An angiogram revealed an extension of the dissection with a functional occlusion of the artery due to a cul-de-sac phenomenon (Fig. 134c). The lesion was redilated, this time with a 3.5-mm balloon. This extended the dissection even more distally but an obstructive

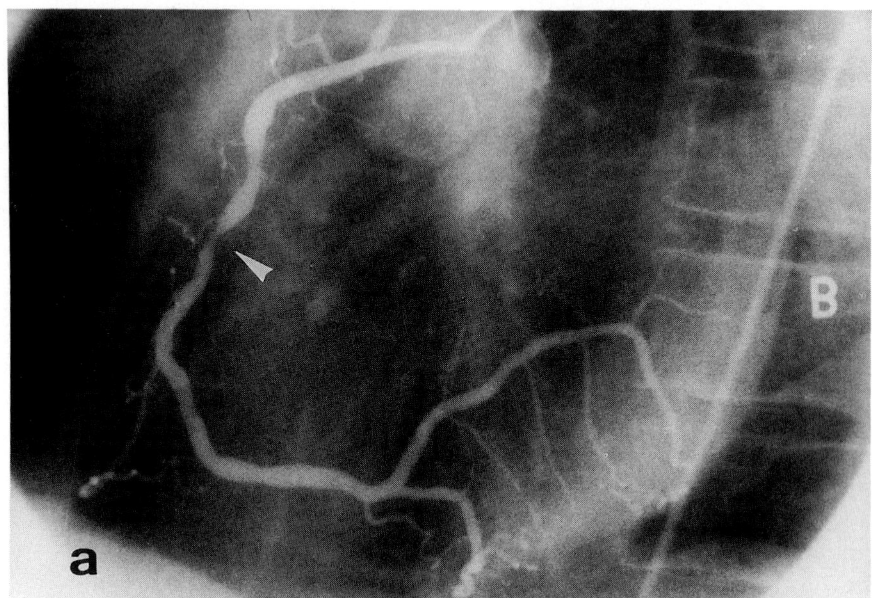

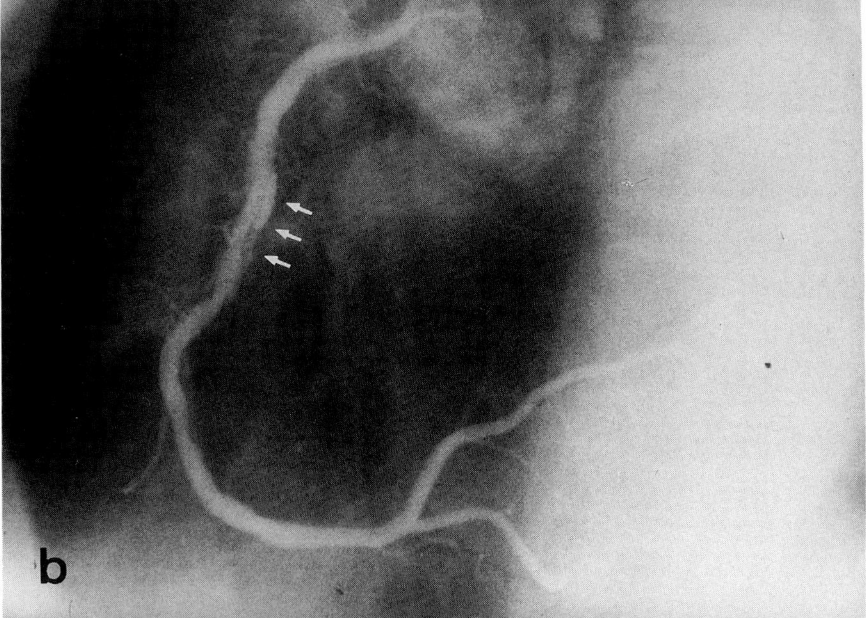

Figure 134

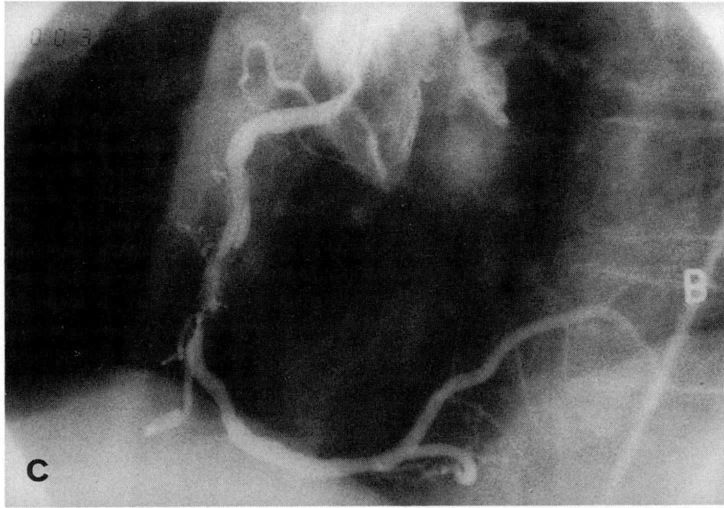

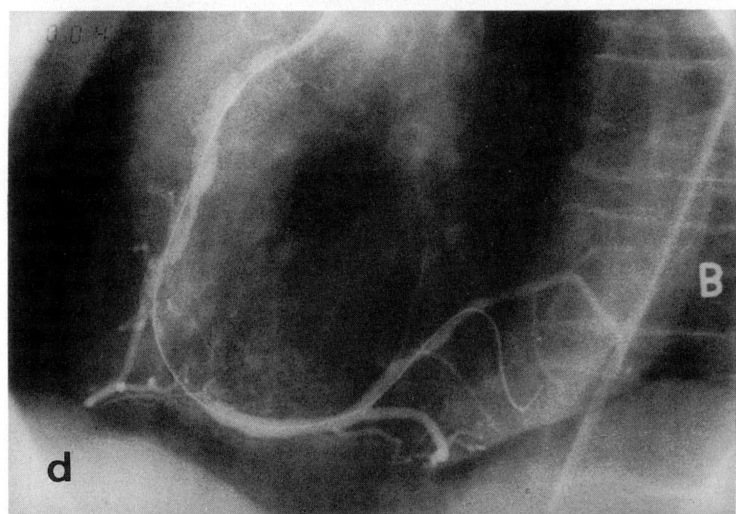

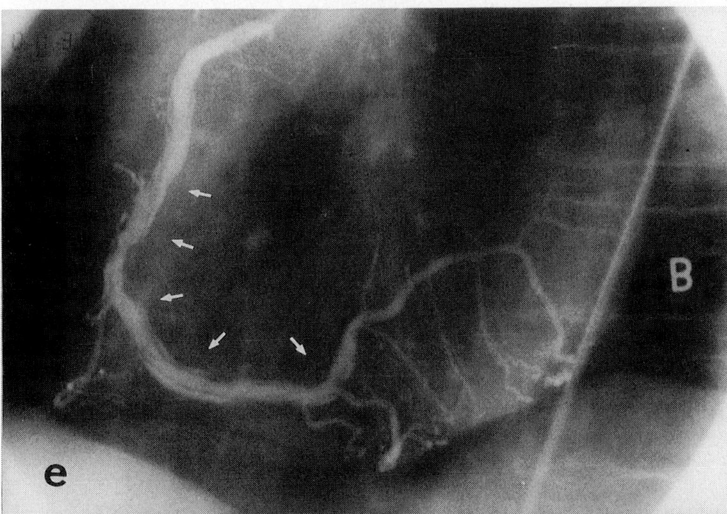

cul de sac formed again at the new end of it (Fig. 134d). The dissection had to be extended farther into the posterolateral branch of the RCA (Fig. 134e) until flow was restored normally. The angioplasty result with a long dissection but normal flow was accepted as the best compromise for the patient, the only alternative being multiple stent implantations. She experienced no further chest pain, and a stress test performed a week later was negative. This example demonstrates how an initially short dissection can extend and cause an acute occlusion, and how making the dissection even longer can be a solution to the problem.

A 39-year-old woman with hyperlipidemia and a smoking habit had a past history of anterior wall myocardial infarction 3 years earlier. She had undergone CABG twice, 3 and 2 years ago, respectively, before she presented with recurrent angina. Angioplasty of an ostial stenosis of the venous graft to the LCx (Fig. 135a) was performed with a good result (Fig. 135b). Two months later, angina recurred, the venous graft was well patent (Fig. 135c). A very proximal stenosis of the RCA was detected (Fig. 135d) and dilated through a 5F diagnostic catheter (Fig. 135e), with a good immediate result. However, the vessel closed abruptly 5 minutes later. The redilatation through a 6F catheter resulted in a long spiral dissection (Fig. 135f). A recurrent cul-de-sac phenomena necessitated more and more distal balloon inflations. Additionally, a tear of the right coronary cusp became apparent (Fig. 135f, curved arrow). Three months later, the patient returned with chest pain. The RCA was seen to be patent, although severely stenosed in its midsegment (Fig. 135g). The tear of the right coronary cusp persisted (Fig. 135g, arrowheads). The mid RCA stenosis was stented with half a Palmaz-Schatz

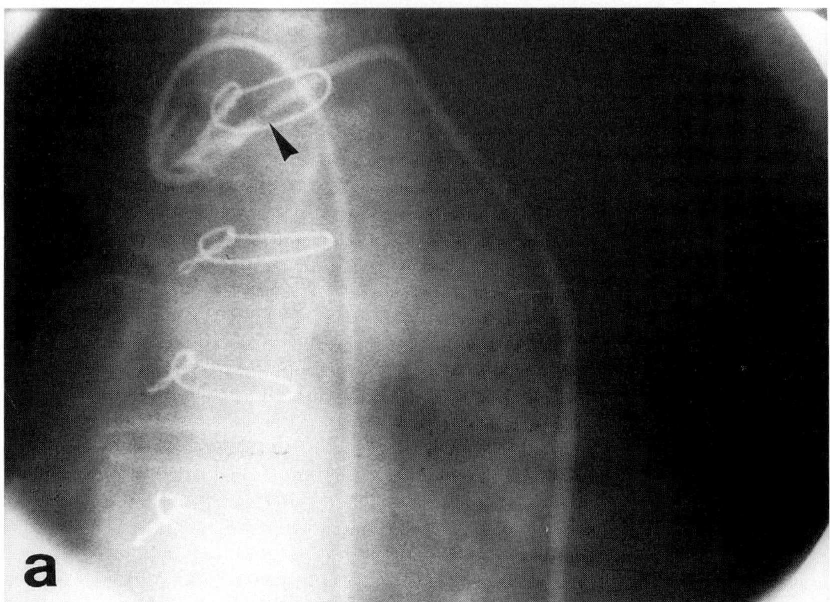

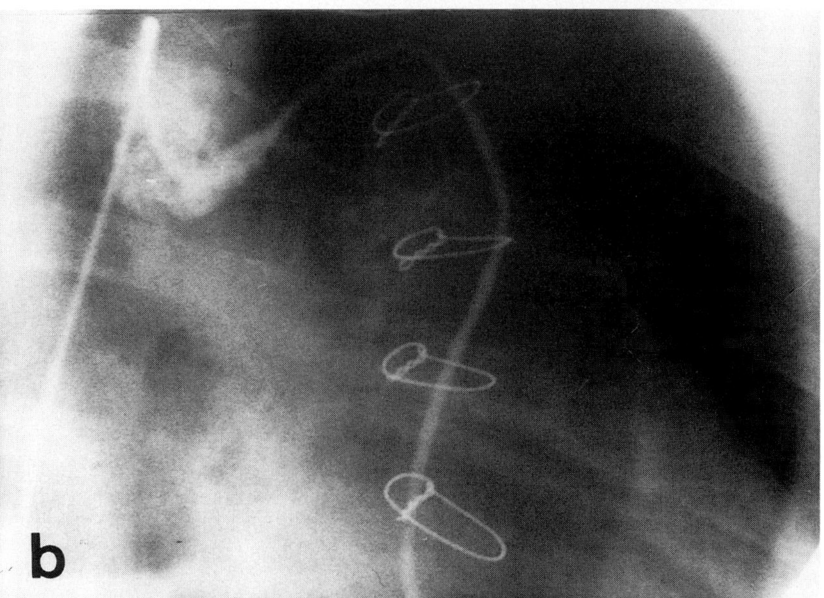

Figure 135

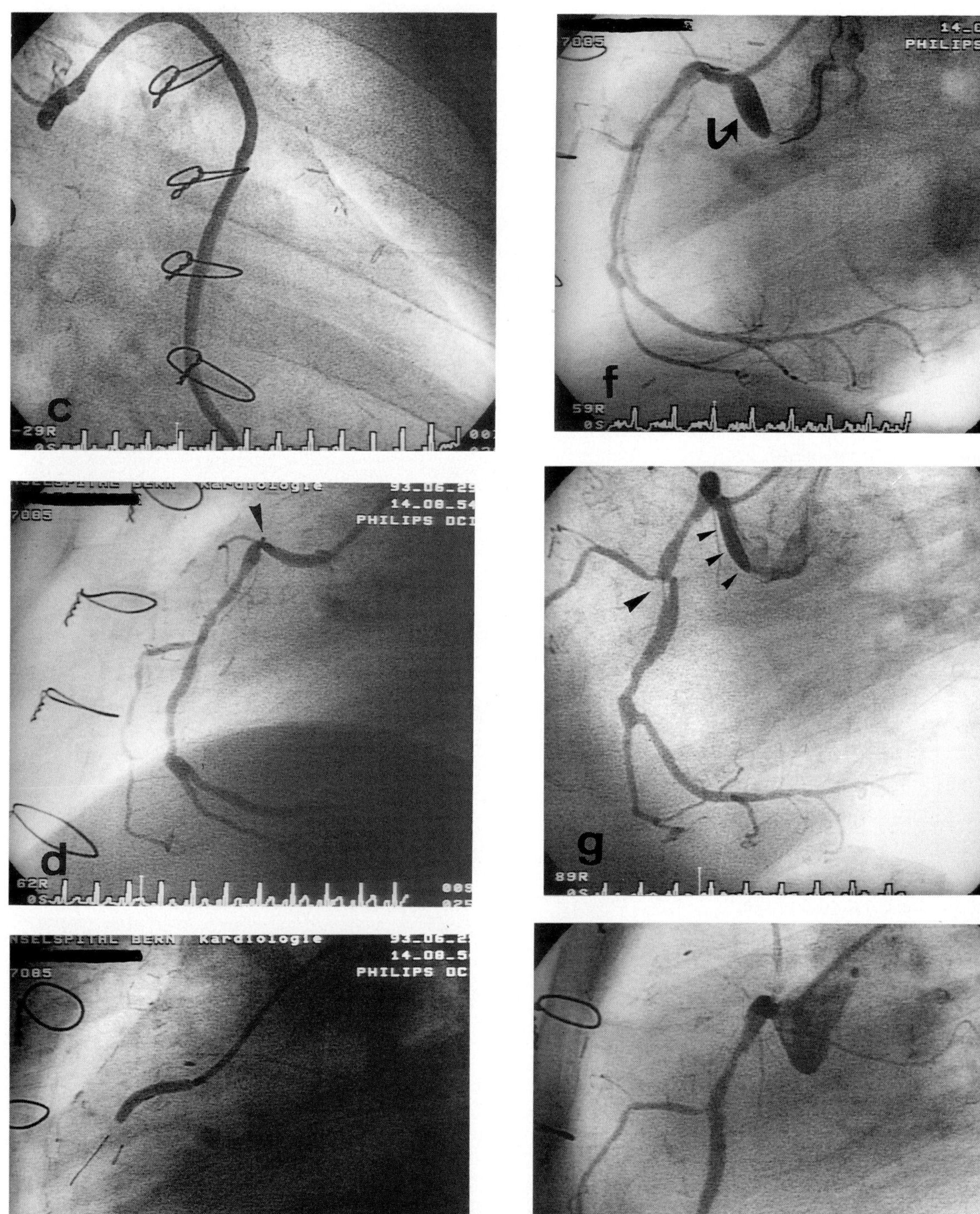
c
f
d
g
e
h

stent, with a good success. Another half stent was implanted at the RCA ostium to seal the cuspal tear with good result (Fig. 135h; the cuspal flap is reduced to a small dark line at the left border of the cusp). Additionally, a stenosis of the anastomosis of the LIMA graft to the LAD was documented (Fig. 135i) and dilated (Fig. 135j) with a good result (Fig. 135k). This case highlights the problems associated with patients with hypercholesterolemia in general and in dealing with spiral dissections after balloon dilatations. In case of stenting such proximal stenoses, care has to be taken that the stent does not protrude too far out into the aortic root. This can render future cannulation of the ostium difficult.

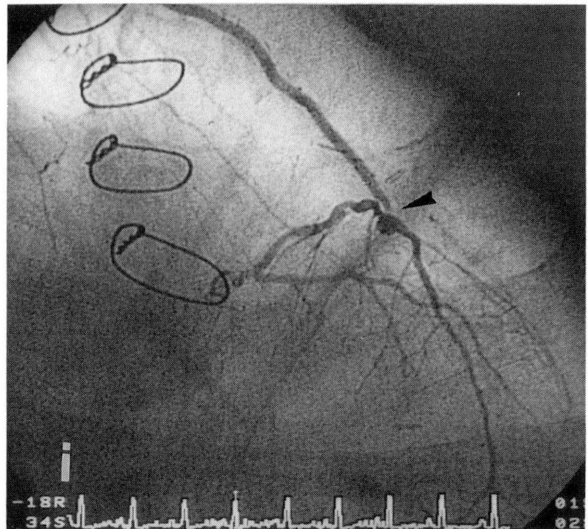

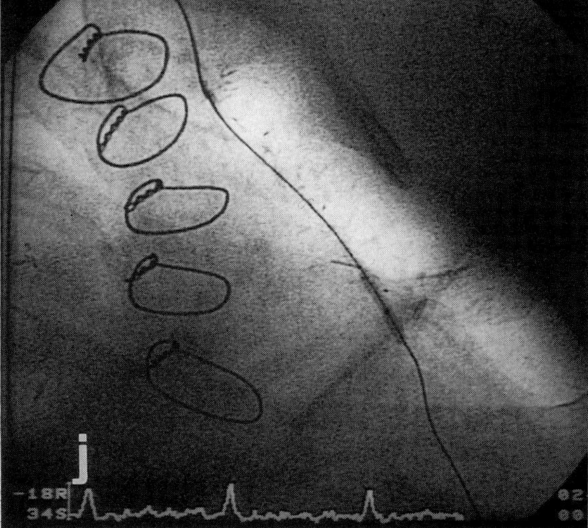

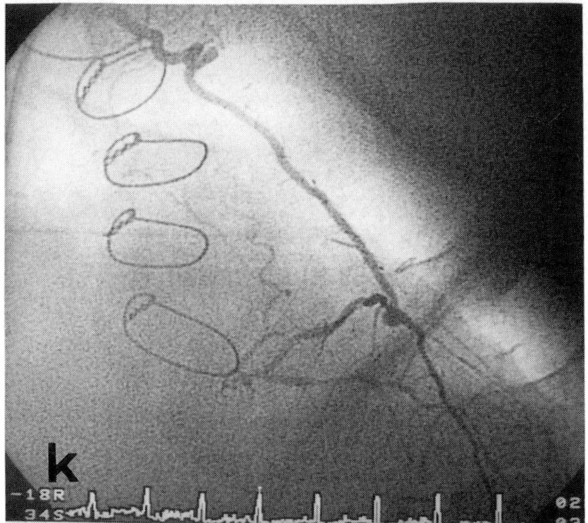

Figure 135 (Continued)

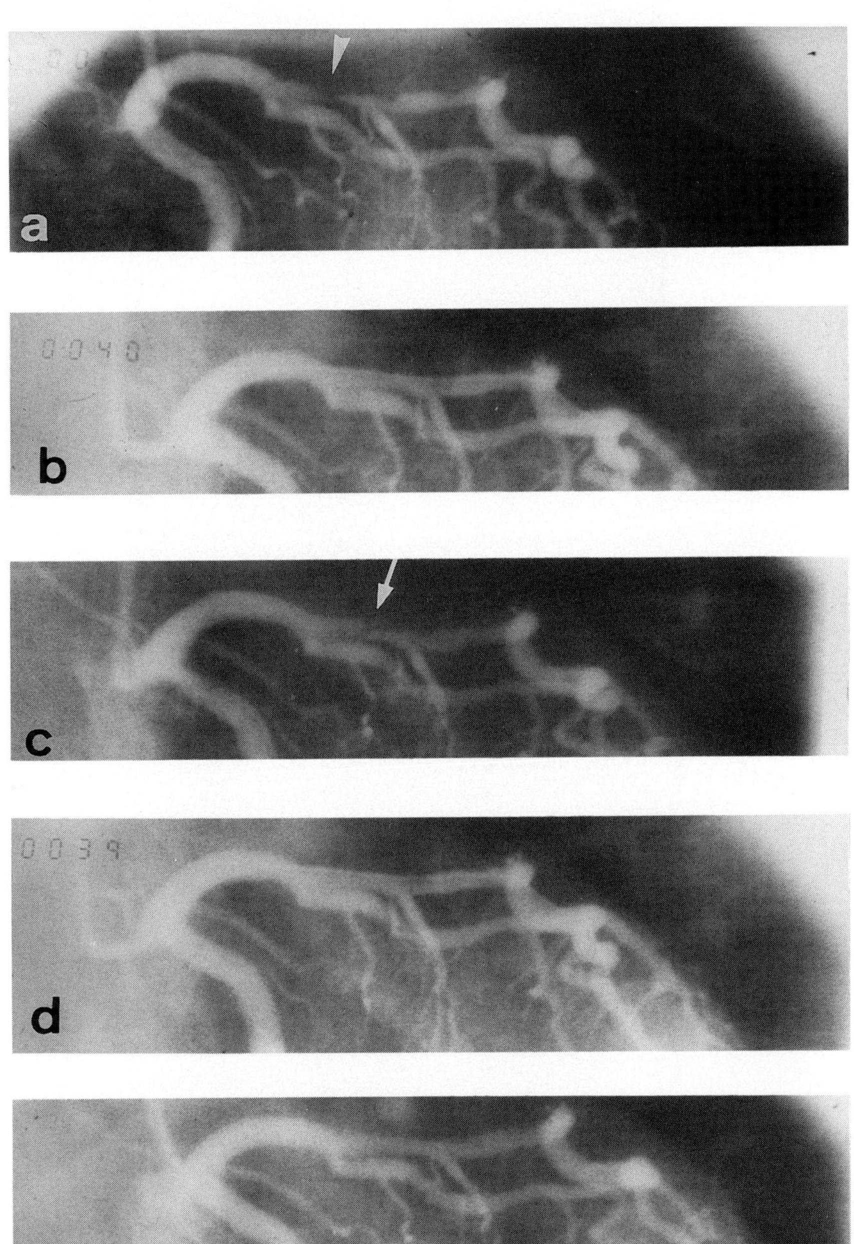

Figure 136

Following PTCA with angiographically visible dissections, it is necessary to assess the result after withdrawal of the guidewire. The guidewire can exert a stenting effect on a dissection, resulting in a spuriously good angiographic picture. A 70-year-old man underwent angioplasty for a mid LAD lesion (Fig. 136a). The result was acceptable (Fig. 136b), with a small local dissection, which remained stable after waiting for 5 minutes. However, on removal of the wire the angiographic aspect deteriorated immediately (Fig. 136c). After reintroducing the wire, the angiographic picture once again looked acceptable (Fig. 136d), the dissection flap being held up (stented) by the wire. The dissection was finally stabilized by a prolonged balloon inflation (Fig. 136e).

If a dissection cannot be stabilized with prolonged balloon inflations or a slightly oversized balloon, it should be stented. A 63-year-old man underwent angioplasty for a long stenosis of the LAD with a spontaneous aneurysm (Fig. 137a) using a long balloon (Fig. 137b). This resulted in a long dissection (Fig. 137c) which could not be stabilized despite a 3-minute inflation using the same long balloon inflated to higher pressure. The balloon was then exchanged for a perfusion balloon, which was inflated for 15 minutes (Fig. 137d). However, despite an initial apparent improvement, the dissection proved unchanged after a few minutes (Fig. 137e). Finally, the lesion was stented using a Palmaz-Schatz stent, with a good result (Fig. 137f). Very long (>10-minute) inflations with perfusion balloons usually do not achieve much over a relatively long (3- to 5-minute) inflation with a normal balloon. As demonstrated once again in this example, it is better to proceed directly to stenting when faced with such a situation rather than investing in a perfusion balloon. Such an approach results in a saving of time and money.

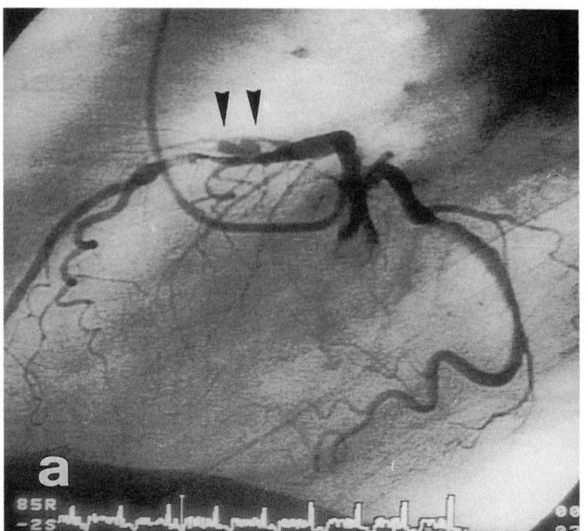

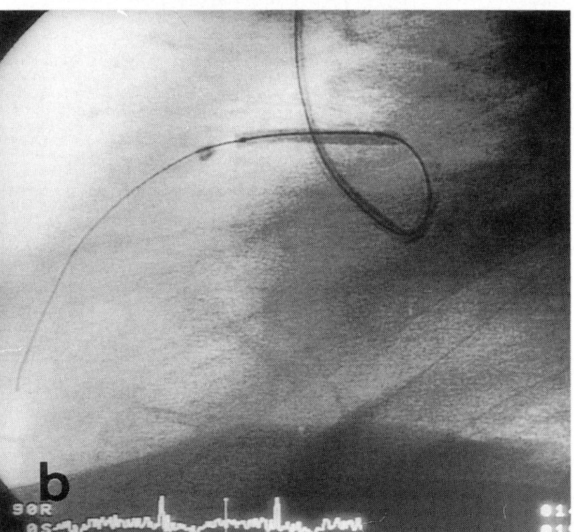

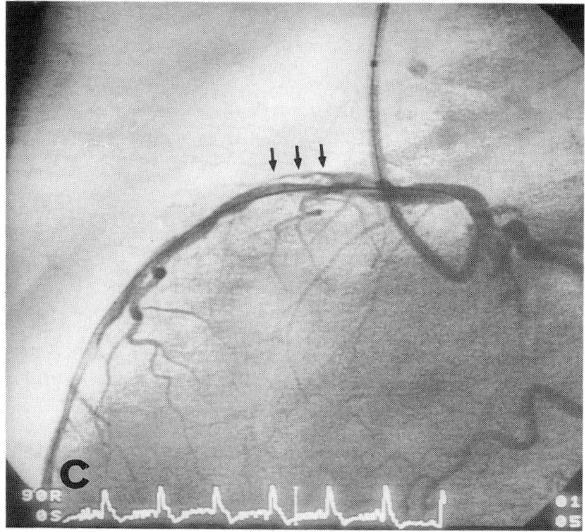

Figure 137

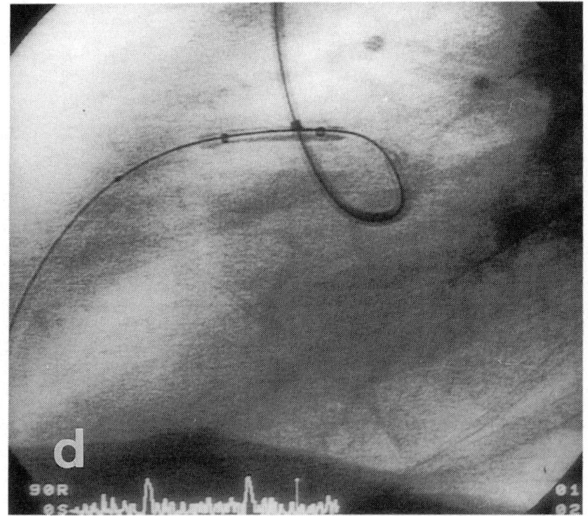
d

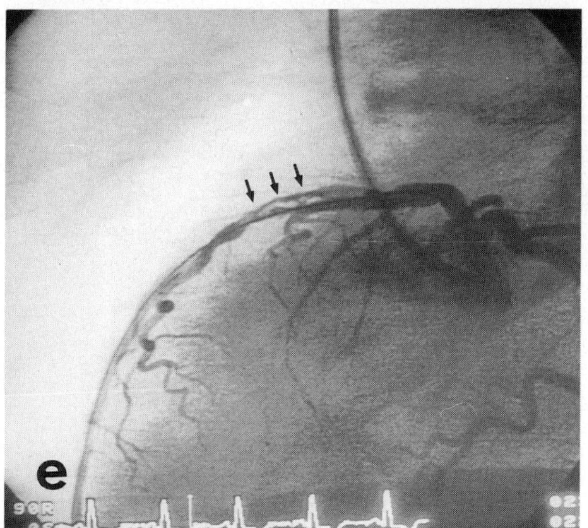
e

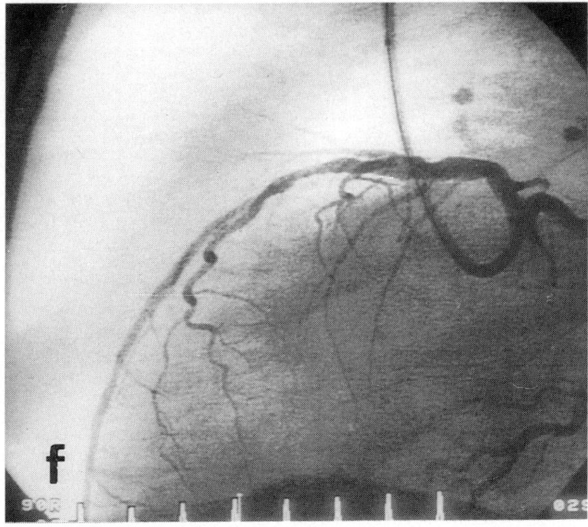
f

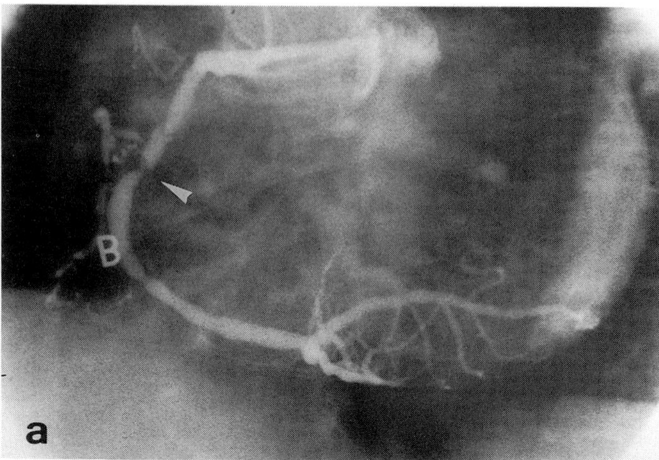

If a dissection occurs in a situation where stenting is not considered a viable option, such as in a small vessel with poor peripheral runoff, or if the periphery is already infarcted, it may be preferable to risk or even allow a "controlled infarction" to occur rather than subject the patient to emergency surgery. Sometimes, the threatening occlusion may not materialize after all. Long dissections, especially if associated with good peripheral runoff, may heal surprisingly well. A 58-year-old man underwent angioplasty for stenoses of the RCA (Fig. 138a), with a resultant dissection with obstructive flow (Fig. 138b). Stenting with a Palmaz-Schatz stent was attempted. However, the balloon–stent assembly could not negotiate the proximal curve of the vessel. Hence the lesion was left unstented. At follow-up 1 month later, the dissection was seen to have healed spontaneously (Fig. 138c).

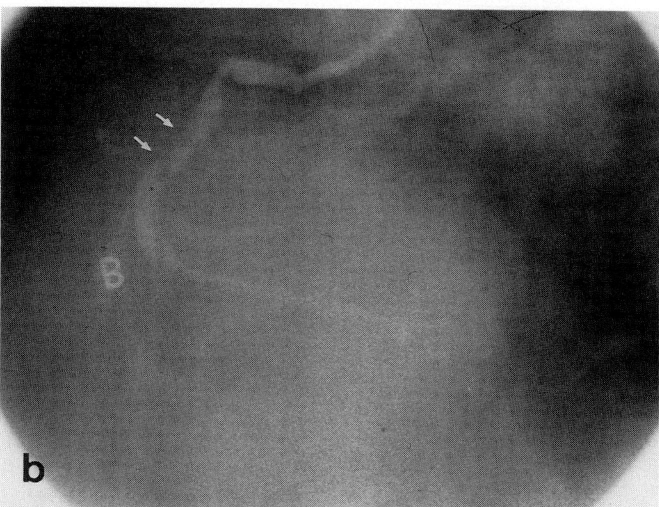

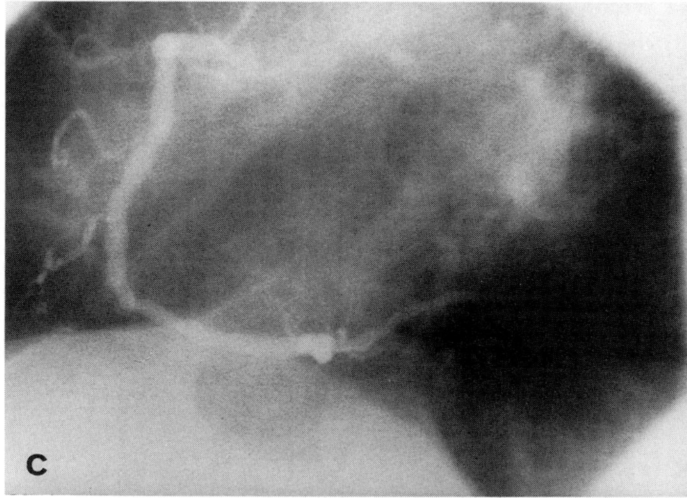

Figure 138

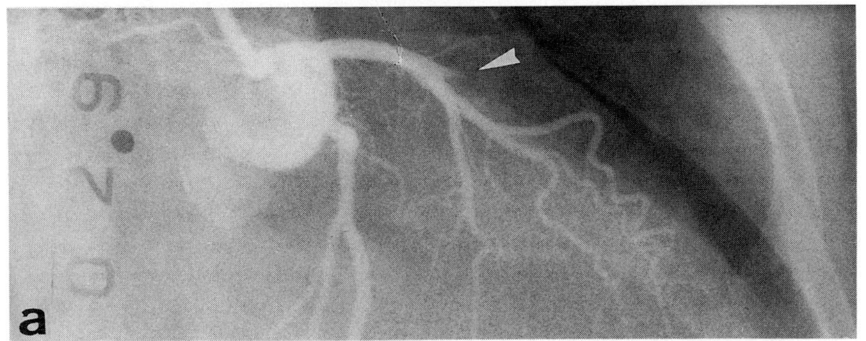

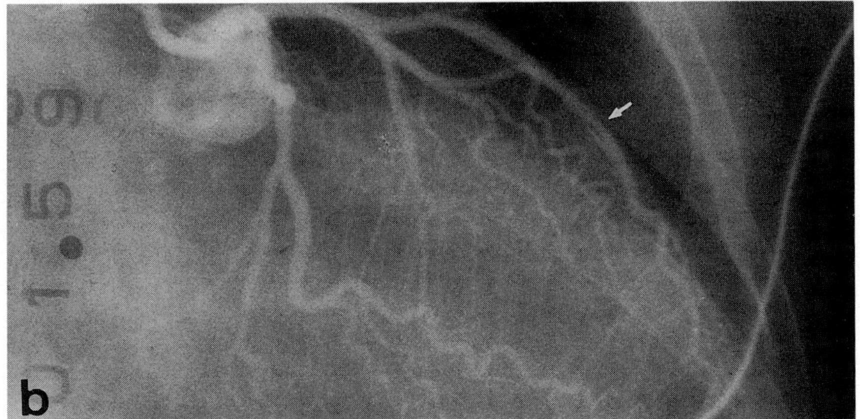

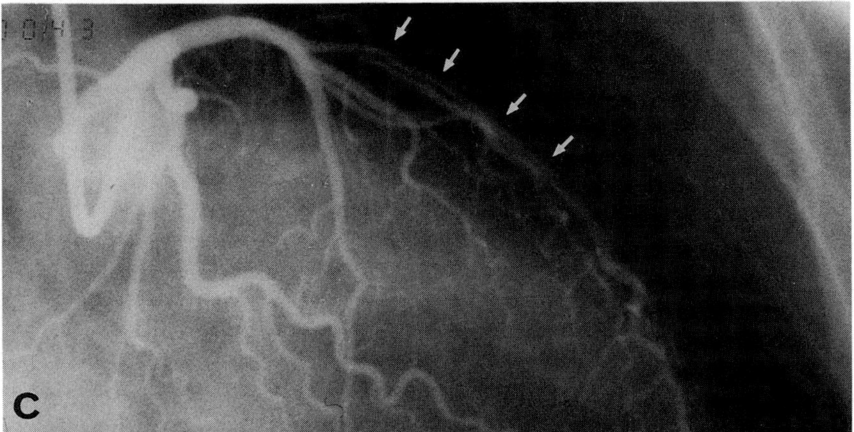

Figure 139

Some dissections may look worse at follow-up and still represent an acceptable long-term result. A 65-year-old male underwent recanalization of an occluded LAD (Fig. 139a) with a good result and only a localized dissection (Fig. 139b). A 6-month follow-up revealed a much longer dissection (double-barrel lumen), but the distal flow was good (Fig. 139c). The patient was asymptomatic, with a normal left ventricle.

Thus, not all dissections are bad, and they need not always be treated aggressively. In fact, some may even prove to be beneficial, as demonstrated by an anecdotal example. A 71-year-old man presented with angina and a positive stress test. Angiography revealed a tight stenosis of the LCx (Fig. 140a). During angioplasty, all attempts to cross the lesion with the wire failed and no balloon was utilized. However, the attempts to cross the lesion with the wire had created multiple dissections, which coincidentally had improved the lesion (Fig. 140b). The procedure was stopped at this stage. The patients symptoms were relieved, and stress tests the following day and 5 months later were negative.

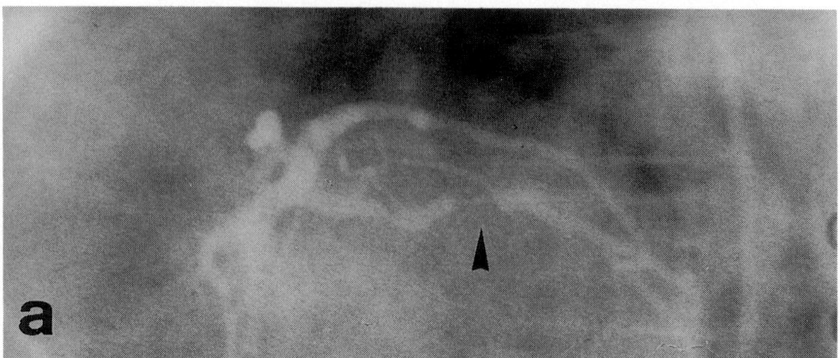

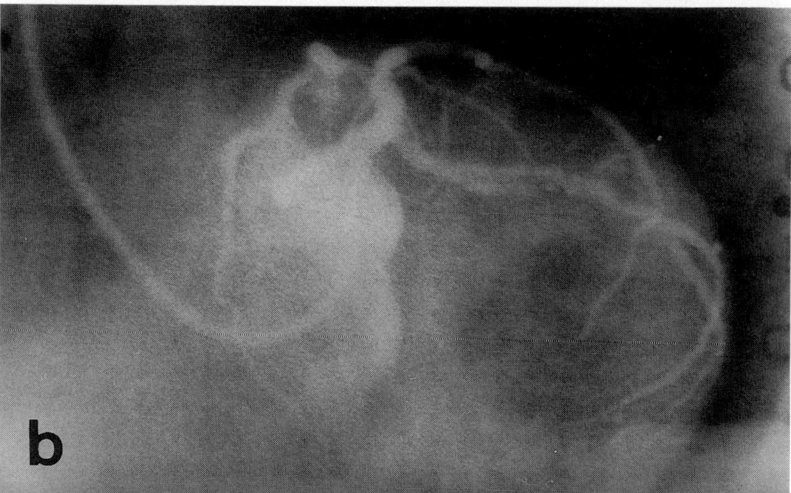

Figure 140

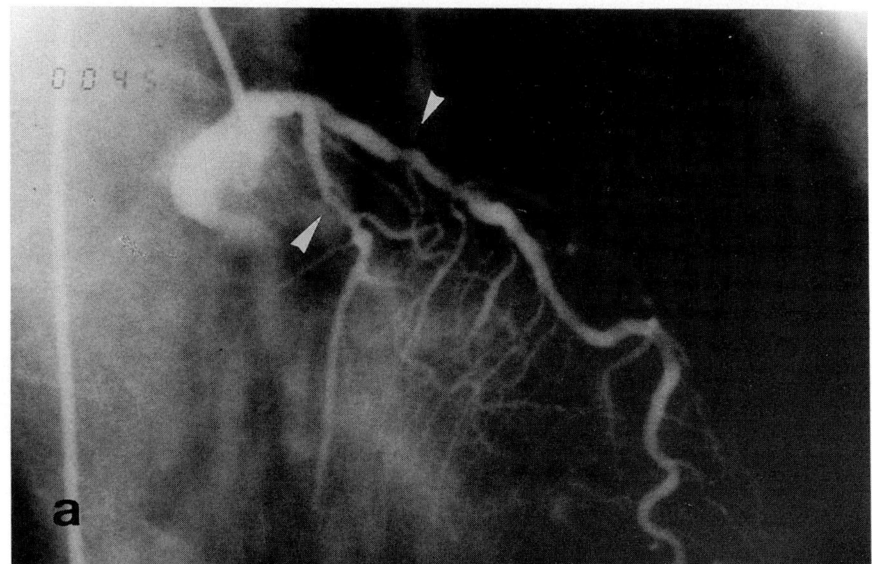

Figure 141

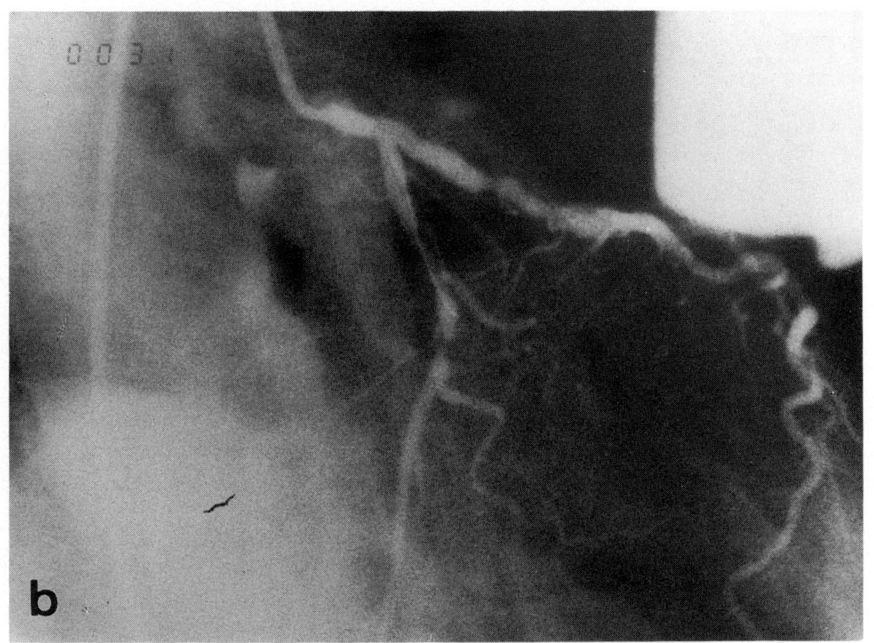

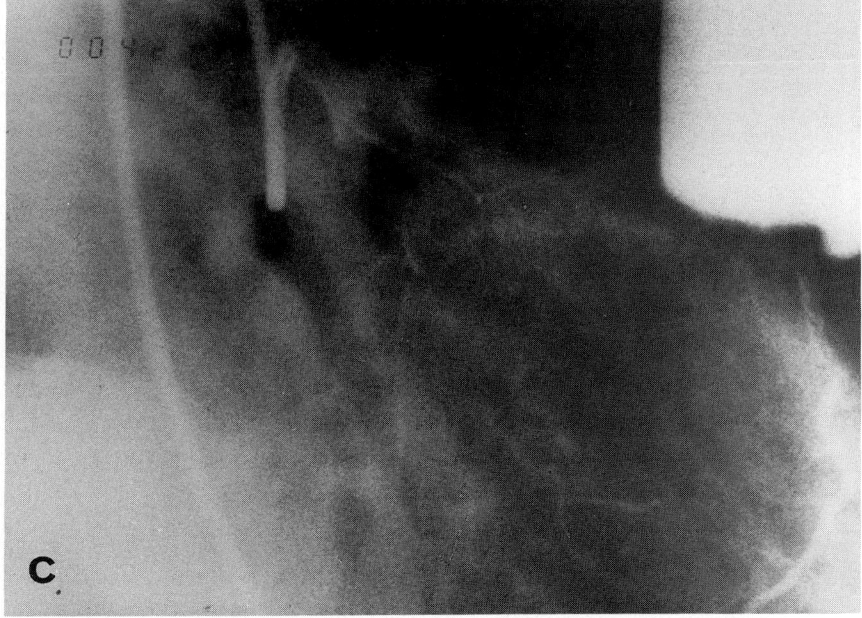

Dissection of the left main coronary artery during angioplasty is one of the most dreaded complications. It calls for ultrarapid measures to save the patient's life. Even these ever so often prove to be in vain. A 75-year-old man presented with stenoses of the LCx and LAD (Fig. 141a). Angioplasty of the stenosis of the proximal LCx artery was attempted using a fixed-wire balloon through the 6F Judkins diagnostic catheter (Fig. 141b), but the balloon could not be advanced through the lesion, possibly due to a subintimal passage of the wire. The guiding catheter was exchanged for an USCI 7 F AL 2 guiding catheter (Fig. 141c). However, after placement of this catheter, a dissection of the left main coronary artery was noticed (Fig. 141d). A control angiogram revealed sluggish flow down the LAD and LCx with holdup of dye in the distal LAD (Fig. 141e). The patient was experiencing severe chest pain, with fall of systolic pressure to 60 mmHg. At this stage, the Amplatz catheter was withdrawn and replaced with a left Judkins catheter. The left main coronary artery was recanalized with a Magnum–Magnarail system (Fig. 141f), which restored flow in the LAD (Fig. 141g) and resulted in the clinical stabilization of the patient. Emergency CABG was performed, leaving the Magnum wire in place during transport for stabilization of the dissection. The patient suffered a myocardial infarction of the circumflex territory without Q-waves. His peak CPK was 3000 units and the subsequent recovery was uneventful. Amplatz catheters offer excellent backup support and are especially well suited for LCx lesions. However, they have the intrinsic disadvantage of tending to get deeply intubated, which may result in wedging or dissections. This tendency may be lesser if smaller 6F rather than 8F and softer guiding catheters (e.g., Pink Power, Schneider) instead of stiffer ones (e.g., USCI) are used.

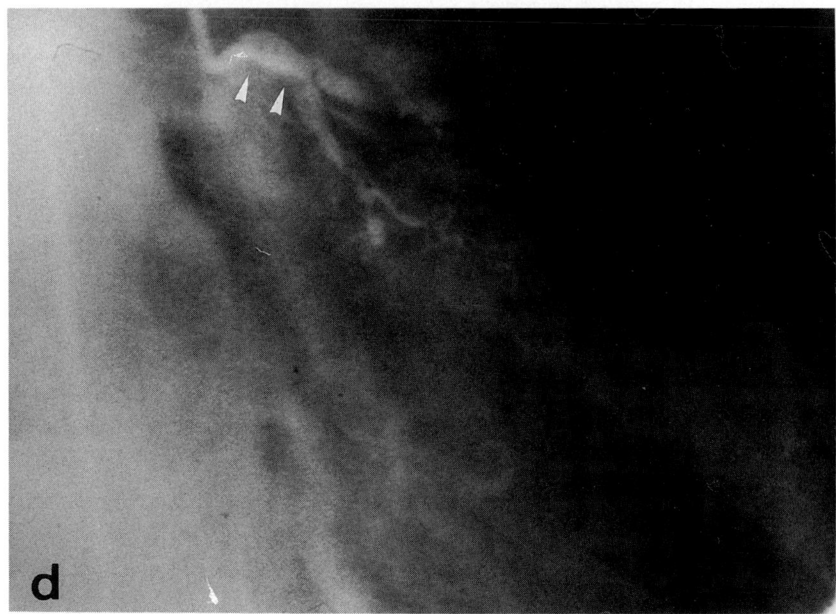

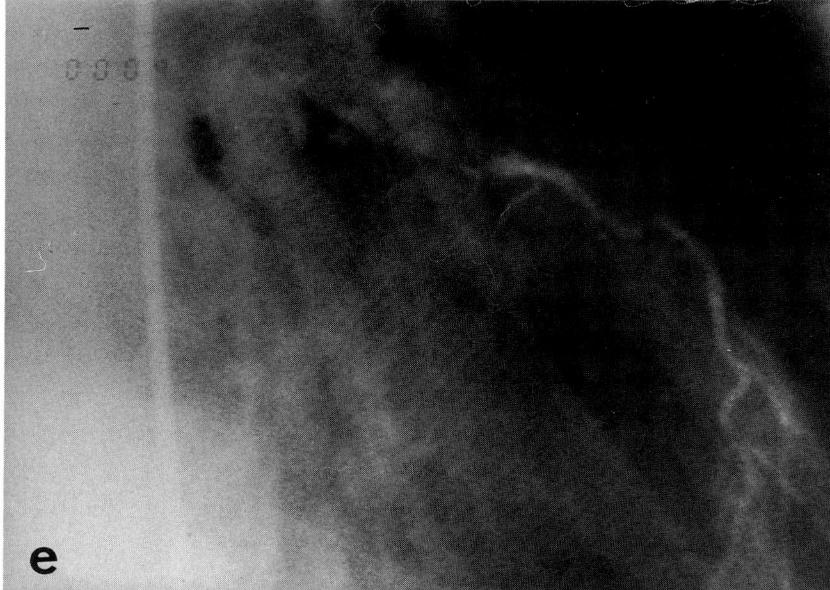

Figure 141 (Continued)

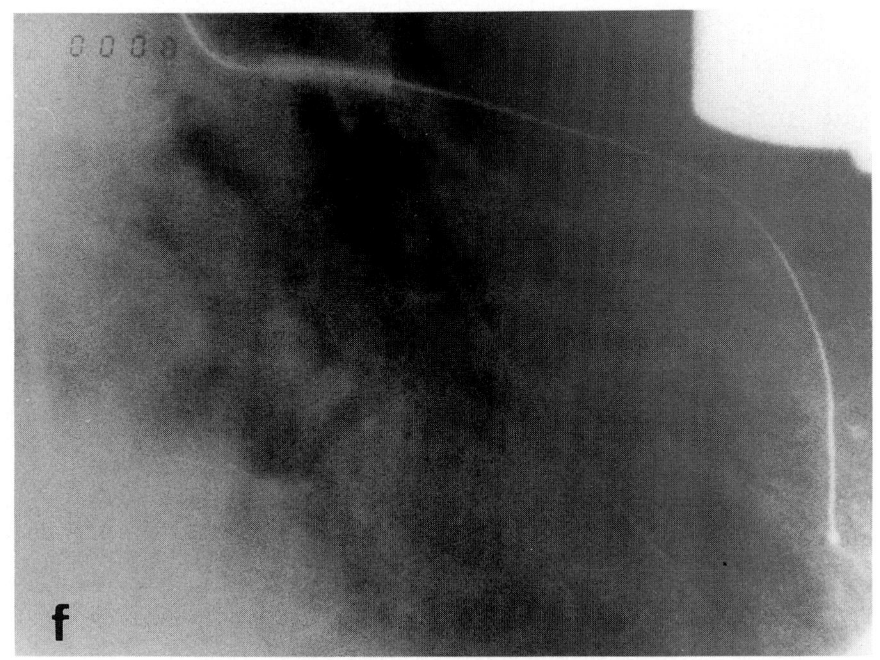
f

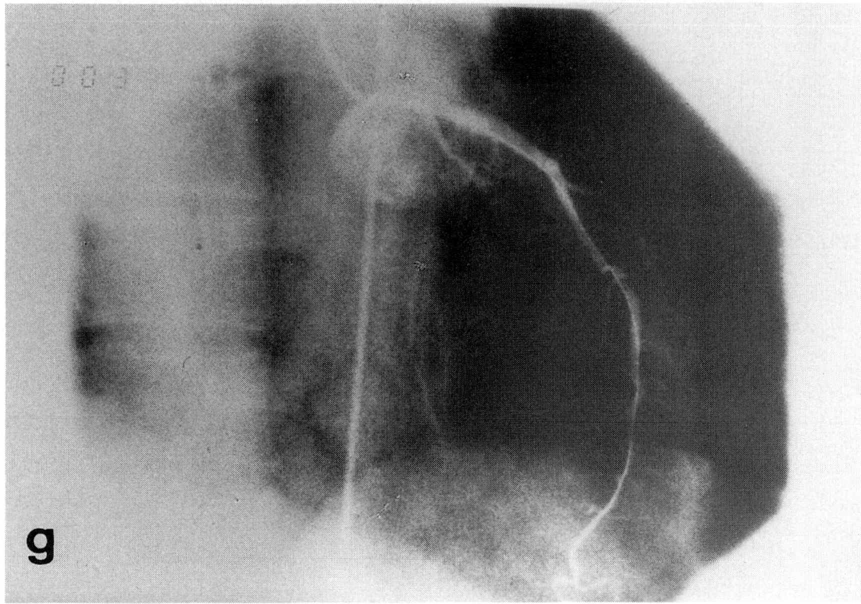
g

All left main dissections are not attributable to Amplatz catheters. A 58-year-old woman had an occluded LAD (Fig. 142a). The attempt to recanalize the vessel using a Judkins left guiding catheter caused a dissection of the distal left main stem extending into the LCx, with occlusion of the LCx (Fig. 142b). Retrospectively, it may be argued that the dissection occurred because the Judkins catheter pointed toward the roof of the angulated left main stem, making the wire exit traumatic, and that an Amplatz catheter would have prevented this. The dissection was stabilized following a balloon inflation, with restoration of distal flow in the LCx. However, there was a long, linear dissection (Fig. 142c) producing an occlusion of the LAD at its origin. The left main stem and LCx were stented with a long Wallstent (Schneider) (Fig. 142d). The patient underwent semi-elective CABG since her primary problem, the chronically occluded LAD with normal anterior wall function, had not been solved and the additional risk of stent occlusion of the LCx had been added.

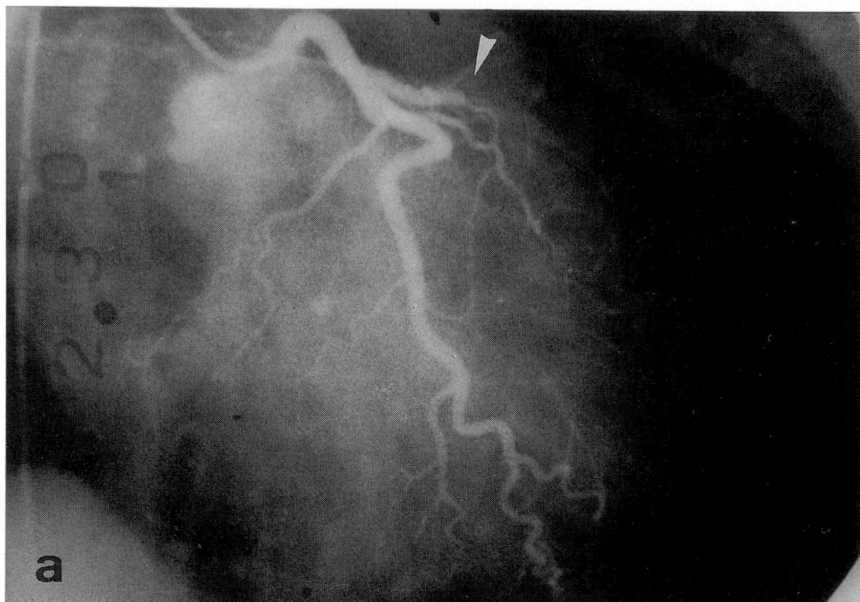

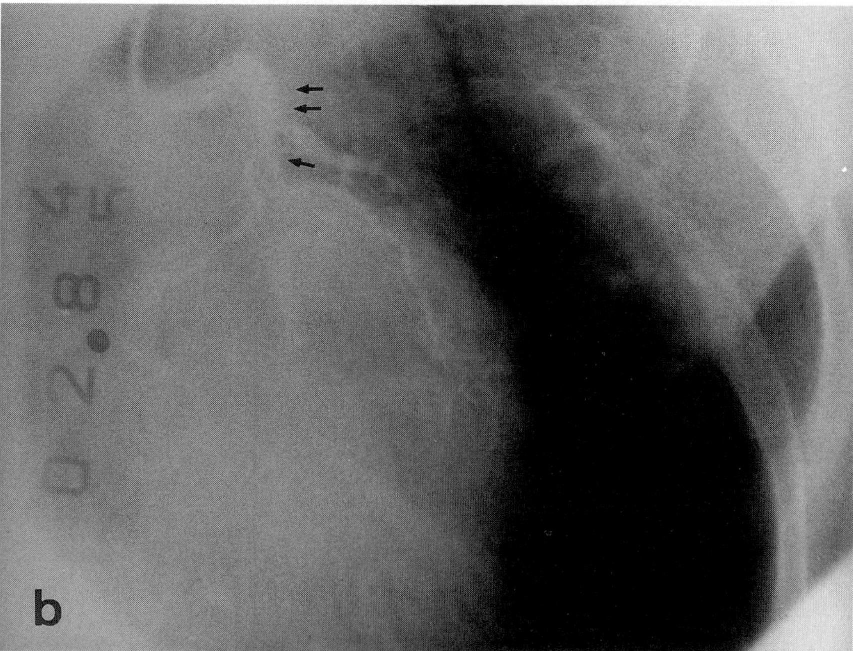

Figure 142

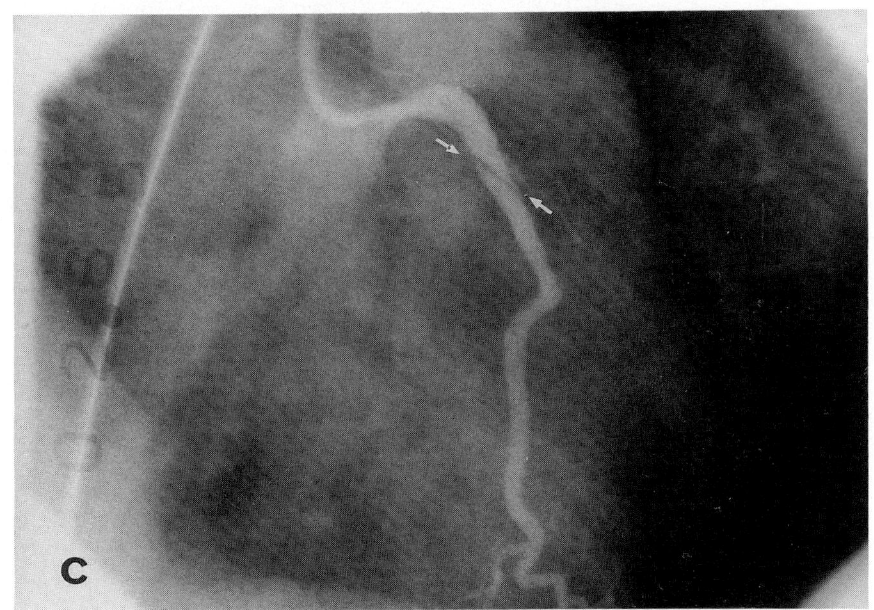
c

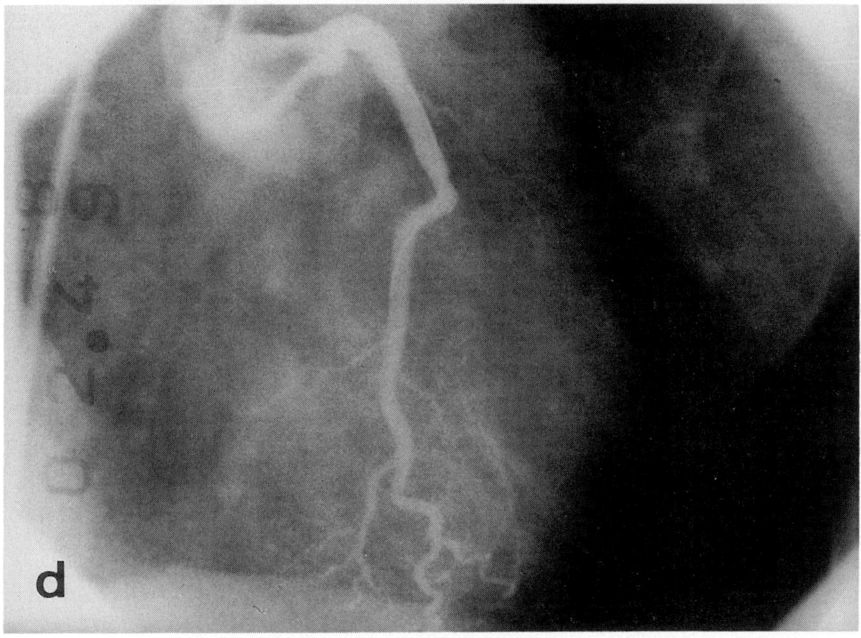
d

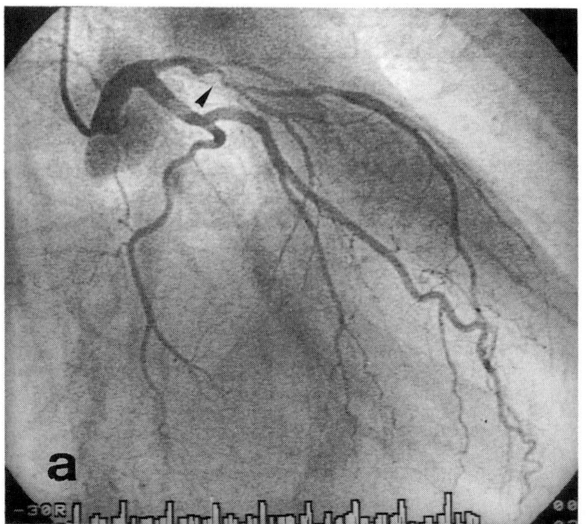

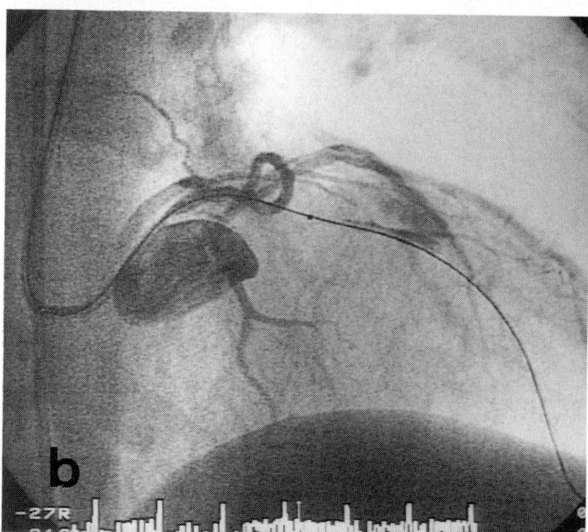

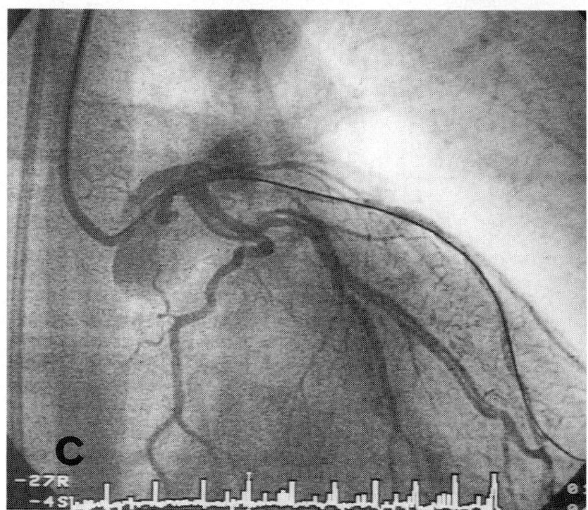

Figure 143

A 63-year-old man underwent angioplasty for a tight stenosis of the LAD (Fig. 143a). After crossing the lesion with a 0.014-in. guidewire, a 3.0-mm balloon could not be advanced across the lesion. This was exchanged for a 1.5-mm balloon, which failed to cross as well; hence the guiding catheter was intubated deeply to afford increased pushing power. The balloon could then be advanced across the stenosis, but a dissection of the left main stem resulted (Fig. 143b). The balloon was withdrawn, leaving the guidewire in place. The dissection was seen to extend into the LAD, the LCx, and its first marginal branch (Fig. 143c). The patient was completely stable, without chest pain or ECG changes. The guiding catheter was removed, leaving the guidewire in place. Emergency CABG was performed. The patient did not suffer a myocardial infarction and had an uneventful recovery. Again, the guidewire was left in place across the left main stem, even though the dissection appeared stable. The wire may have some stenting effect. Additionally, it enables rapid access for further intervention with a perfusion balloon or stent, in case of a deterioration of the clinical situation.

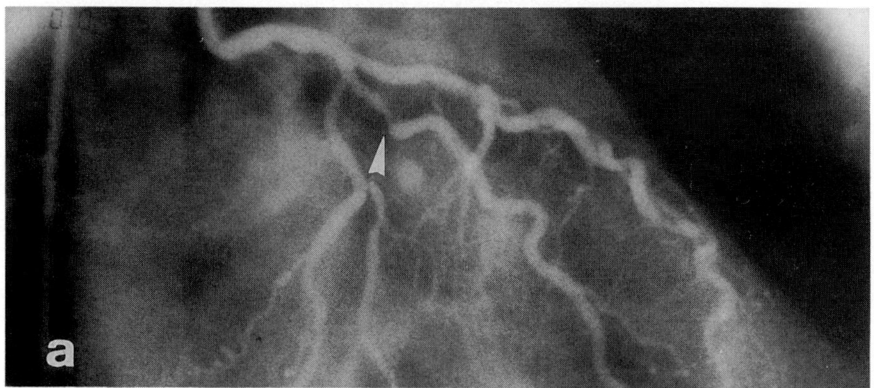

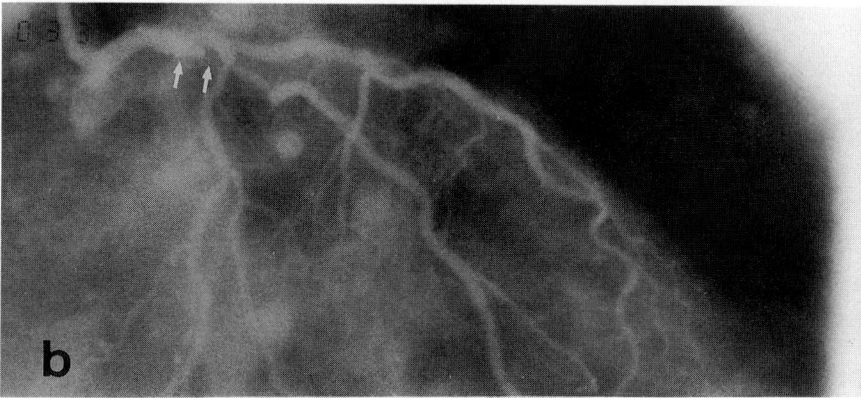

Figure 144

A dissection of the left main stem can on some rare occasions be treated conservatively, although such an approach needs a cautious estimate of inherent risks. A 56-year-old man underwent PTCA for stenosis of a marginal branch of the LCx (Fig. 144a). During the procedure, the Judkins left guiding catheter caused a dissection of the left main stem (Fig. 144b). The dissection was observed in the catheterization laboratory for several minutes and deemed stable. The patient was not subjected to surgery. A 2-month follow-up evaluation revealed a healed dissection, with a nonsignificant left main stem stenosis (Fig. 144c). A repeat study performed 8 months later for angina revealed progression of the left main lesion. The marginal branch, the reason for PTCA, was free of restenosis (Fig. 144d). The patient underwent elective CABG.

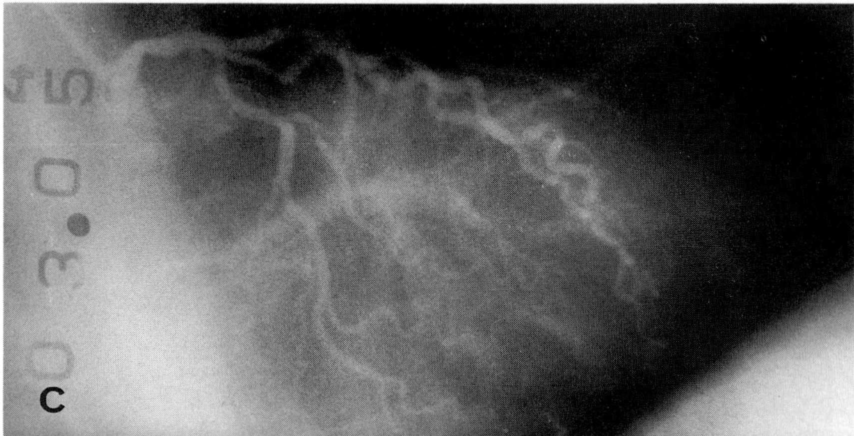

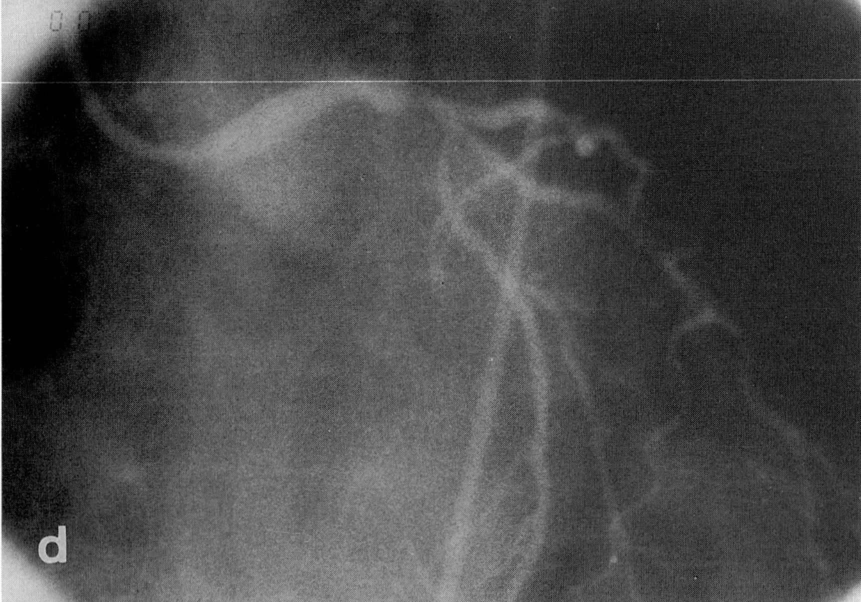

Figure 144 (Continued)

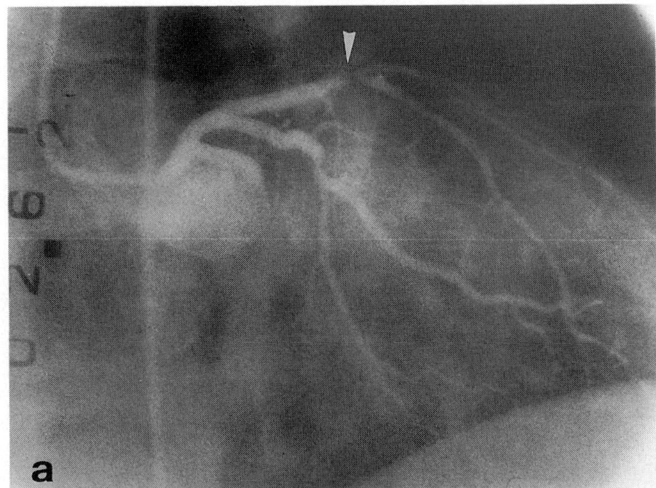

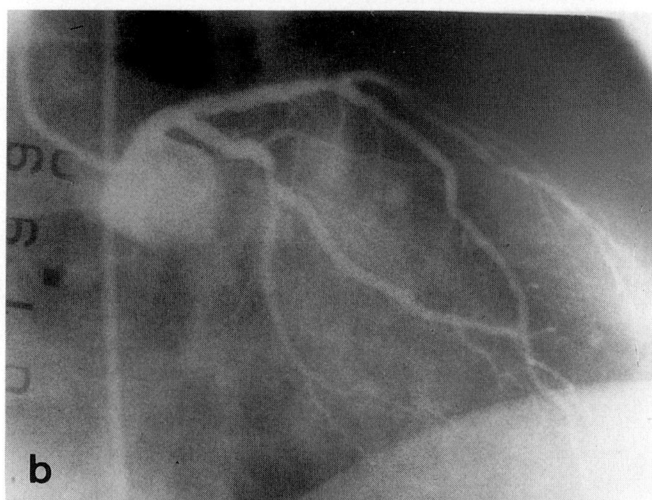

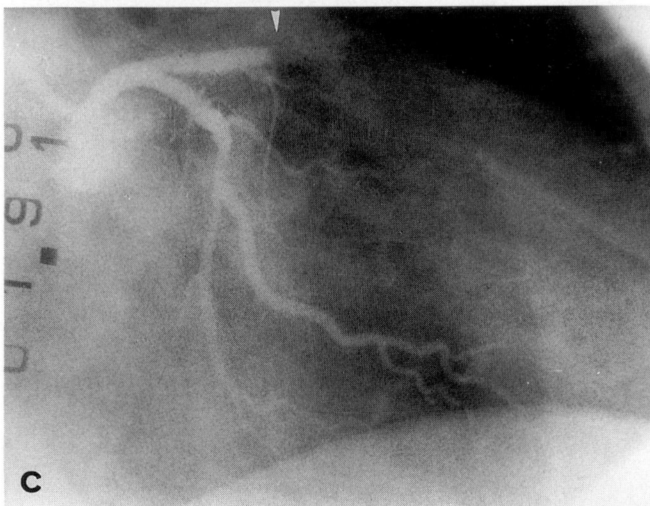

Figure 145

5.2 ACUTE OCCLUSION

The incidence of acute occlusion following angioplasty remains at around 5%. The risk of acute closure is highest during the first few hours after angioplasty. If prolonged heparin is administered, the risk of acute occlusion may be postponed until the heparin is discontinued. Acute occlusions occurring during PTCA can generally be stabilized with prolonged inflations or stents. Those occurring later when the patient has left the catheterization laboratory are more troublesome, often resulting in an infarction or necessitating a repeat angioplasty. A 53-year-old man underwent angioplasty for an LAD stenosis (Fig. 145a), with a good result (Fig. 145b). Two hours later, an acute occlusion of the vessel occurred (Fig. 145c), which was redilated successfully. The long-term result was good, and a 4-year follow-up examination showed no restenosis (Fig. 145d). However, at that time he had a progession of the RCA disease, with a tandem stenosis (Fig. 145e) that was dilated with a 3.0-mm balloon with a resultant dissection (Fig. 145f). A few minutes later the vessel acutely occluded (Fig. 145g). The lesion was stented with a Palmaz-Schatz stent on a 4.0-mm balloon (Fig. 145h). The next morning the patient had acute chest pain, with ECG changes and a rise in CPK. Repeat angiography revealed an occlusion of the posterolateral branch of the RCA distal to the stent (Fig. 145i). This was successfully dilated (Fig. 145j). A 6-month reevaluation for chest pain revealed a restenosis of the distally dilated site (Fig. 145k), which was successfully redilated (Fig. 145l). It is possible that some patients are more prone to dissection and acute occlusion, although no parameters exist to identify them.

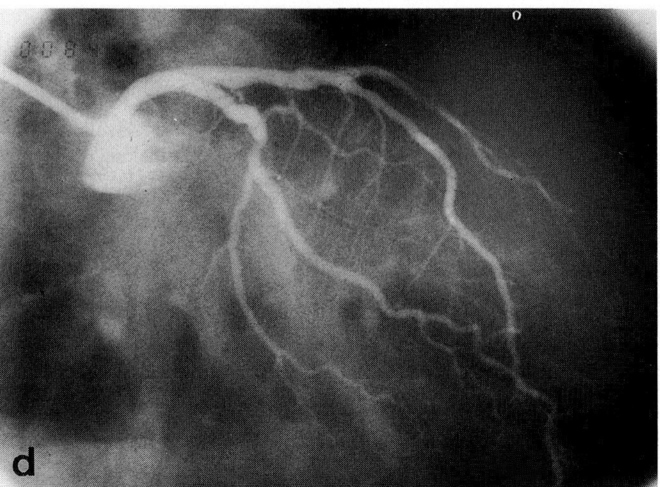

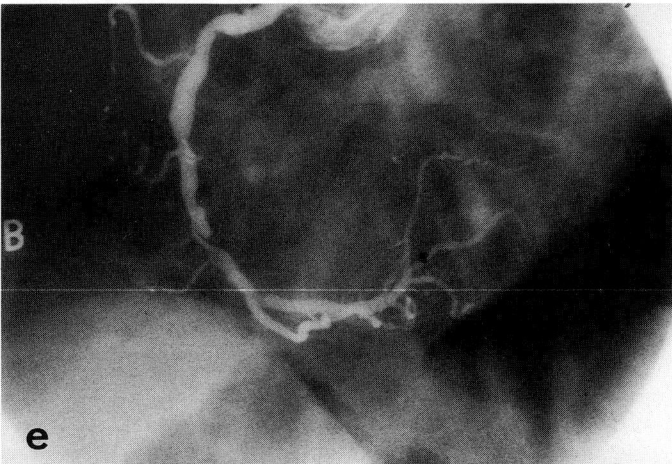

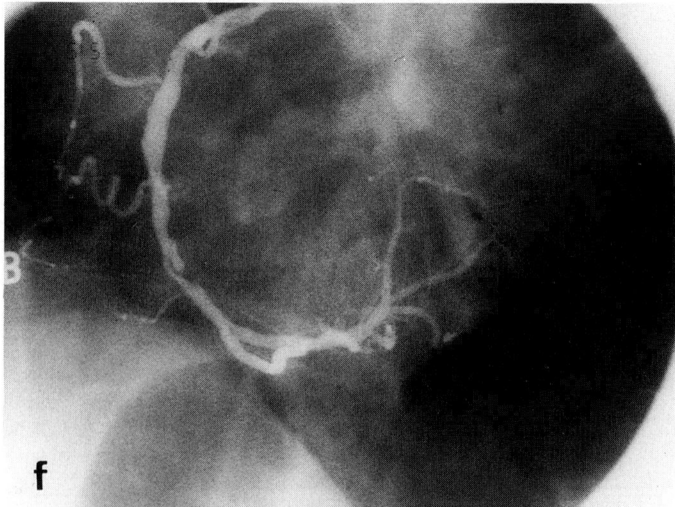

Figure 145 (Continued)

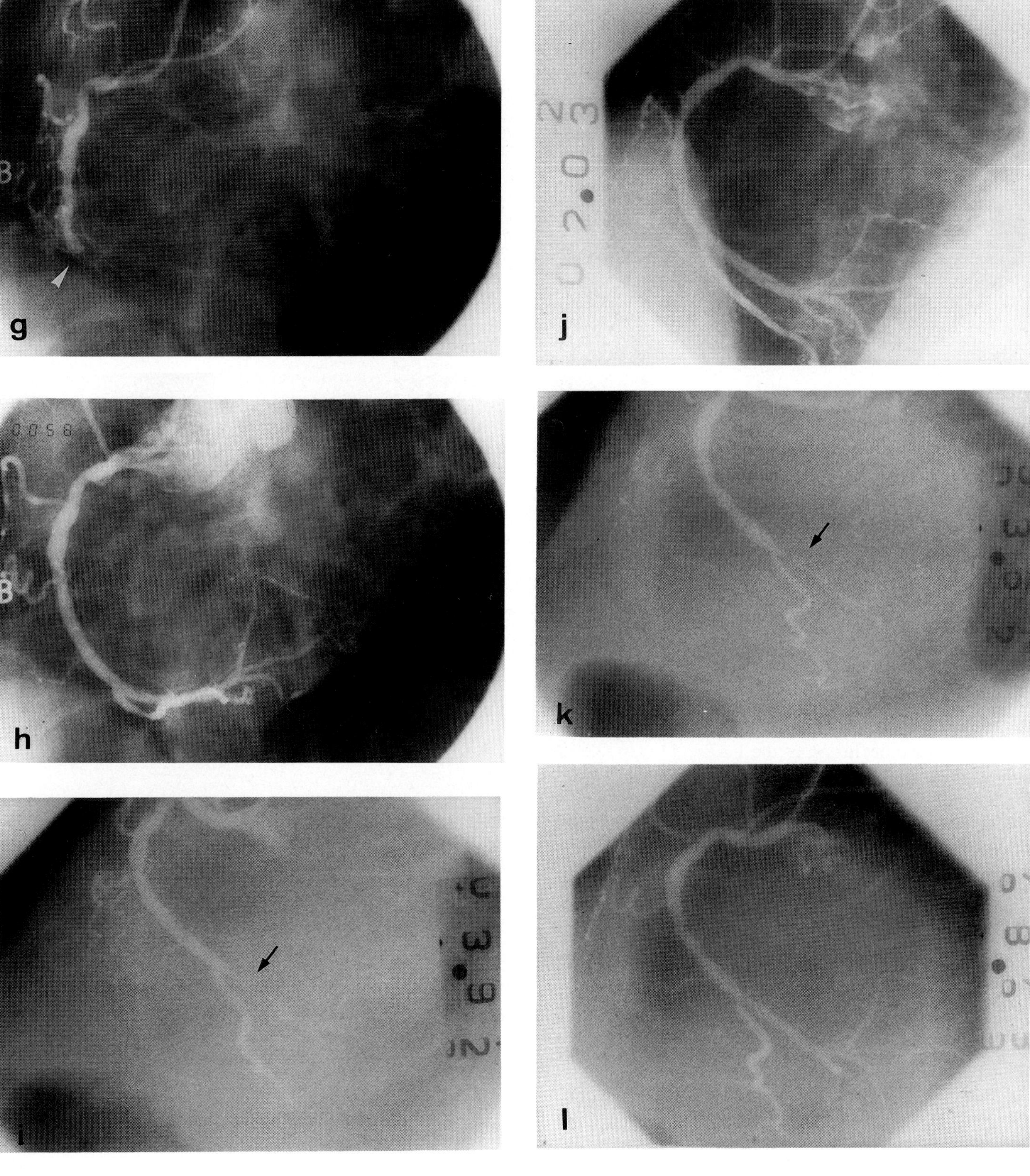

A 57-year-old man underwent angioplasty for a proximal LAD stenosis (Fig. 146a), with a good result (Fig. 146b). Six hours later, the femoral sheath was removed. The patient had a vagal episode during groin compression. Atropine was administered, to which the patient overreacted. His heart rate rose to 170 beats per minute and remained so for roughly 20 minutes. Finally, he slowed down but at the same time complained of chest pain. The ECG revealed ischemic changes in the anteroseptal leads (Fig. 146c). An emergency coronary angiogram revealed an acute occlusion of the LAD (Fig. 146d), which was redilated suc-

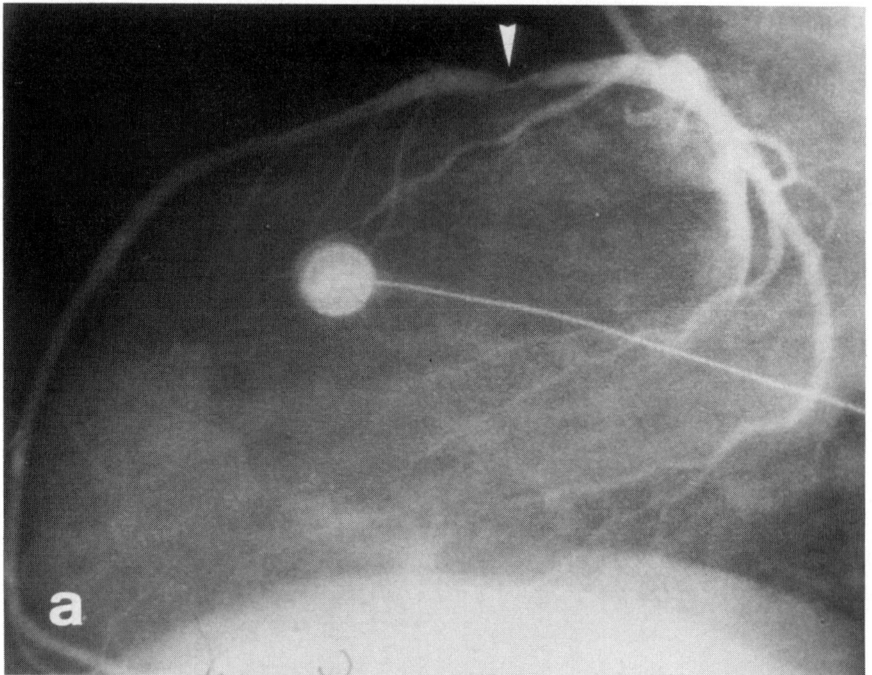

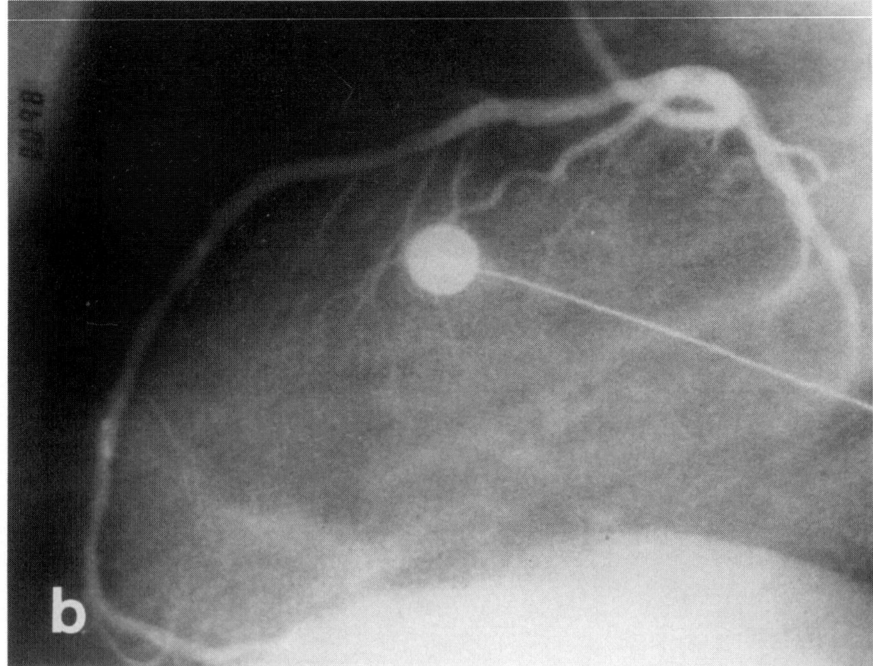

Figure 146

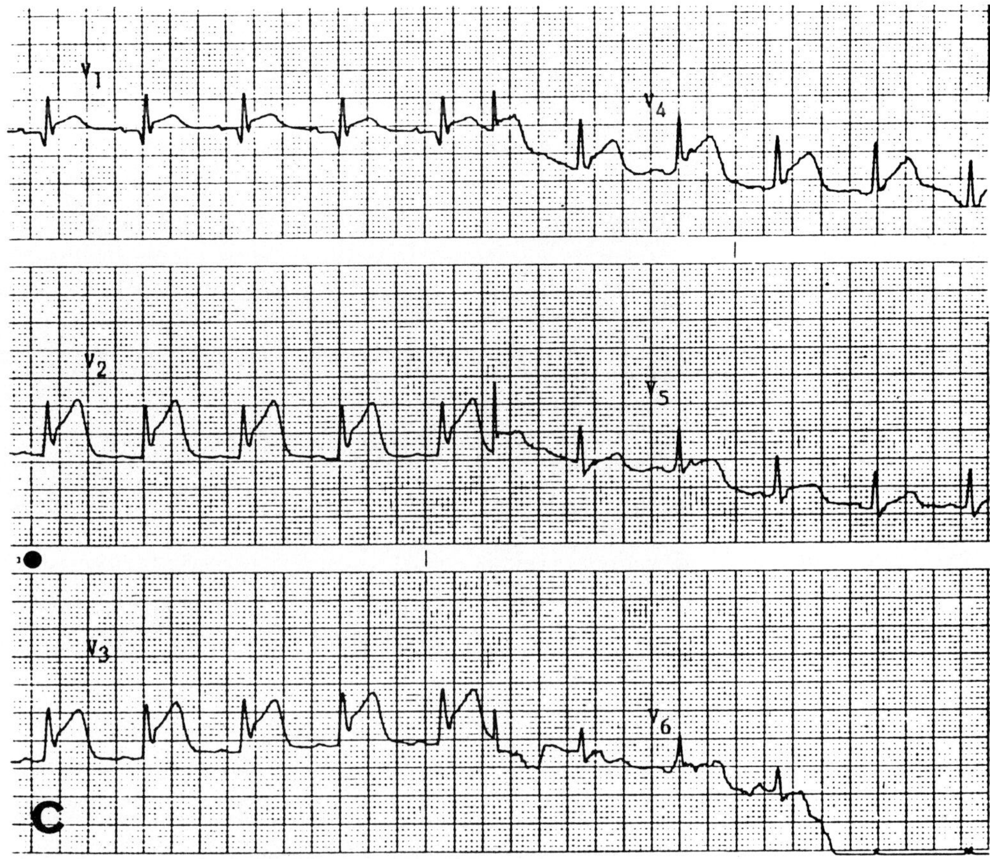
V1
V4
V2
V5
V3
V6
c

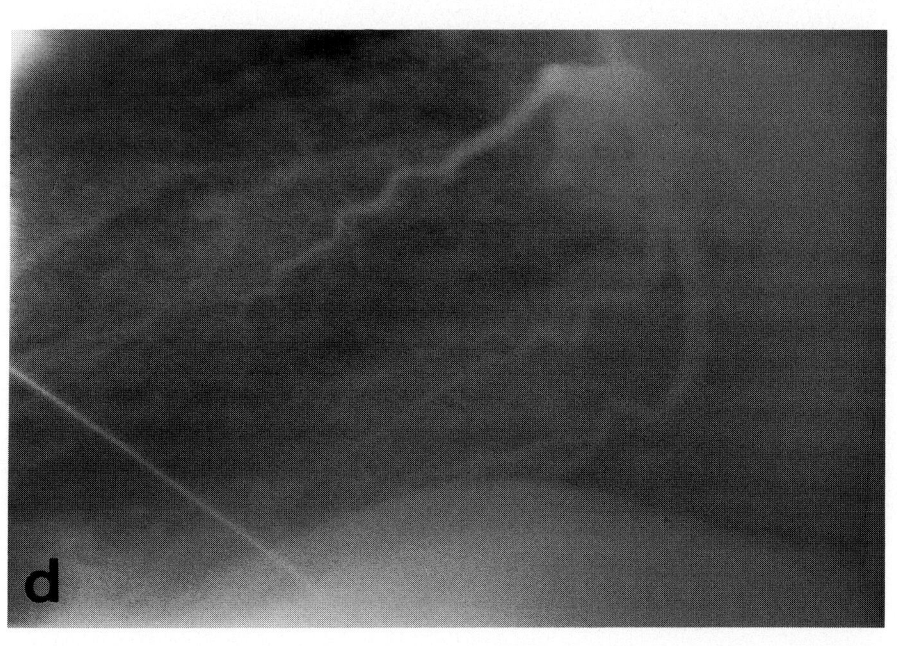
d

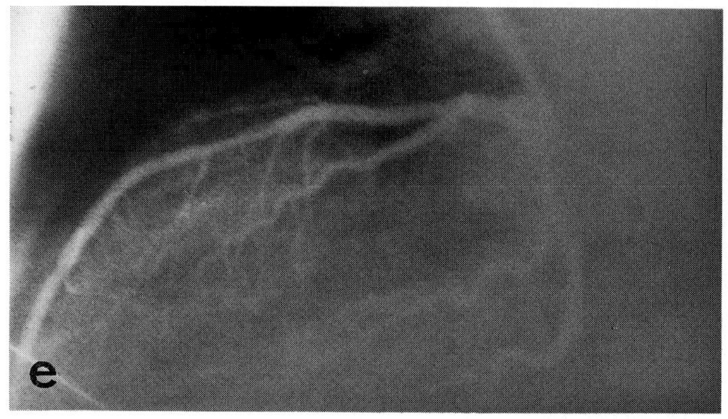

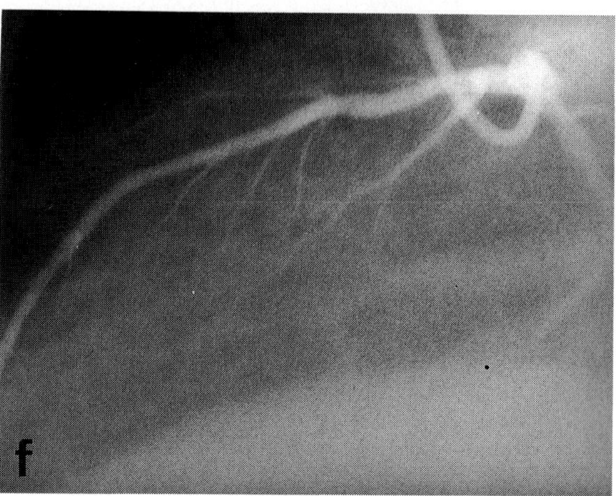

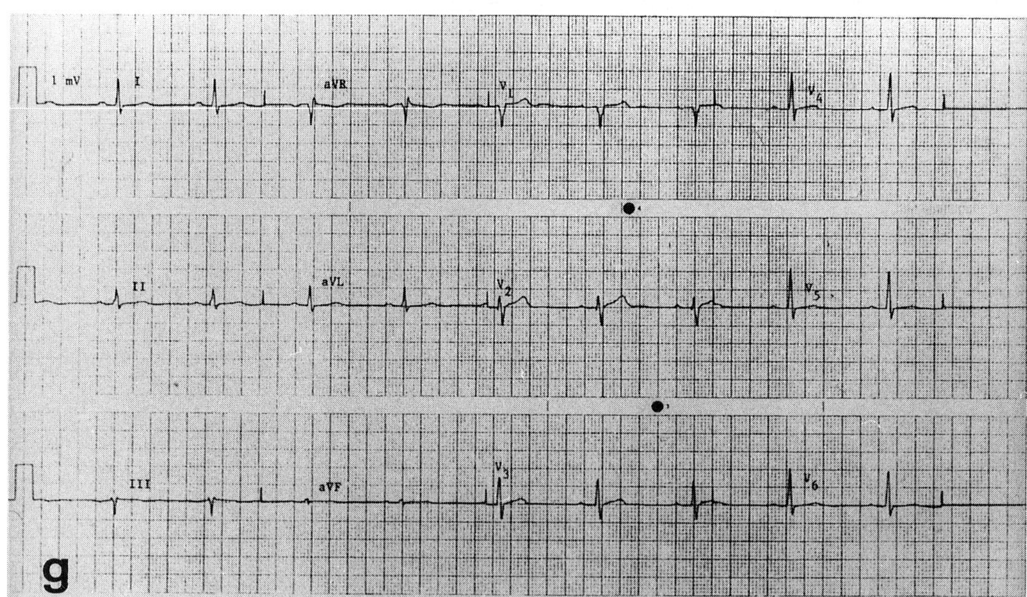

Figure 146 (Continued)

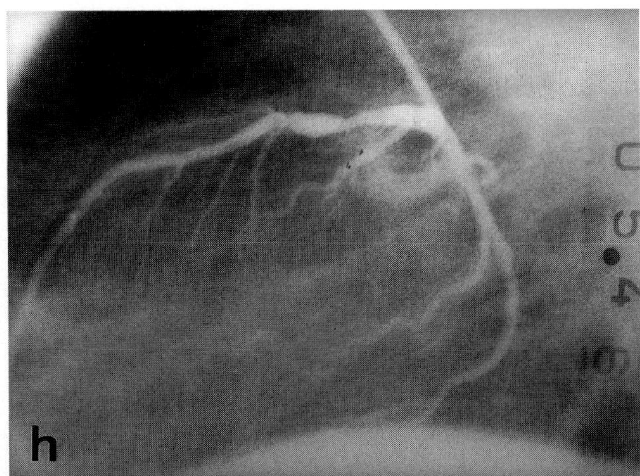

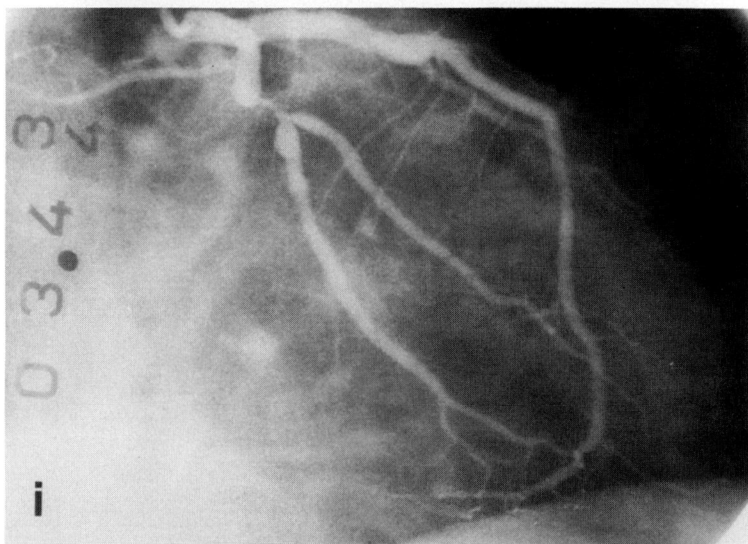

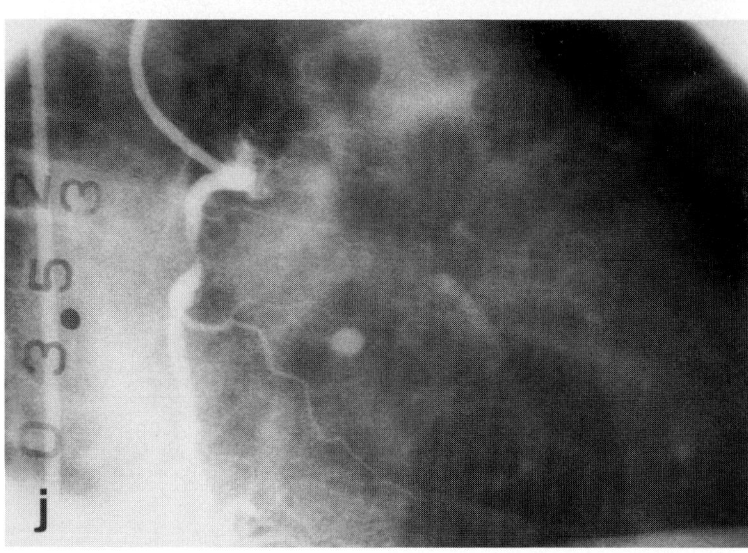

cessfully (Fig. 146e). The patient experienced a non-Q-wave myocardial infarction, with a peak CPK of 1800 units. A follow-up angiogram 2 days later showed a widely patent vessel (Fig. 146f). At a follow-up examination 3 months later the ECG was normal, with no evidence of the infarction (Fig. 146g), and the LAD was well open (Fig. 146h). A 4-year follow-up still showed the LAD in perfect condition (Fig. 146i). However, he had progressive disease of the LCx (Fig. 146i, arrowhead) and the RCA (Fig. 146j) for which he underwent CABG. Acute vessel occlusion is frequently a consequence of vagal hypotension secondary to groin, back, or bladder discomfort following PTCA. However, it may also occur due to inappropriate tachycardia following atropine administration, as illustrated in this case. This may be an argument against routinely administering atropine before femoral sheath removal. One of the assets of PTCA through an upper limb approach (axillary, brachial, or radial) is that it allows for immediate ambulation and is devoid of problems associated with best rest and groin complications.

5.3 SPASM

Coronary spasm can be initiated by the guiding catheter, balloon, or guidewire. A spasm occurring at or near the coronary ostium is usually guiding catheter related. A spasm at the dilated site is caused by mechanical irritation of the balloon, and a spasm distal to the dilated site is commonly attributable to the guidewire. Spasm may be localized, or diffuse, and appears commoner in the RCA. It may result in ongoing angina after balloon deflation or appearance of new stenoses, and it may confound the analysis of the angioplasty result.

Spasm can be reversed rapidly by the intracoronary administration of nitrates (e.g., nitroglycerin 0.2 mg), or calcium antagonists (e.g., nifedipine 0.2 mg), which have an additive effect

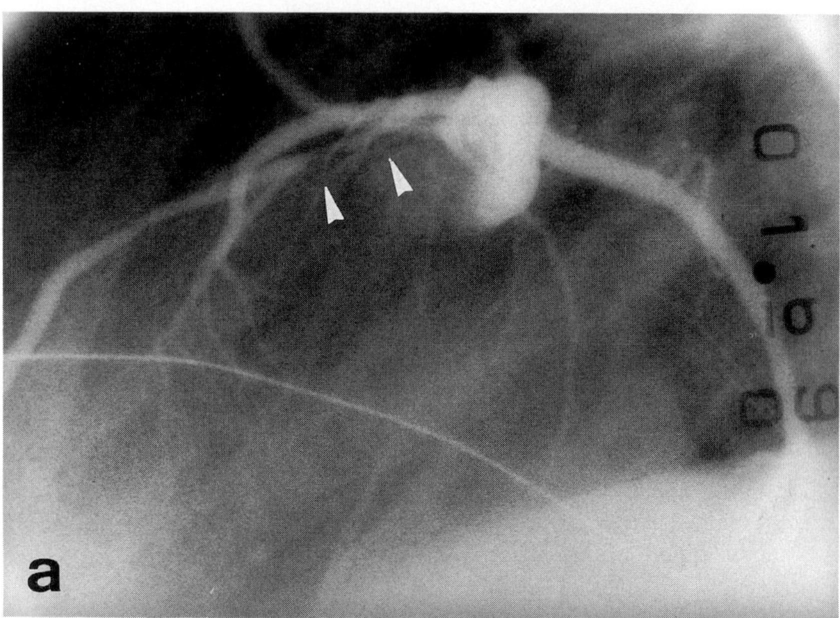

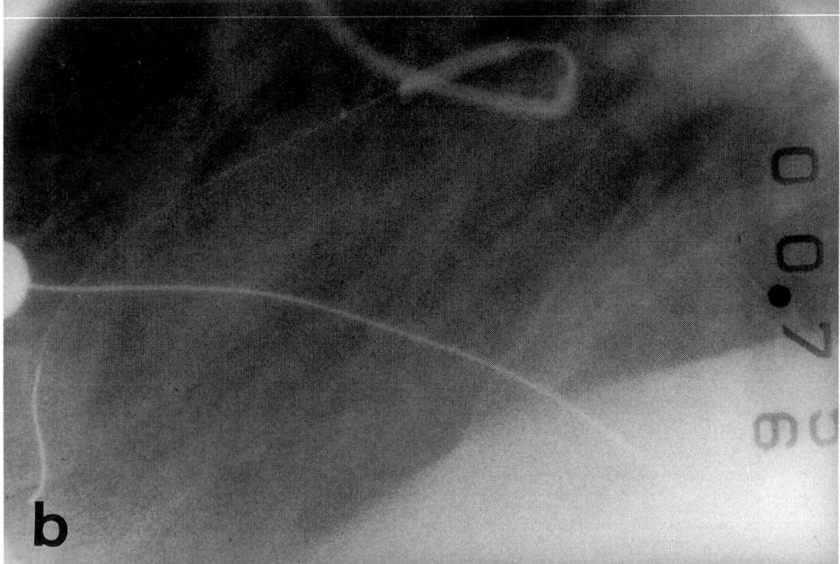

Figure 147

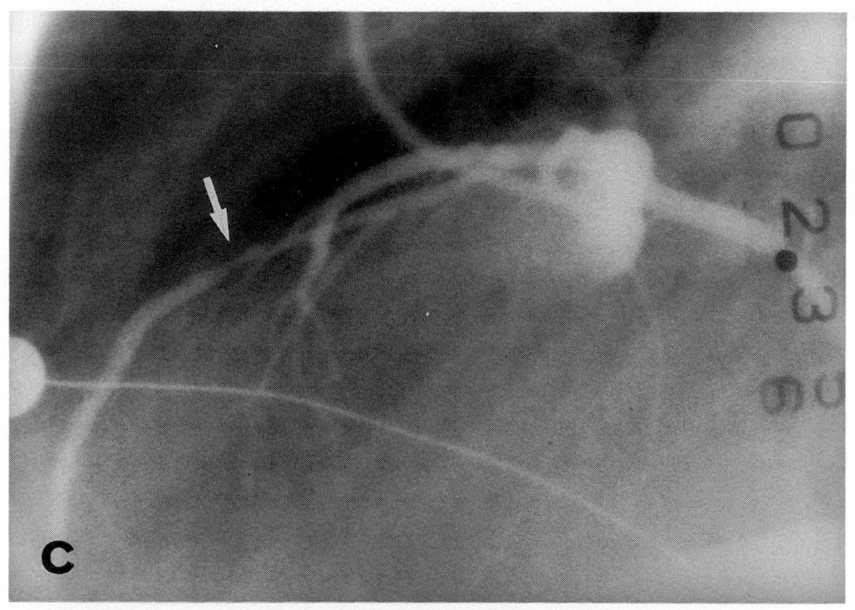

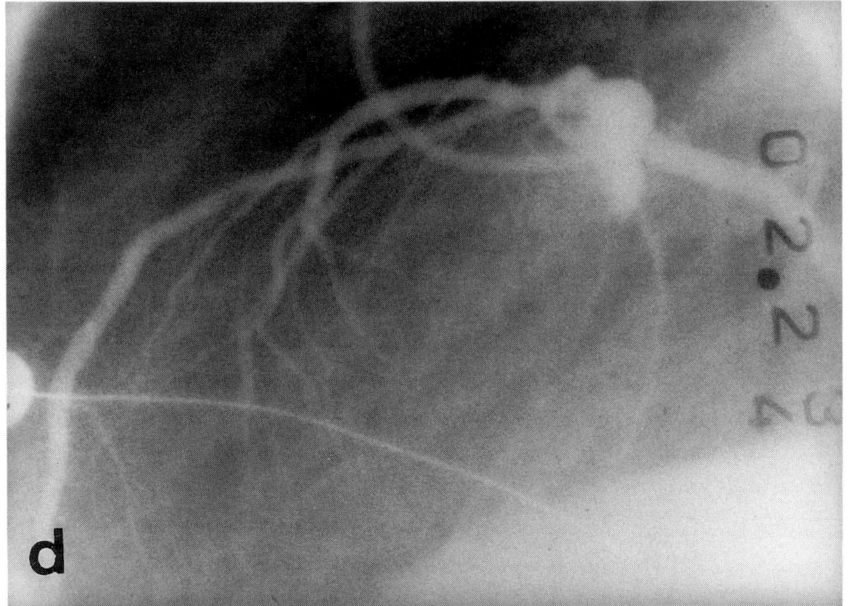

on nitrates. The solution of nifedipine is alcoholic. Hence its intracoronary injection is painful. If the guiding catheter is wedged during the administration of nifedipine, it has a propensity to induce ventricular fibrillation. Intracoronary nifedipine should therefore be flushed through with dye under fluoroscopic control to ensure that the coronary flow is not impaired. A 54-year-old man underwent angioplasty of a proximal LAD stenosis (Fig. 147a) with an over-the-wire system (Fig. 147b). After withdrawal of the wire, a stenosis was seen distal to the dilated site (Fig. 147c, arrow), which had not been present on the diagnostic film (Fig. 147a). Spasm was identified by the disappearance of the lesion following 0.2 mg of intracoronary nitroglycerin (Fig. 147d). To reduce the occurrence of spasm, all patients should receive nitrates prior to angioplasty.

A 50-year-old man with a stenosis of the first diagonal branch of the LAD (Fig. 148a) underwent angioplasty with an ACS floppy wire, which coiled distal to the stenosis (Fig. 148b). After successful angioplasty of the lesion, a spasm was seen distal to the dilated site (Fig. 148c), corresponding to the place where the wire had coiled. The spasm responded to 0.2 mg of intracoronary nifedipine (Fig. 148d).

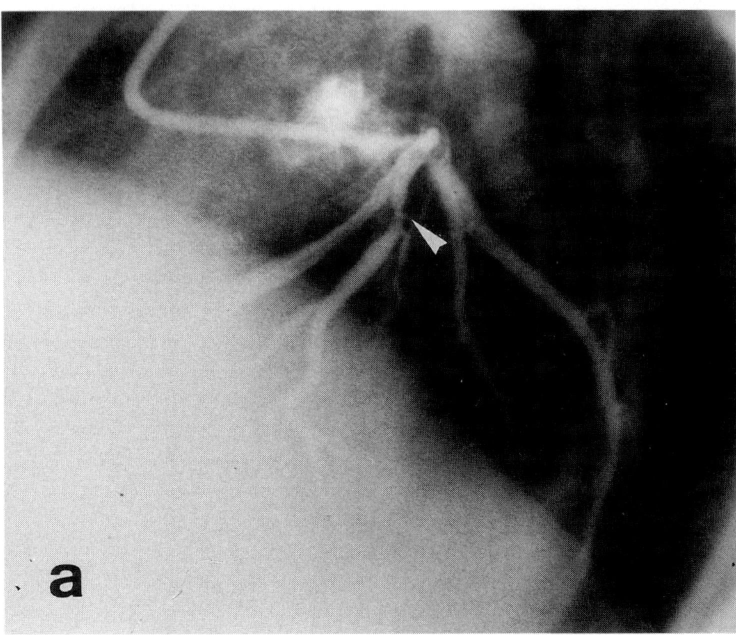

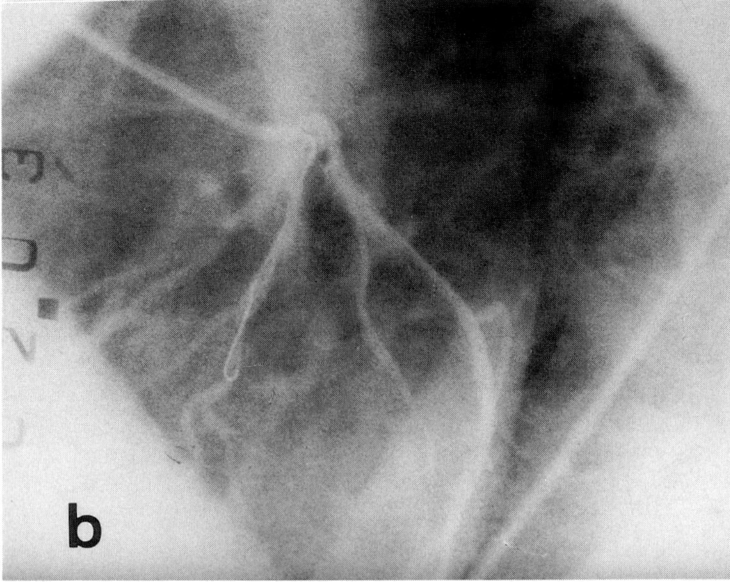

Figure 148

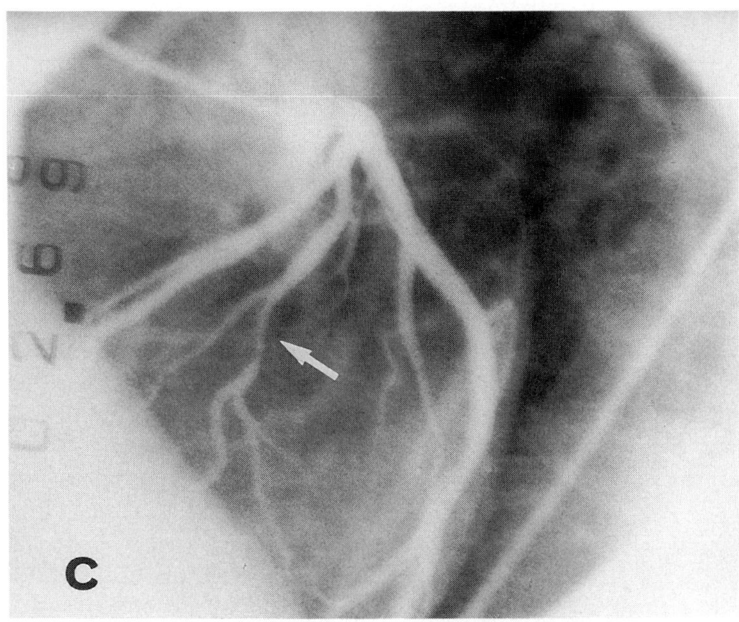
c

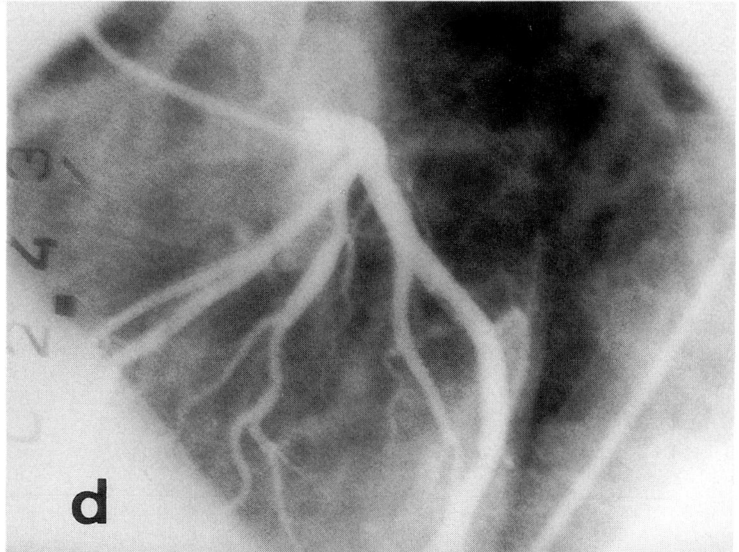
d

Occasionally, the entire vessel may be spastic, as in this patient following angioplasty of a tight LAD stenosis (Fig. 149a). The droplike thrombus distal to the stenosis in this setting is a benign finding and does not increase procedural risks, unlike other thrombus-containing lesions. Its contribution to the ensuing spasm is unlikely. Following angioplasty the entire LAD filled poorly (Fig. 149b). A differential diagnosis of such a picture is long dissection. However, in this case the cause was spasm, as evident by the good result following an intracoronary injection of nitroglycerin (Fig. 149c).

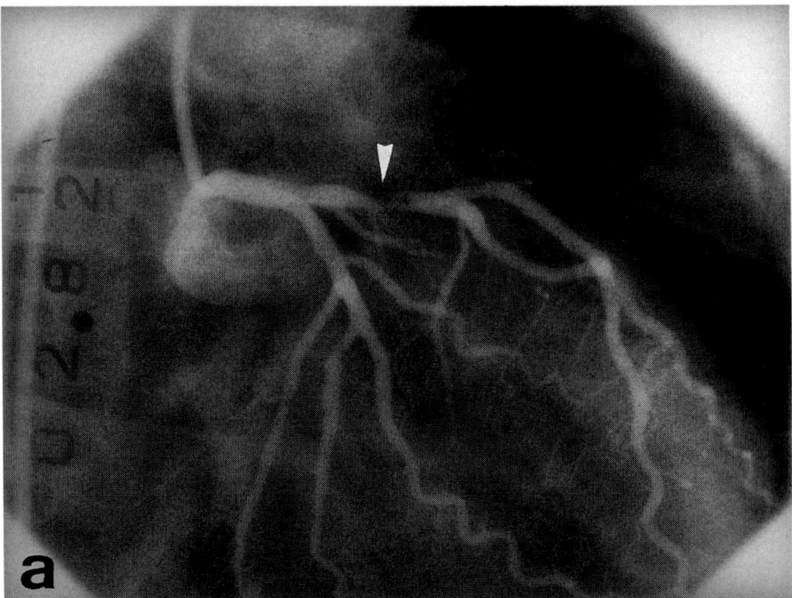

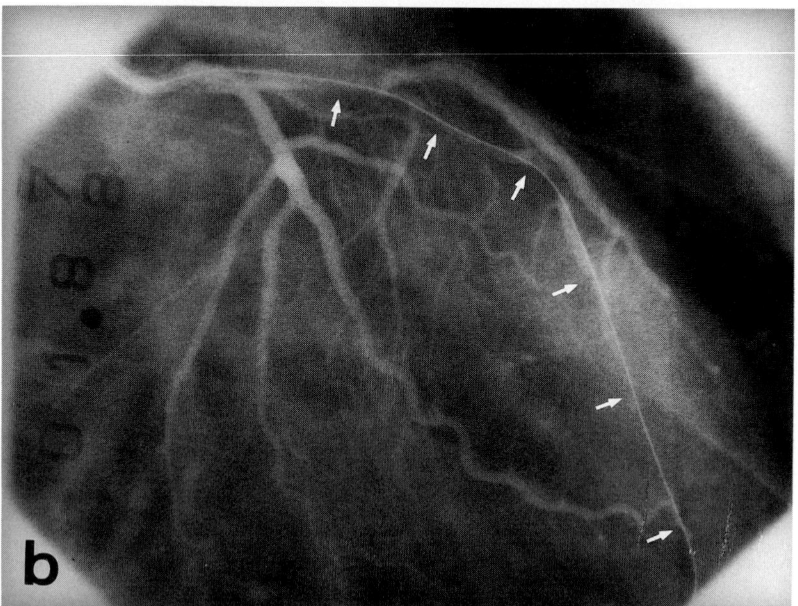

Figure 149

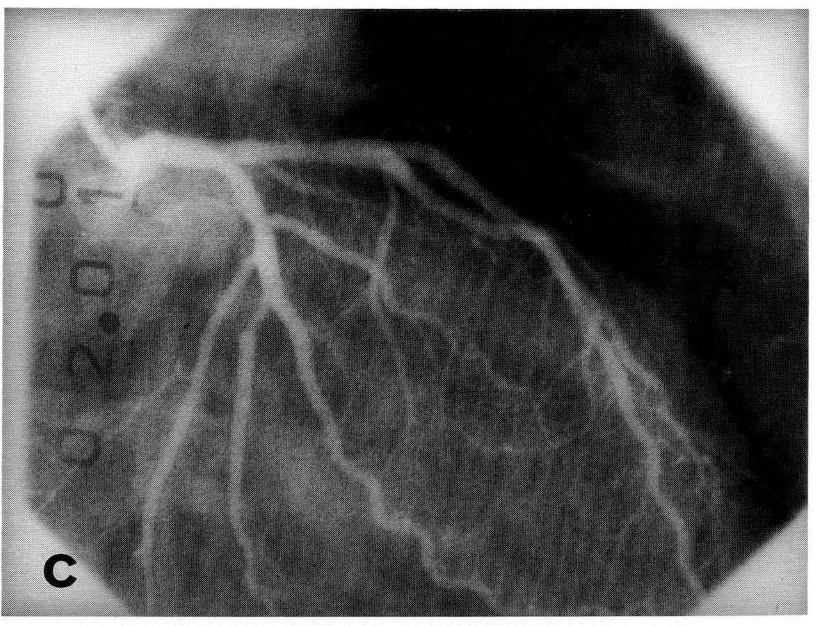

Figure 149 (Continued)

5.4 SIDE BRANCH OCCLUSION

Almost half of all angioplasties will involve a side branch, which will be overlapped by the balloon catheter. Balloon inflations generally do not adversely affect side branches that are not involved in the stenosis. Side branches that do occlude have a high potential for spontaneous recanalization. An infarction may nevertheless take place but it is generally small and often inconsequential. The risk of side branch occlusion is higher if the stenosis of the target vessel involves the origin of the side branch. A large side branch in this setting may need to be protected with a kissing wire or a kissing balloon technique (see Section 3.11). A 62-year-old man underwent angioplasty for an LAD stenosis, located just distal to the first diagonal branch (Fig. 150a). The LAD result was good, but the diagonal branch occluded (Fig. 150b). The patient suffered a small myocardial infarction (peak CPK 540 units), with minor ECG changes. A 16-month follow-up examination showed a good long-term result of the LAD lesion, and the side branch had recovered (Fig. 150c).

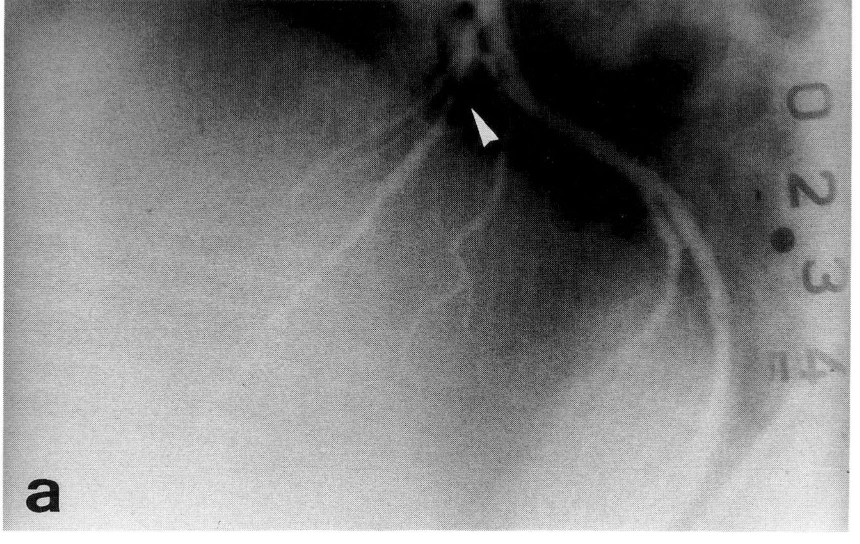

Figure 150

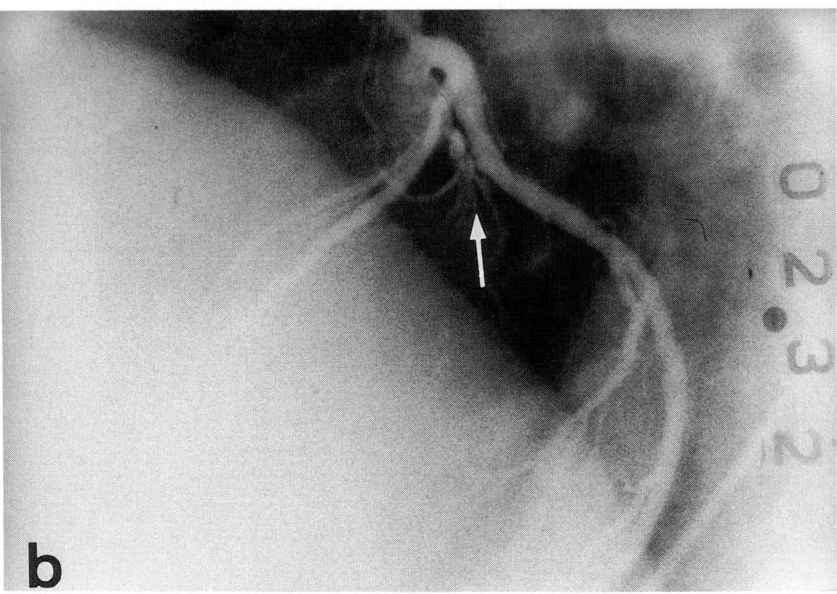

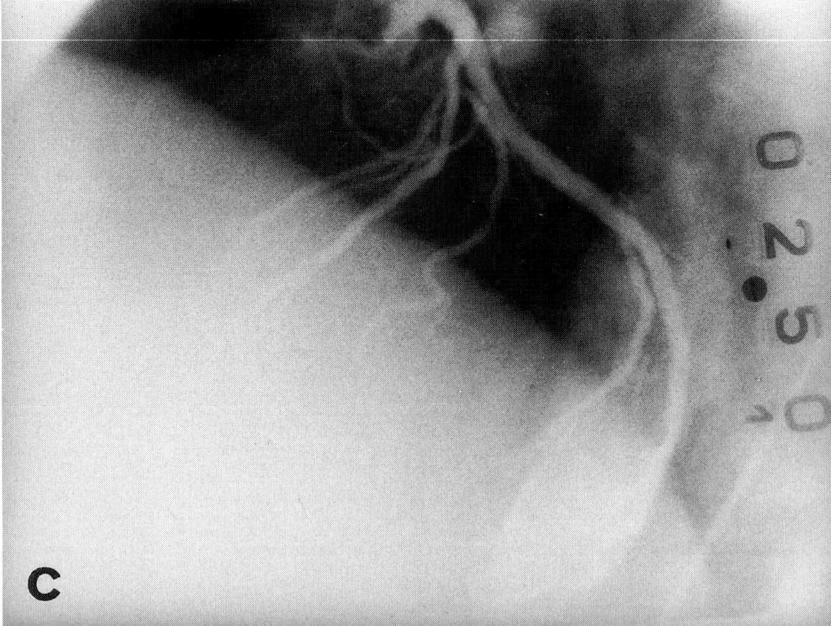

Figure 150 (Continued)

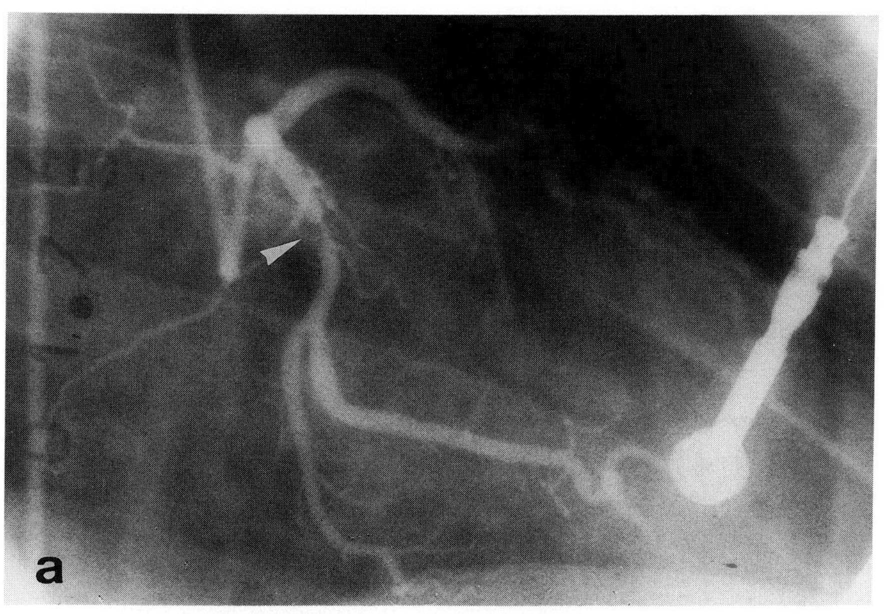

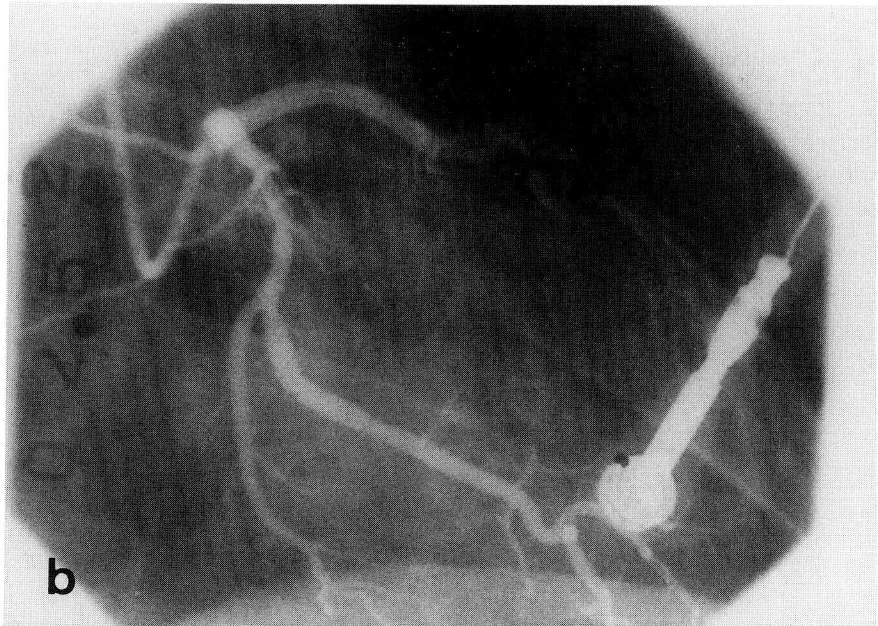

Figure 151

Occlusion of side branches can sometimes occur at a distance to the angioplasty site secondary to long dissections. Fortunately, this almost invariably involves branches that are downstream of the lesion. A 50-year-old man underwent angioplasty for a proximal LCx stenosis (Fig. 151a) with a good result (Fig. 151b). One hour following the procedure he experienced an acute occlusion of the vessel (Fig. 151c). Repeat angioplasty resulted in reopening of the vessel, but the LCx artery distal to the major marginal branch was occluded (Fig. 151d), probably related to distal extension of the dissection. However, the patient did not experience a myocardial infarction. He either had collaterals from the RCA, prompt spontaneous recanalization, or both. A 3-month follow-up study revealed restenosis at the angioplasty site (Fig. 151e), and reappearance of the distal LCx which had previously been occluded (curved arrow). Figure 151f shows the left ventricle in systole preangioplasty and at 3-month follow-up (Fig. 151g), revealing no regional wall motion abnormality.

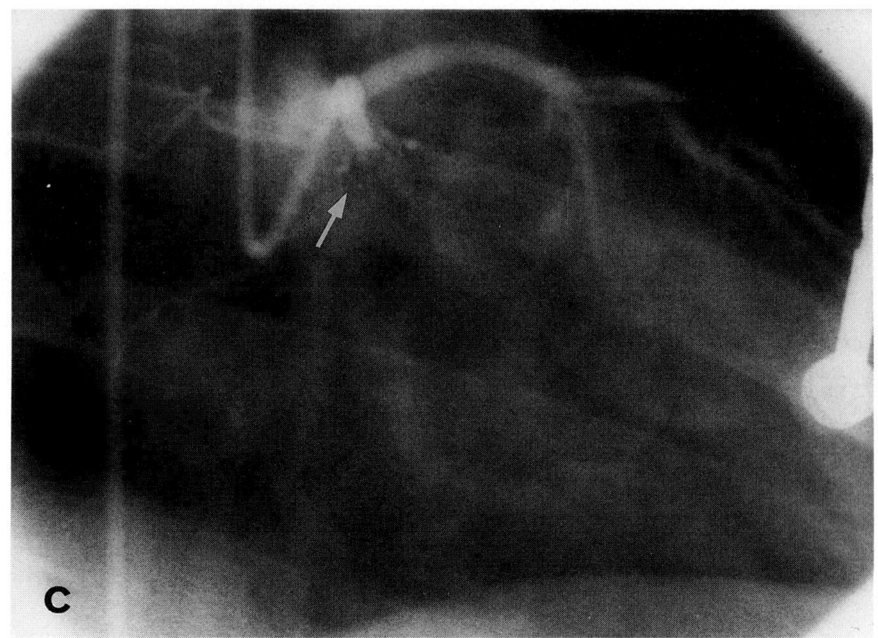

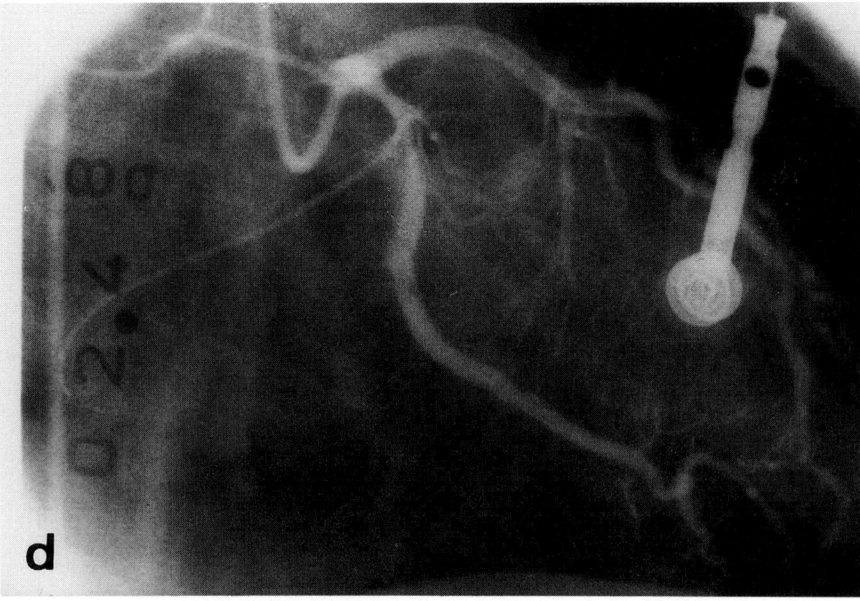

Figure 151 (Continued)

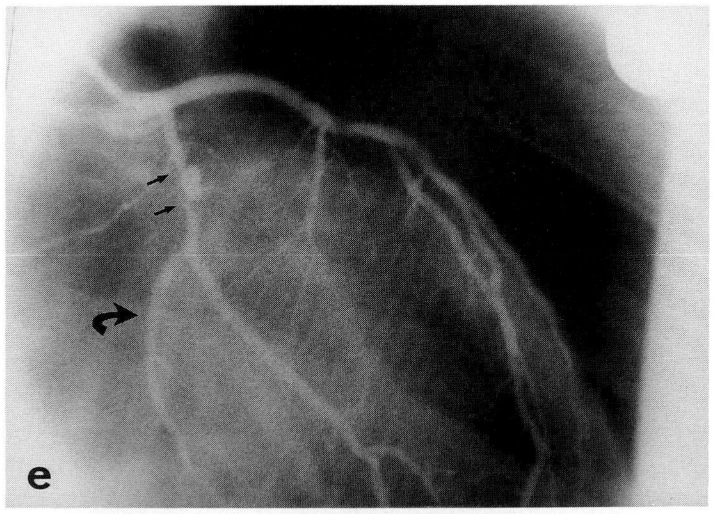
e

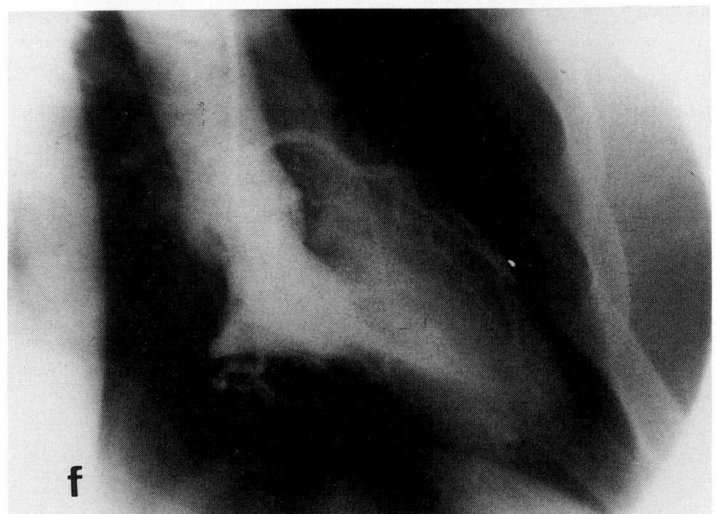
f

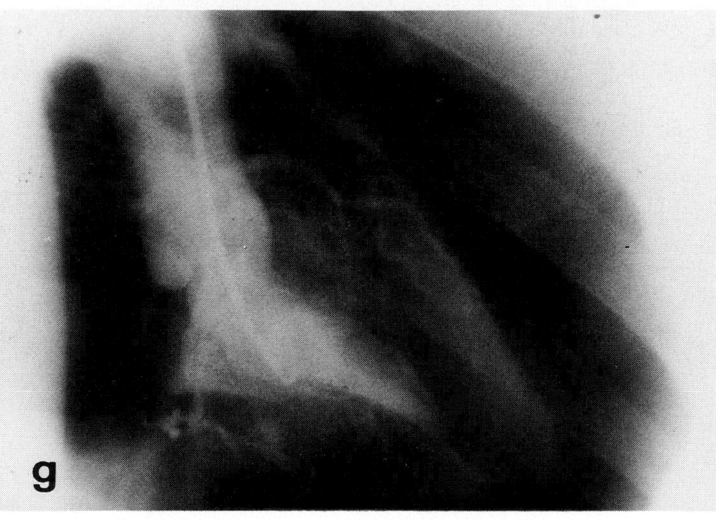
g

5.5 THROMBOSIS

Thrombosis is a rare complication since generous heparinization is routine during angioplasty. We administer 20,000 units of heparin routinely to all PTCA patients at the beginning of the procedure. Others start with smaller doses and add heparin to maintain the activated clotting time (ACT) above 350 seconds. However, thrombosis remains a hazard with poor flow and may occasionally occur with adequate flow if administration of heparin is erroneously omitted or given in inadequate dosage. Patients with unstable angina or recent myocardial infarction tend to require higher heparin doses. Rarely, a thrombus may form in the guiding catheter tip and embolize distally.

Another mechanism is embolism from a thrombotic plaque as in unstable angina, acute infarction, or old venous grafts. Such a thrombus can sometimes embolize into a vessel other than the one dilated. A 58-year-old man underwent angioplasty for a recently occluded diagonal branch of the LAD (Fig. 152a). The procedure was successful; however, once the balloon was withdrawn the patient started

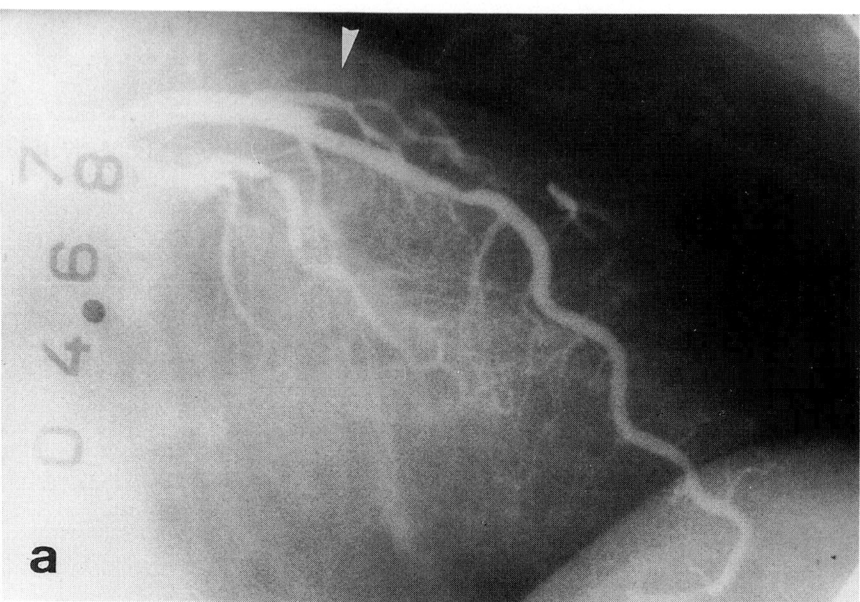

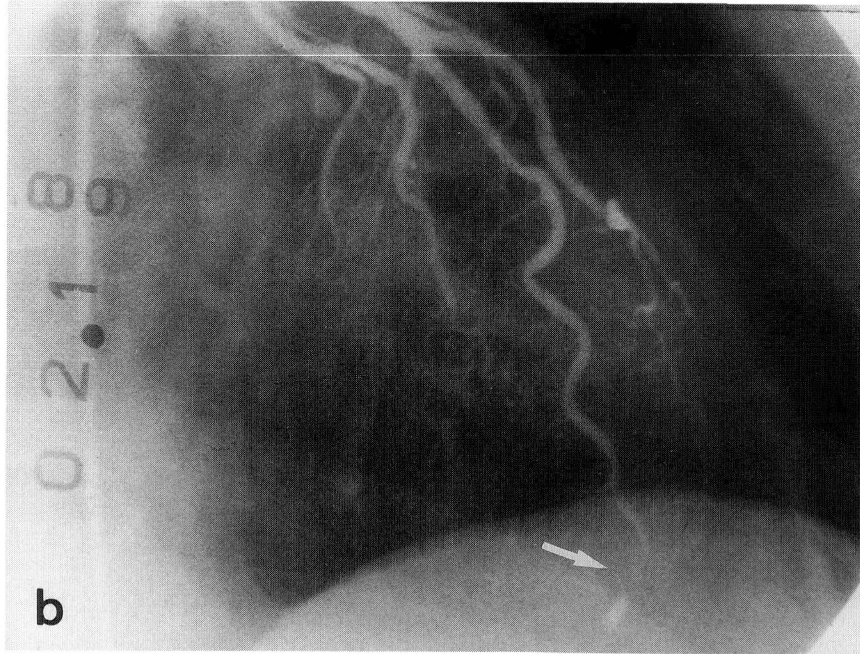

Figure 152

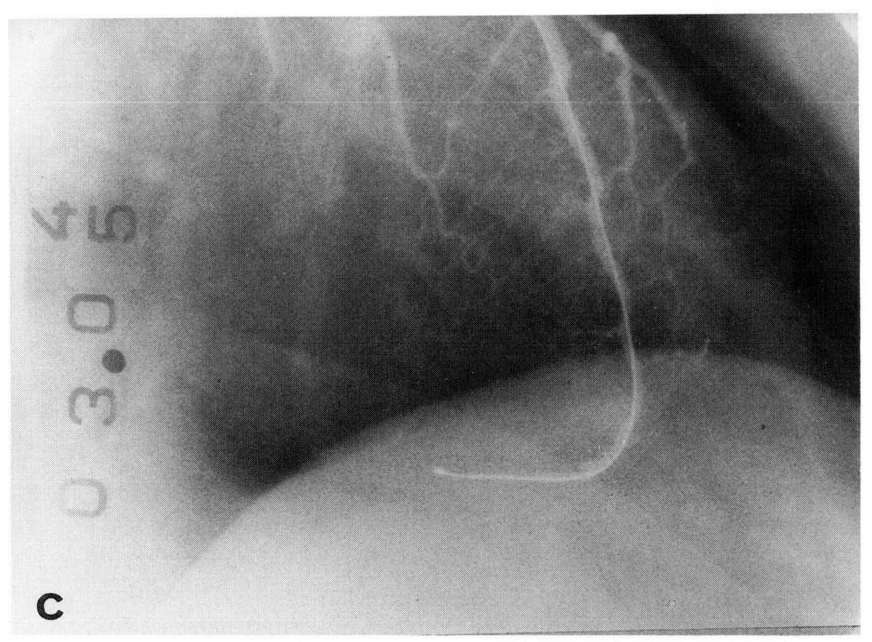

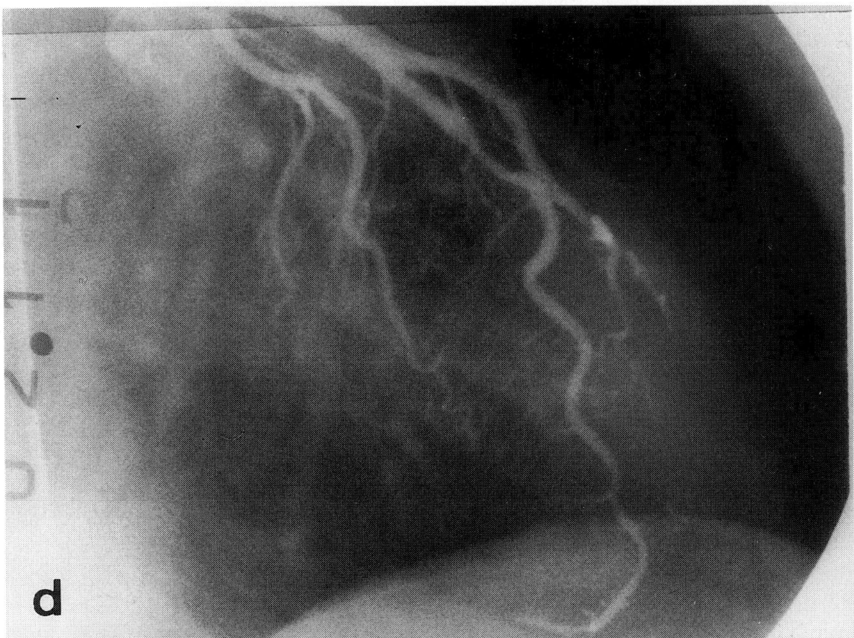

complaining of chest pain. An angiogram revealed occlusion of the distal LAD (Fig. 152b). This event probably occurred because the thrombus associated with the diagonal occlusion was pulled back by the balloon, and subsequently embolized down the LAD. This embolism was treated by advancing the Magnum guide wire down the LAD (Fig. 152c), thereby pushing the thrombus distally (Fig. 152d). The patient suffered only a small rise in CPK, with no ECG changes. This case demonstrates one way a thrombus can embolize, and a possible treatment for this event. A thrombus may also embolize down the dilated vessel. However, this event is generally less dangerous than embolization down another, uninvolved vessel. Pushing the thrombus down the vessel thereby fragmenting it is usually sufficient to solve the problem. Adjunctive thrombolytic therapy may also be administered if the thrombus is assumed to be fresh.

Other rare thromboembolic complications of angioplasty are a thrombosis of the femoral artery at the puncture site, or even rarer, an occlusion of a distal leg vessel by an embolus. A young patient benefited from a successful coronary angioplasty. An 8F femoral introducer sheath was left in place overnight while the patient received intravenous heparin. The next morning, heparin was stopped and the sheath was removed 4 hours later. The patient complained about claudication in his right calf upon mobilization. He was not taken seriously until a few weeks later a physician noticed absent right pedal pulses. An embolic occlusion of the right popliteal artery was documented (Fig. 153a) and treated with angioplasty with a good angiographic (Fig. 153b) and clinical result. A thrombus had probably formed in the introducer sheath and had been milked out during sheath removal and embolized down the leg. This speaks in favor of not routinely leaving sheaths overnight unless necessary, and of using sheaths that do not get squeezed upon removal. Another way of preventing this sort of accident is to reinsert the obturator into a sheath that is to be left in place. This, however, harbors risks more important than the one it should prevent. The iliac artery may be perforated during reintroduction of the obturator unless a safety wire is used, and the obturator may have been contaminated on the table during the case and cause infection. Some companies provide an additional, blunt-tipped soft obturator along with the femoral sheath for this purpose. Use of such an obturator may prevent these complications.

5.6 AIR EMBOLISM

Air embolism is preventable, but it happens to all invasive cardiologists. Air may stem from leaks in the contrast injection system or from rupture of a balloon containing air. The presence of an air bubble may be seen clearly during a contrast injection, and readily explains subsequent pain and ECG changes. However, if air has been injected unnoticed (e.g., during flushing of the catheter system, from a ruptured balloon, etc.), its sequelae can be a vexing diagnostic problem. Occasionally, a large vessel may get occluded by the air bubble, in which case a sharp cutoff is seen. In others, especially if the air has migrated distally, the presence of air can be suspected by sluggish coronary blood flow in selected vessel areas. Air will ultimately get dissolved in the blood, but a bubble of air that impairs blood flow may persist for a long time. Although small amounts of air are relatively harmless, larger air emboli can be fatal.

A 49-year-old male underwent angioplasty for a proximal LAD stenosis with a 3.5-mm fixed-wire balloon. The balloon burst at 14 bar, following which the patient complained of severe chest pain. An angiogram revealed an abrupt cutoff of the LAD (Fig. 154a, arrowhead) distal to the dilated site (arrow). Embolism of the air trapped within the balloon was diagnosed, and 0.2 mg intracoronary nifedipine administered. This resulted in rapid disappearance of the chest pain, and the control angiogram revealed a normal patient LAD (Fig. 154b).

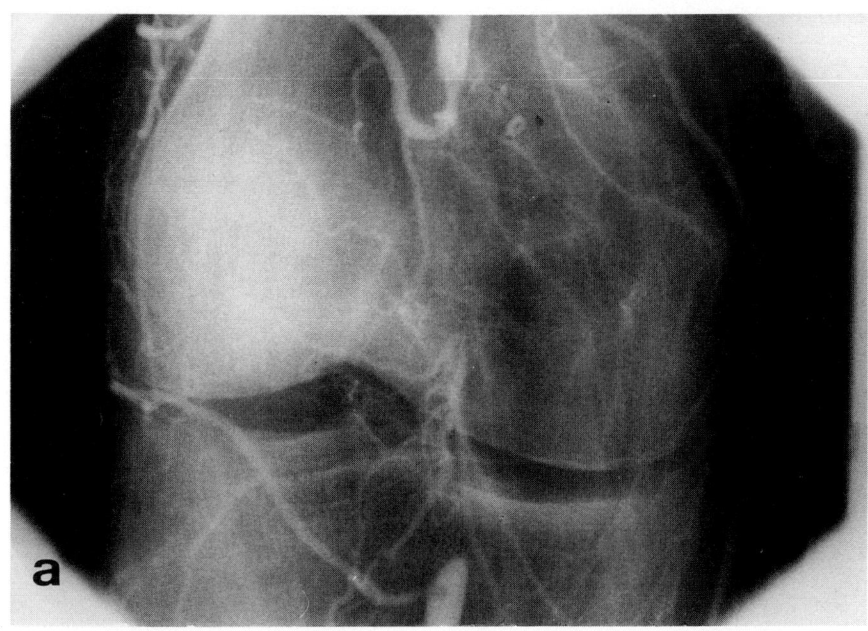

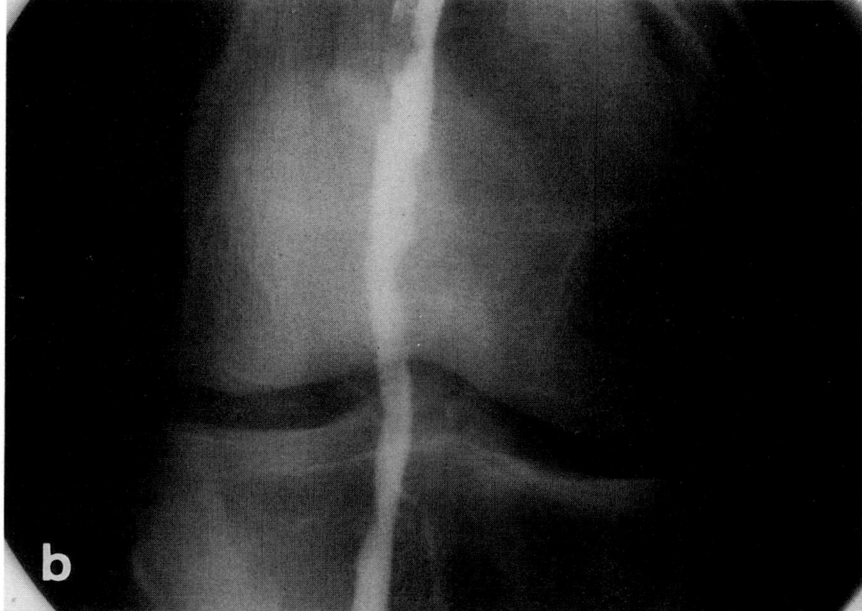

Figure 153

The consequences of air embolism are reversed more quickly if the affected vessel is vigorously flushed. Administration of vasodilators increases coronary blood flow and speeds up dissolution of the trapped air. In case of hypotension or bradycardia, cardiac massage may become necessary to "pump" the air through the coronary arteries. If this does not succeed, because large amounts of air have been injected, an end-hole catheter or a non-Monorail balloon can be utilized to aspirate the air.

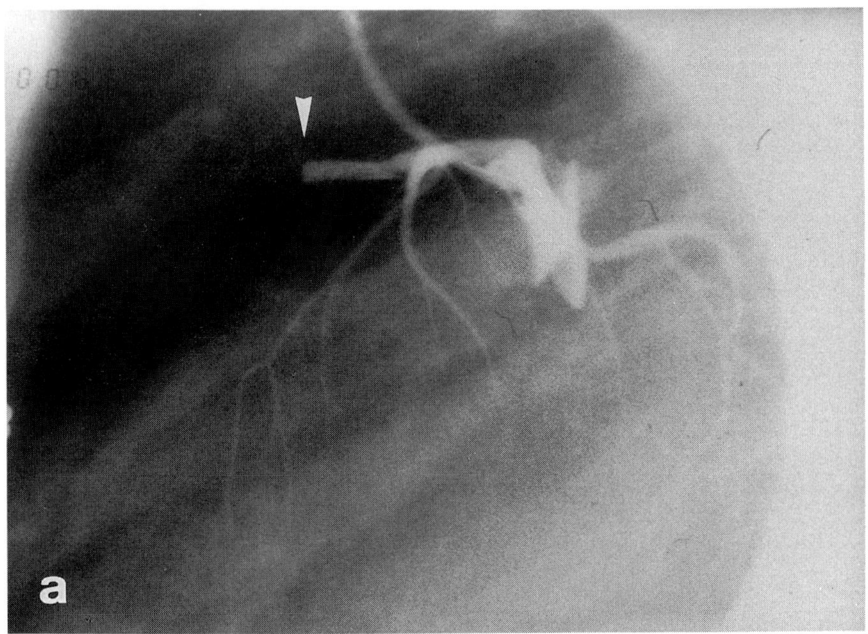

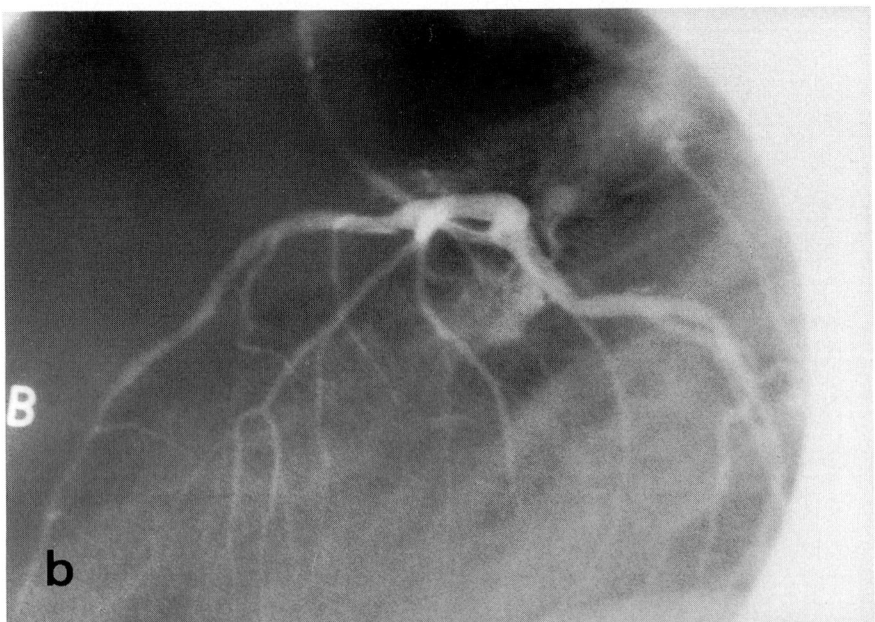

Figure 154

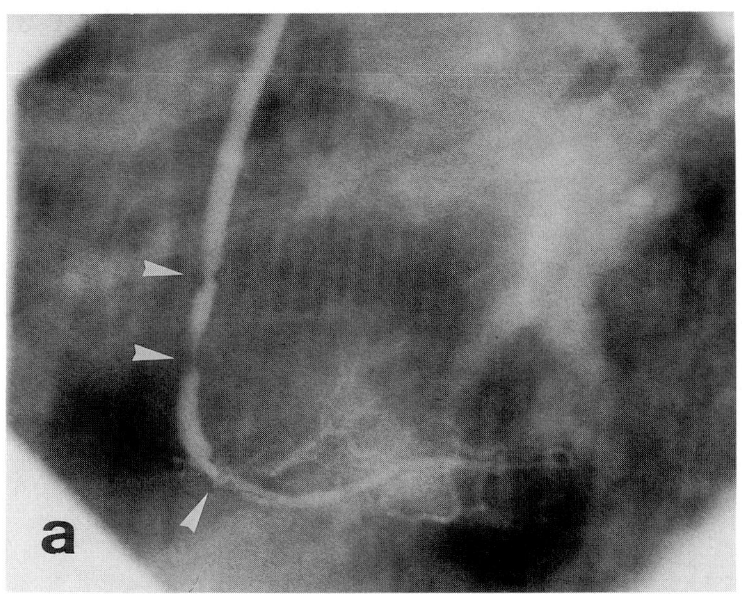

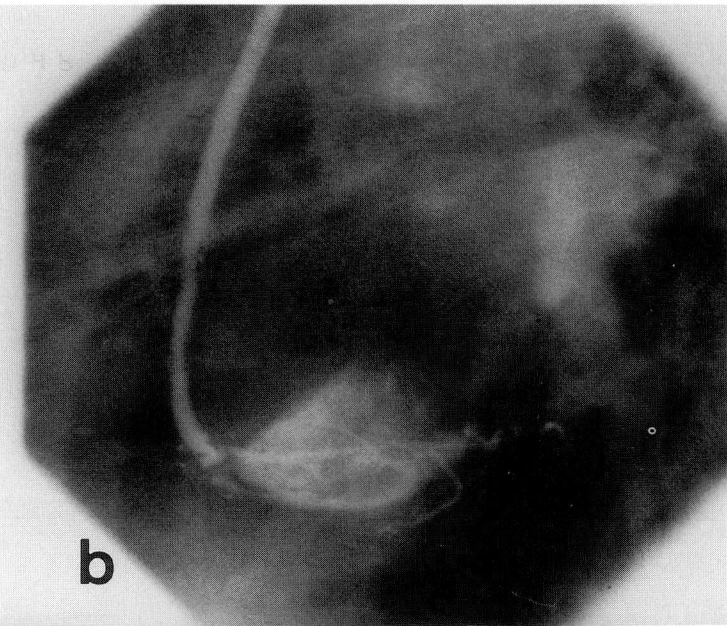

Figure 155

5.7 PERFORATION AND RUPTURE

Perforation of a vessel by the coronary guidewire may go unnoticed. More dangerous is a vessel rupture secondary to balloon inflation. A rupture or pinhole of the balloon, or dilatation with an oversized balloon, may lead to extravasation of dye without clinical sequelae. A 72-year-old man underwent angioplasty for a diseased venous graft to the RCA (Fig. 155a). Attempts to dilate a tough stenosis at the distal anastomotic site with the 3.5-mm balloon used for the graft and a high balloon pressure led to balloon rupture and dye extravasation (Fig. 155b). In such a situation, the danger of hemopericardium and tamponade is small, especially if the dye remains localized to the same site over several minutes of observation. The patient was observed in the intensive care unit. An echocardiogram ruled out the presence of pericardial fluid, and subsequent recovery was uneventful.

6
Stenting

6.1
BAIL-OUT STENTING

Bail-out stenting refers to a situation where stent is utilized to improve on an inadequate angioplasty result. The stent provides mechanical support to the vessel and helps to tack up a dissection. Indications include dissections that cannot be stabilized by prolonged balloon dilatations, inadequate results due to a thrombus at the dilated site, and immediate relapse of the dilated stenosis. A variety of stents have been developed, the most widely used being the Palmaz-Schatz stent (Johnson & Johnson). Stents have had a tremendous influence on the management of menacing dissections and acute closures. Their utilization is bound to increase markedly, as it emerges that coumadin treatment may not be as essential as thought initially and that restenosis rates are significantly reduced by stents. The prospect of making the dilated lesion look perfect in a predictable manner by implanting a stent, having the patient leave the hospital the next day on antiplatelet therapy alone, and having a reduced risk of recurrence is highly appealing.

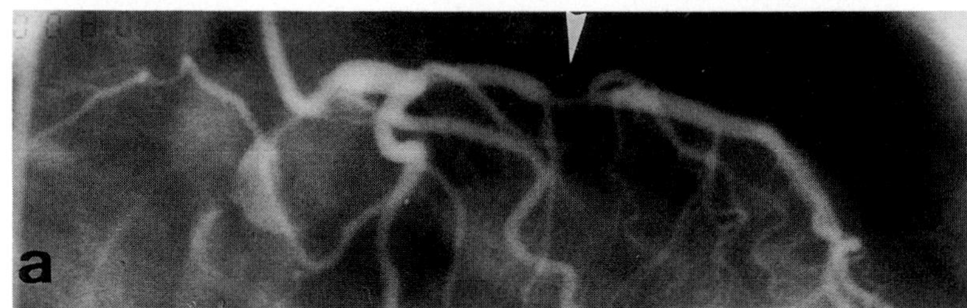

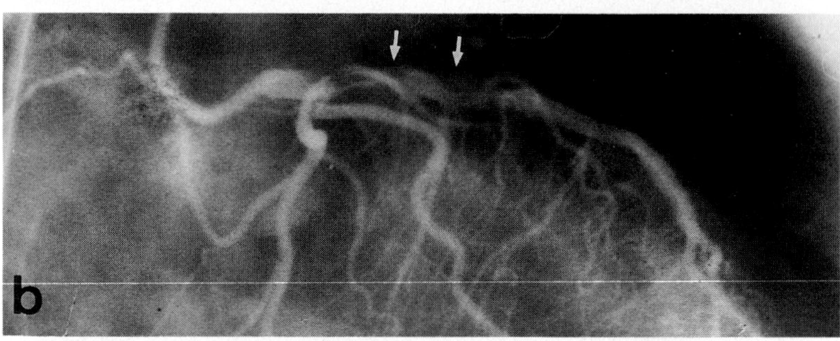

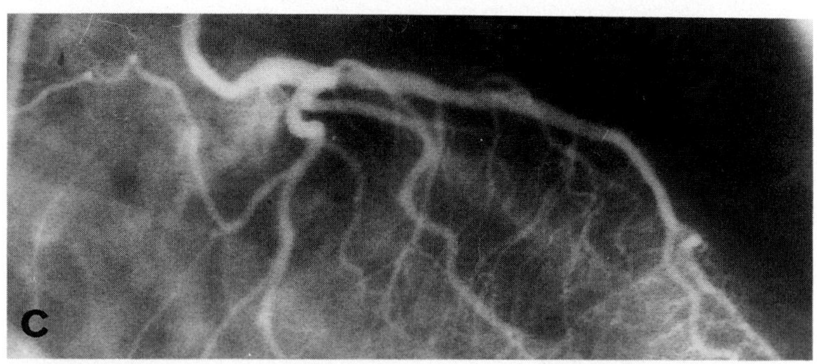

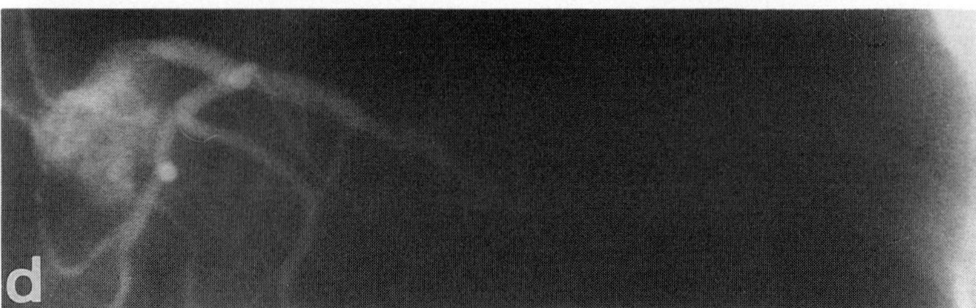

Figure 156

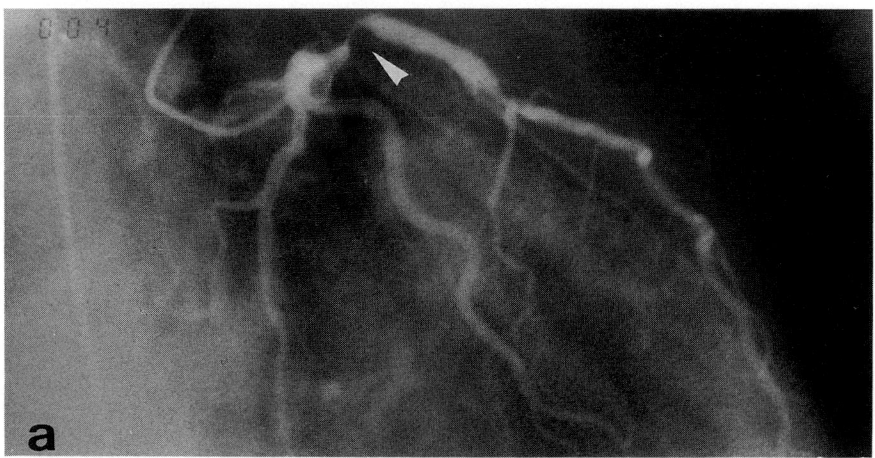

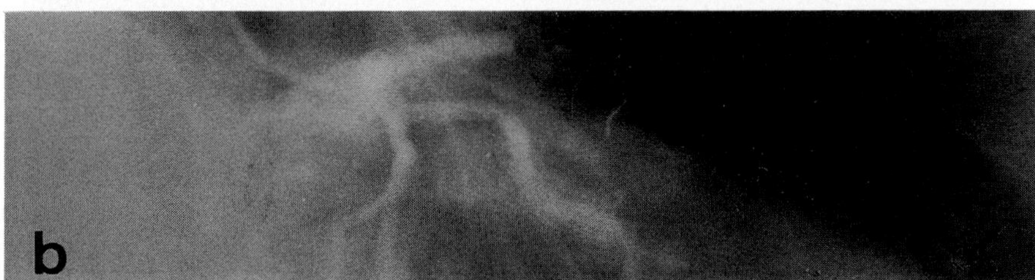

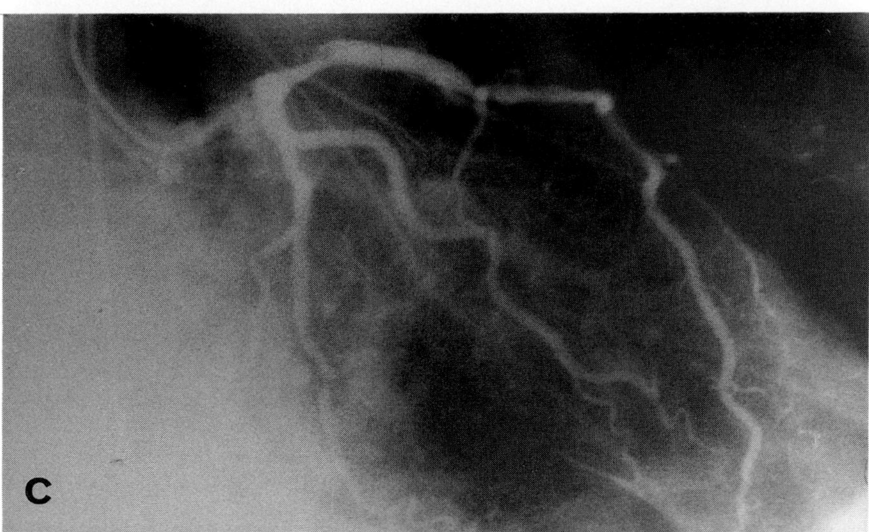

Figure 157

The primary use of stents is in bail-out situations, following a dissection in a vessel undergoing angioplasty. A 61-year-old woman underwent angioplasty of a mid LAD stenosis (Fig. 156a). The result after balloon inflation revealed a long dissection, with sluggish flow, and dye hold up in the dissection, these signs being predictors of an unstable dissection (Fig. 156b). A Gianturco-Roubin stent (Cook) was implanted over a 3.0-mm balloon, and the lesion stabilized (Fig. 156c). A repeat angiogram 1 week later revealed a good result (Fig. 156d). Stents in these situations are invaluable, reducing the dependence of the angioplaster on the surgeon. However, stenting for bail-out situations is no panacea because even with strict anticoagulation, acute or subacute thrombosis occurs in a significant percentage of patients. It is commoner in smaller vessels, with poor distal runoff and with imperfect results. This speaks in favor of using stents early before the dissection has extended too far, and to reserve stenting for larger vessels. In addition, if anticoagulation is strictly maintained, groin bleeding complications have to be expected. This is exemplified in a 83-year-old patient, who underwent angioplasty of a tight proximal LAD stenosis (Fig. 157a) through a 4F catheter using a fixed-wire balloon (Fig. 157b) with an acceptable result (Fig. 157c). Twenty minutes later the patient experienced chest pain, and the angiogram revealed an acute occlusion of the LAD (Fig. 157d). Bail-out stenting with a Palmaz-Schatz stent on a 3.0-mm balloon was performed, with a good result (Fig. 157e). The patient received routine poststent anticoagulation and died following a retroperitoneal bleed a week later. The stent was patent on necropsy. Whether a lenient anticoagulation regimen with antiplatelet therapy alone that is currently being adopted for routine stenting can be extended to high-risk stent cases has yet to be evaluated.

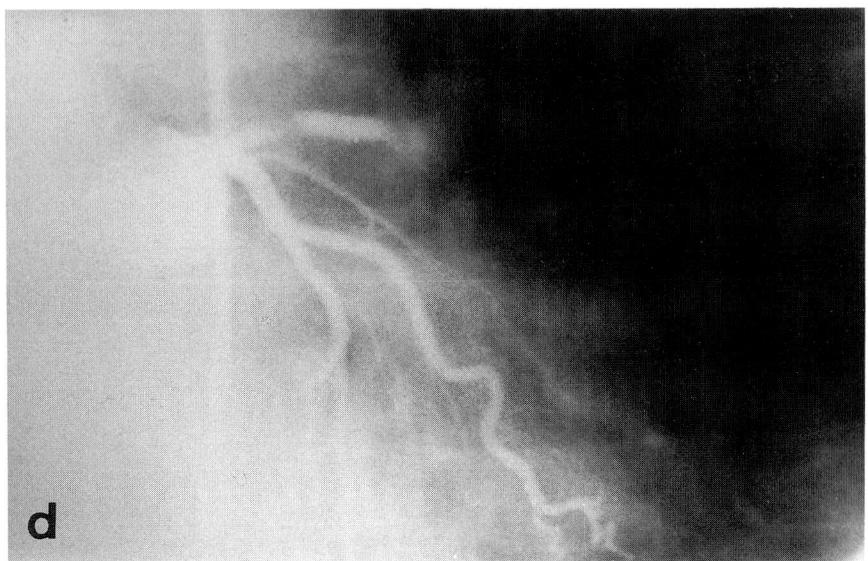

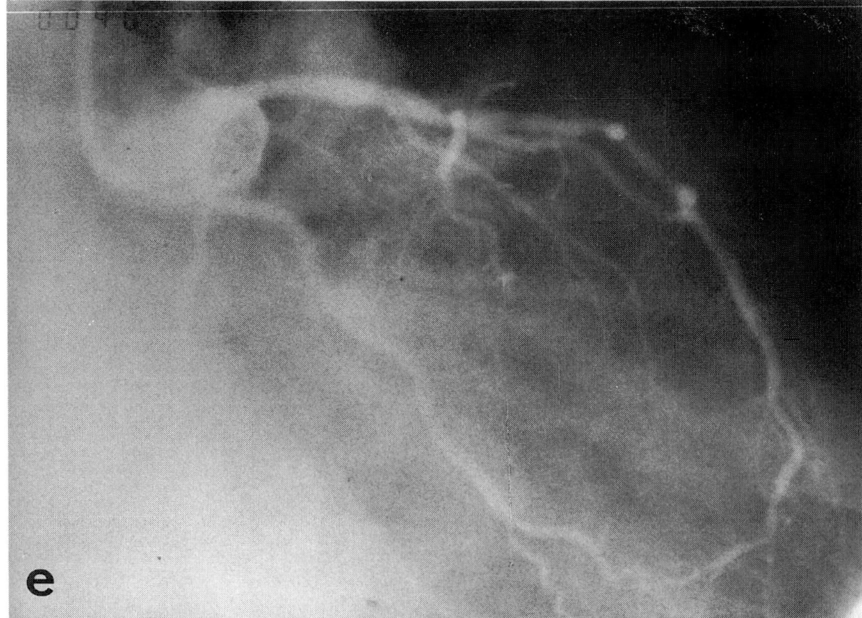

Figure 157 (Continued)

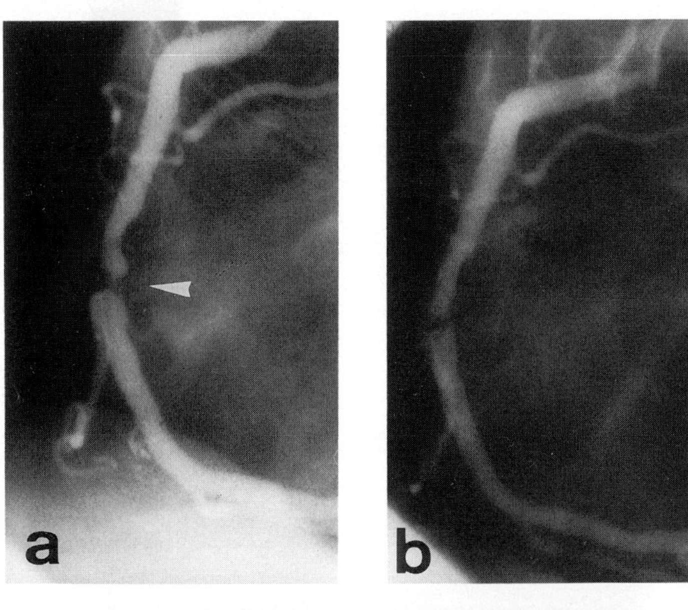

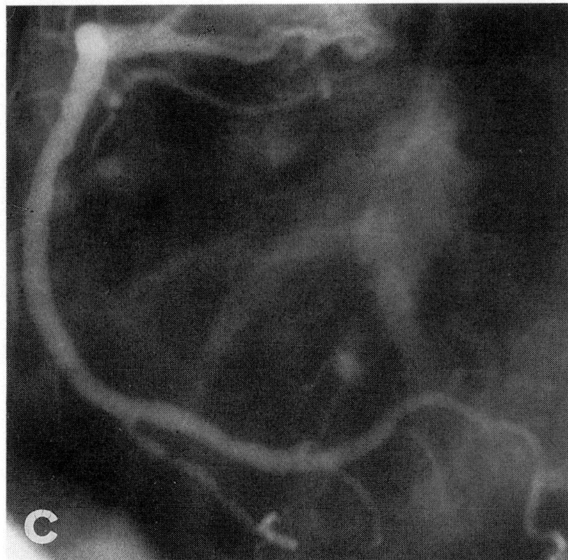

Figure 158

For short, discrete lesions with a suboptimal result after balloon inflation, a half (disarticulated) Palmaz-Schatz stent may be utilized. The advantage of such an approach is that the amount of metal in the artery is reduced, thus limiting the risk of thrombosis. Moreover, the implantation of such a short stent may have less deleterious consequences on vessel compliance and laminar intravascular blood flow. These factors may play a role in reducing acute stent thrombosis, and also possibly the incidence of restenosis. Additionally, since only half a stent is used, vessel negotiation is facilitated and cost is reduced by 50%. A patient underwent angioplasty for a lesion in the mid RCA (Fig. 158a), which relapsed after dilatation with a 4.0-mm balloon (Fig. 158b). Half a Palmaz-Schatz stent was implanted with an excellent result (Fig. 158c). The patient was discharged the next day on 100 mg of aspirin alone after completing a negative stress test.

A 57-year-old man presented with angina and a positive stress test. An LAD stenosis was seen (Fig. 159a), and angioplasty performed with a 3.5-mm balloon (Fig. 159b). The post-angioplasty result was unsatisfactory, owing to a relapsing intimal flap (Fig. 159c, arrow). Half a stent was implanted, and the effect was good (Fig. 159d). Again, the patient was treated with oral aspirin alone. No further anticoagulation was administered. The sheath was removed the same evening, and the patient was discharged the next morning. Such an approach of stenting without anticoagulation is reasonable with short stents in a large vessel (≥3 mm in size) with good peripheral run-off and an excellent angioplasty result. Its use with longer and multiple stents is under investigation.

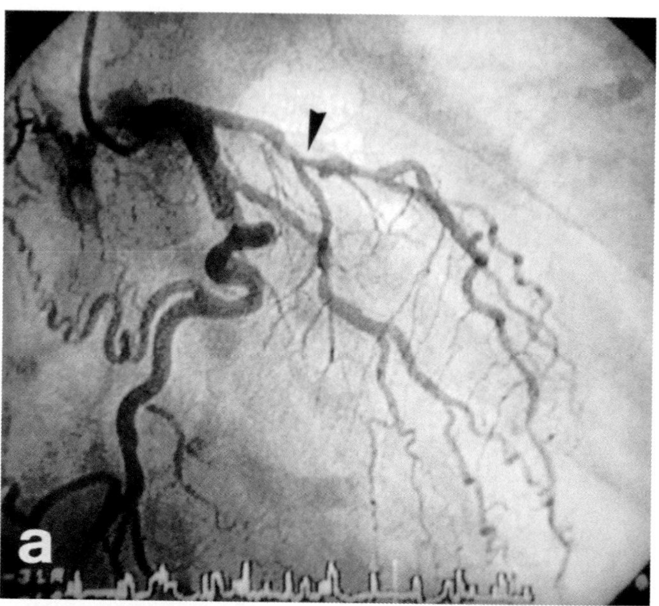

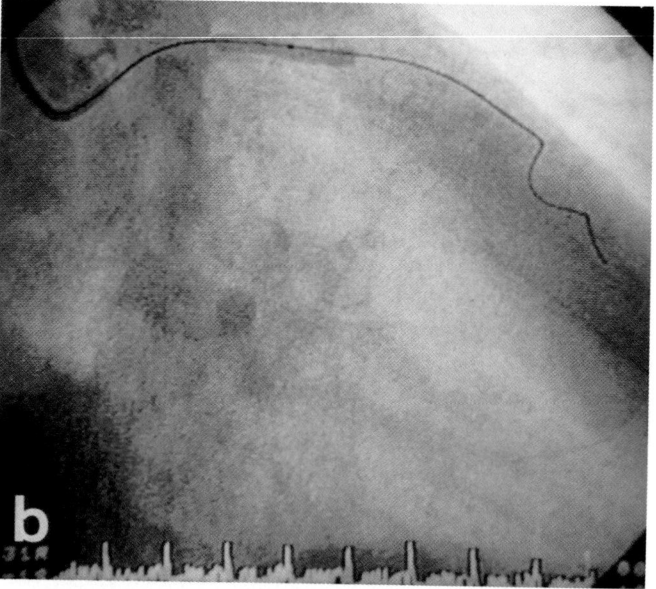

Figure 159

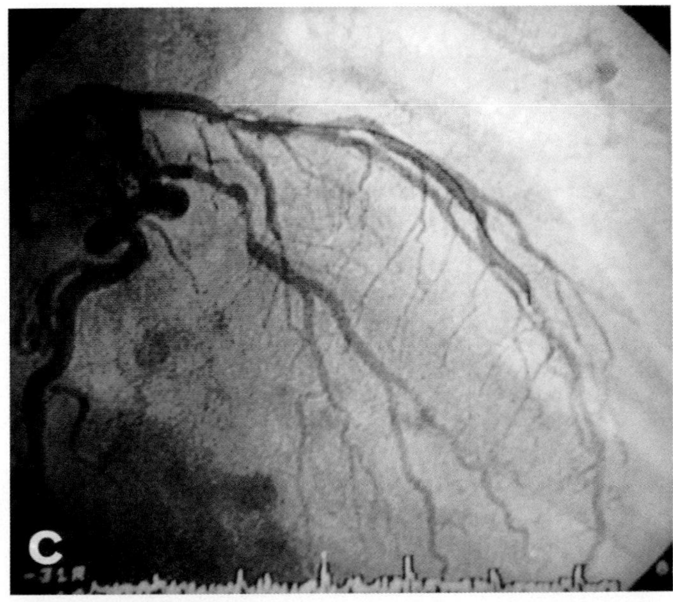
c

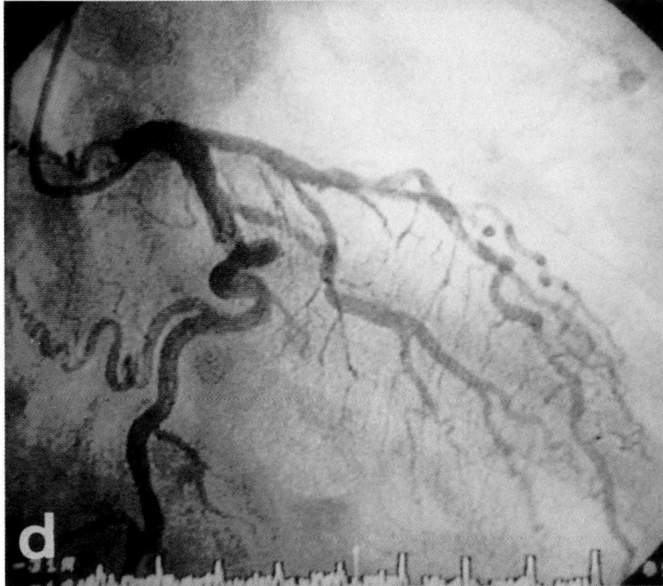
d

Although stenting is useful for the management of acute dissections and may reduce restenosis, it does not eliminate it. A 57-year-old man underwent angioplasty of a proximal LAD stenosis (Fig. 160a). A 3.5-mm balloon was used, with a resultant dissection (Fig. 160b). The lesion was stented, using a Palmaz-Schatz stent mounted on the same balloon, with a good result (Fig. 160c). The lesions in the distal LAD (Fig. 160a, black arrow) and the LCx (Fig. 160a, white arrow) were not addressed. The patient presented 7 months later with recurrent symptoms and restenosis (Fig. 160d). It was decided to redilate the stented site and also to dilate the distal LAD and LCx

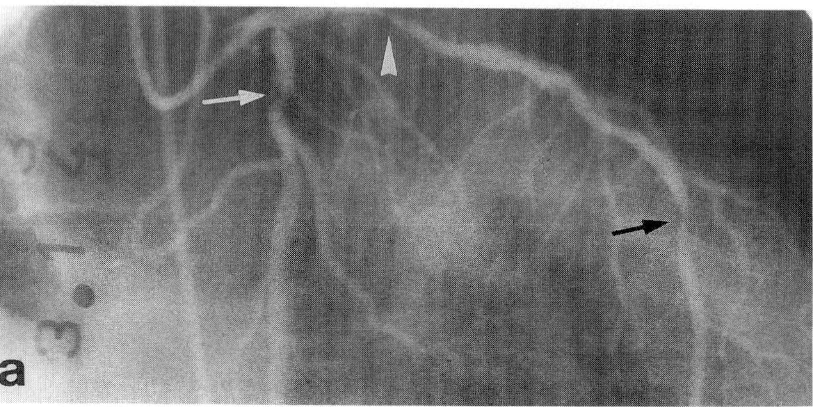

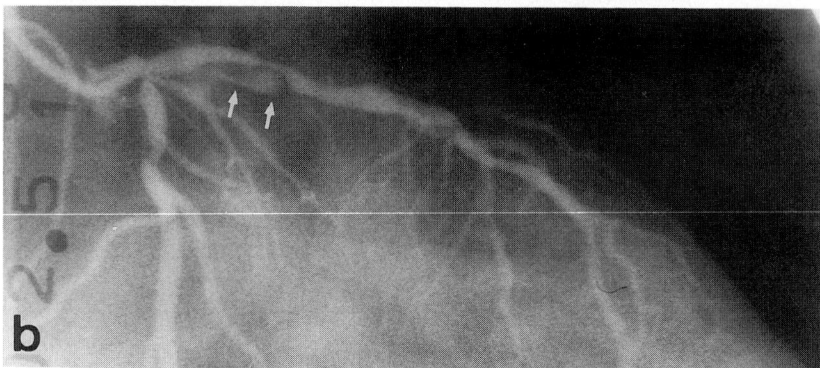

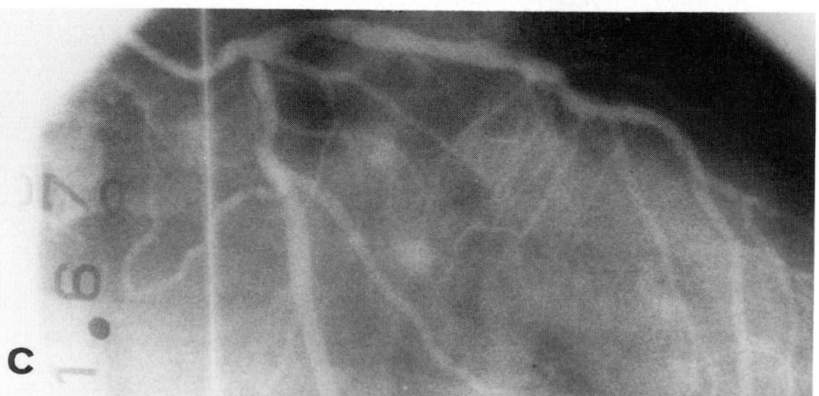

Figure 160

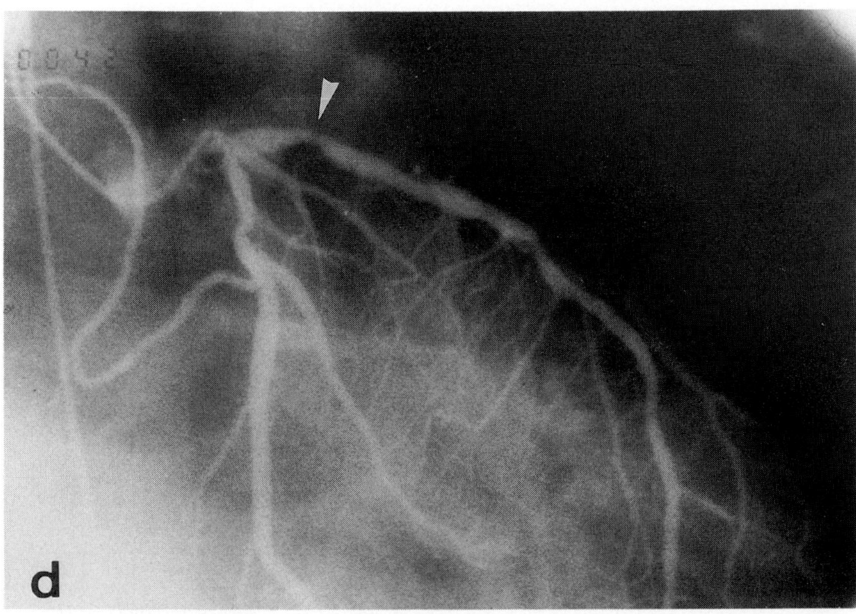

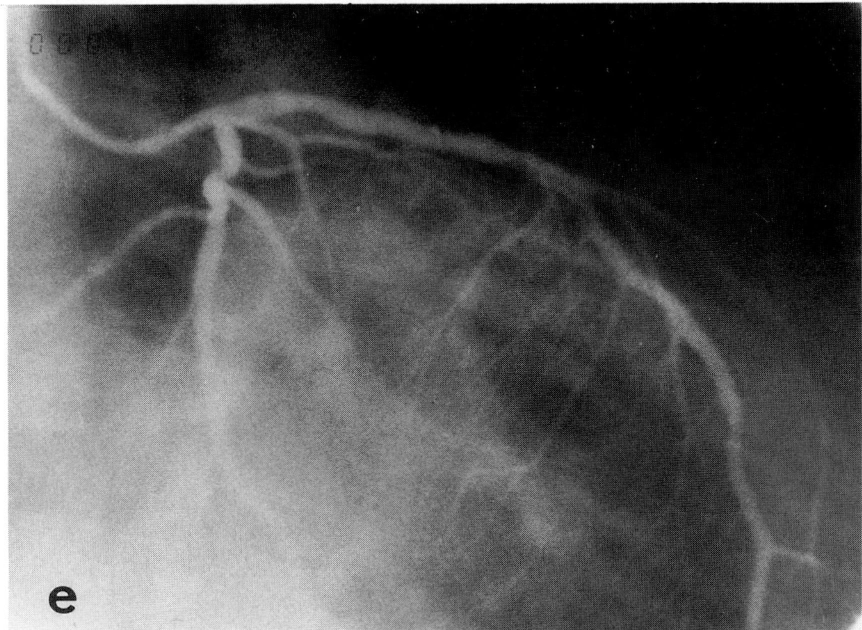

lesions. A compliant 3.0-mm balloon was selected this time. The distal LAD and the LCx lesions were dilated with low pressures (4 to 6 bar), and the proximal lesions with 10 to 12 bar, thereby achieving good angioplasty results of all segments (Fig. 160e). This example demonstrates:

- That stent restenosis can be adequately managed by redilatation
- How a compromise of balloon size can be used to dilate lesions in vessels of different sizes at low cost, making use of the property of a compliant balloon to expand at greater pressures

6.2 ELECTIVE STENTING

Elective stenting refers to stenting of a stenosis at primary intent rather than to remedy a poor angioplasty result. Such an approach is often adopted for recurrent restenoses or diffusely diseased venous grafts. Although restenosis also occurs after elective stenting of primary lesions, the Benestent and STRESS studies show a trend toward lower restenosis rates in electively stented vessels.

A 46-year-old woman underwent angioplasty for a proximal LAD stenosis (Fig. 161a) with a good immediate result (Fig. 161b). She presented 2 months later with chest pain and restenosis (Fig. 161c) and underwent successful re-PTCA (Fig. 161d). Symp-

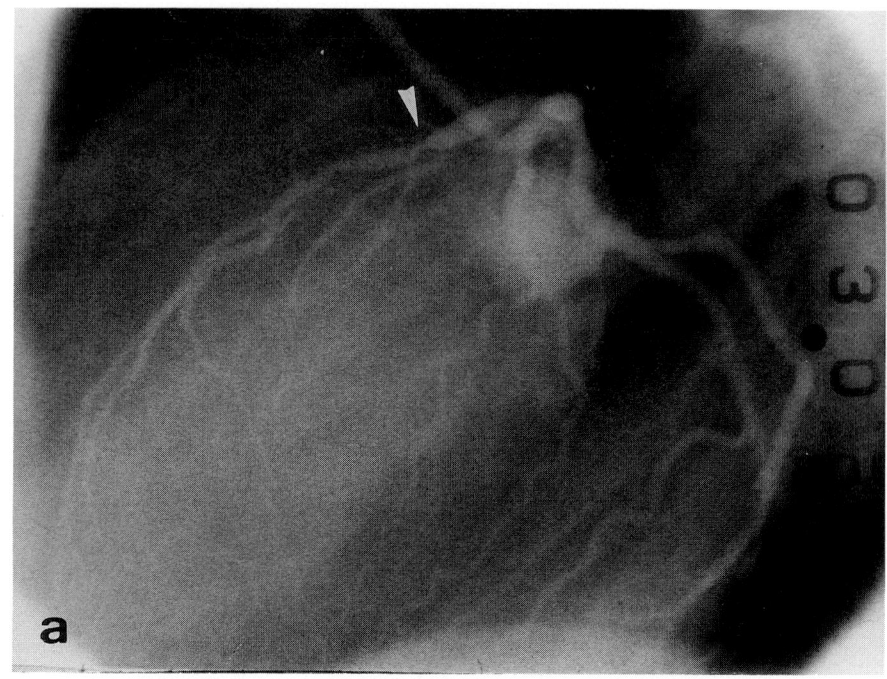

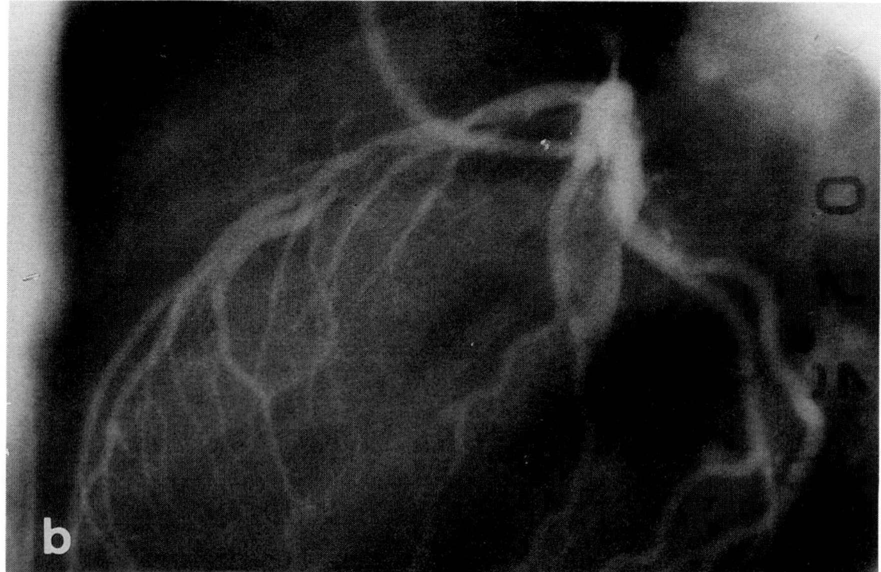

Figure 161

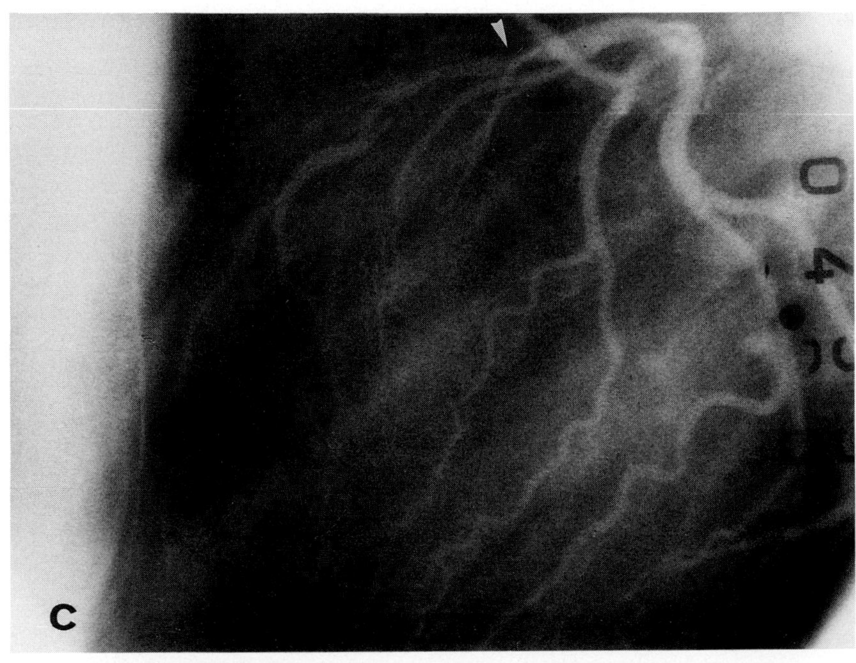

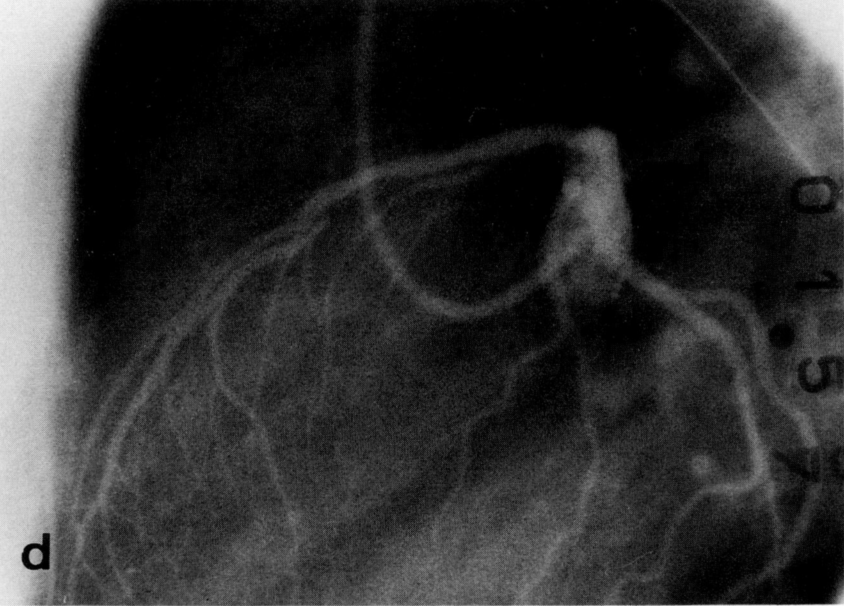

toms recurred 3 months later, and restenosis was again discovered (Fig. 161e). A third angioplasty performed (Fig. 161f). The patient presented once again 3 months later with restenosis (Fig. 161g). It was now decided to electively stent the recurrent restenosis. A 3.5-mm Wallstent (Schneider) was implanted, although the initial balloon dilatation had yielded a perfect result (Fig. 161h). The final angiographic result is shown in Fig. 161i. Figure 161j shows the stent in place (arrows). The patient remained asymptomatic and a follow-up angiogram 6 months later revealed no evidence of restenosis (Fig. 161k). Although the absence of restenosis in this case cannot be attributed unequivocally to the stent, it is reasonable to electively stent a restenotic lesion, especially if the lesion has recurred several times. Unless a self-expanding stent is used as in this case, a larger balloon diameter than that used for the angioplasty attempt is advisable and permits achievement of a larger initial lumen.

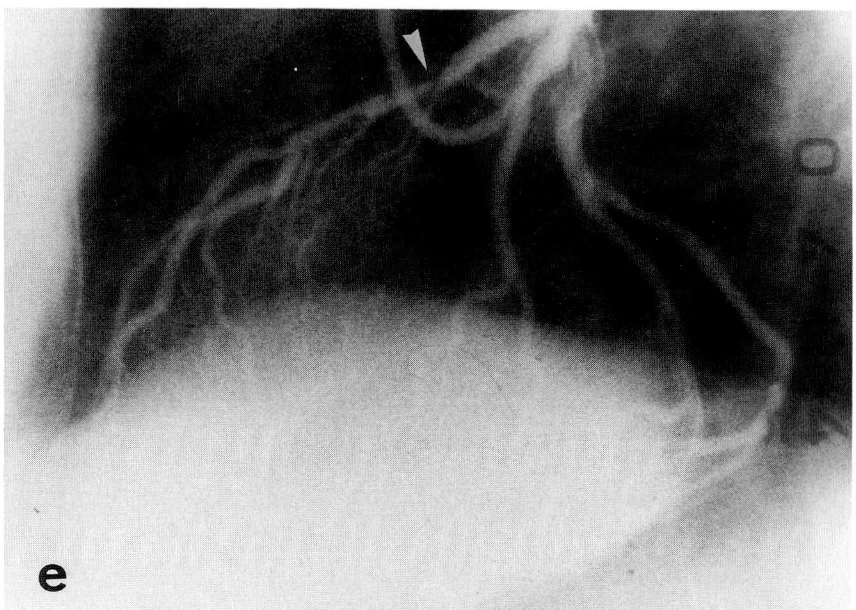

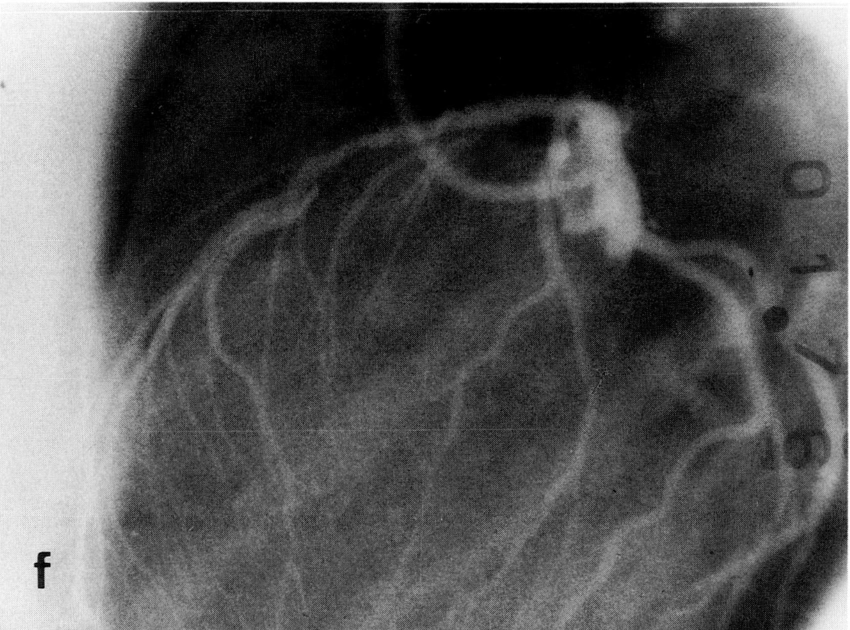

Figure 161 (Continued)

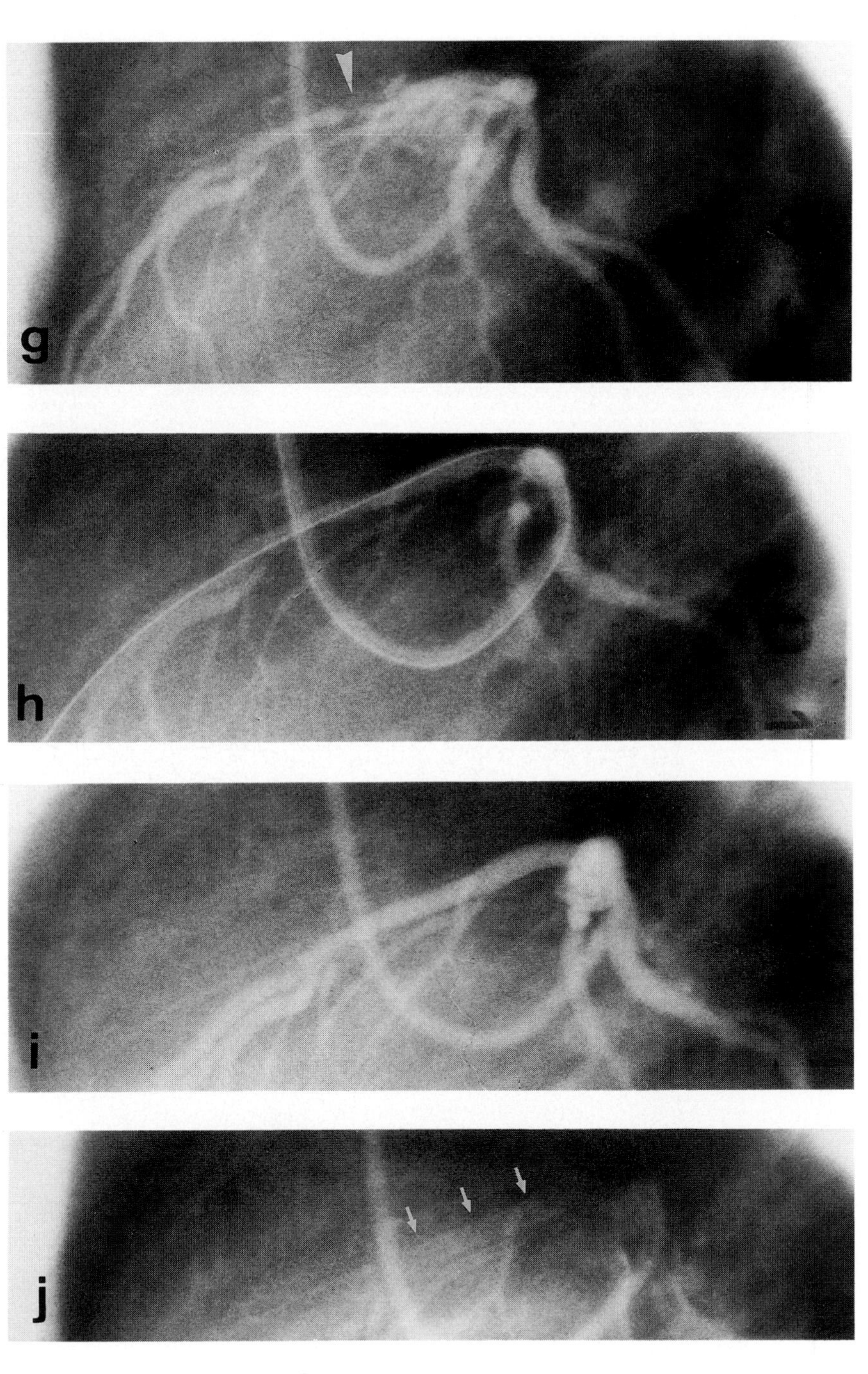
g
h
i
j

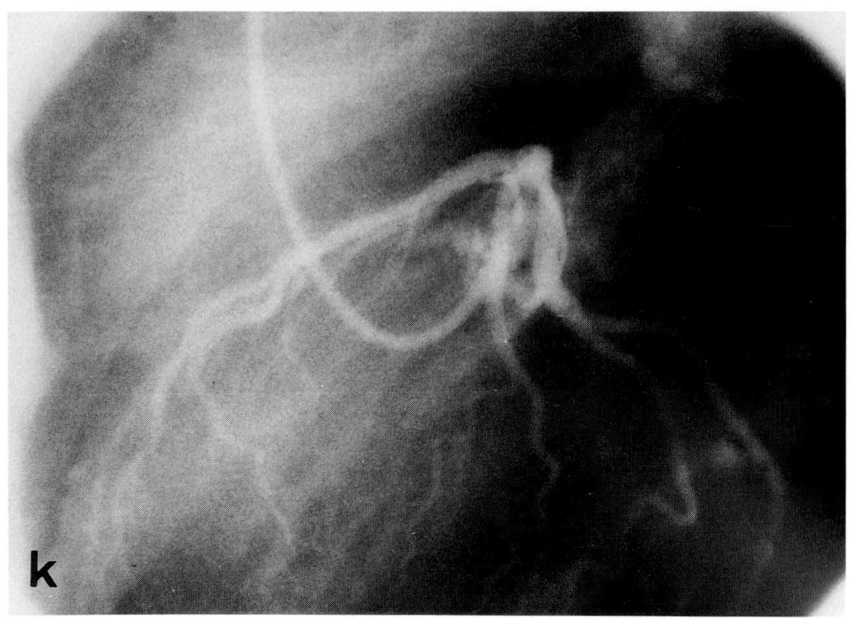

Figure 161 (Continued)

Elective stenting is a good policy when dealing with venous grafts. A 59-year-old man with triple-vessel disease had undergone CABG 3 years prior, and presented with angina. A discrete graft body stenosis of the venous graft to the LAD was seen (Fig. 162a). In view of the mediocre long-term results of angioplasty of graft body stenoses, and the discrete nature of the stenosis, it was decided to primarily stent the lesion. Stenting was performed using a half (disarticulated) Palmaz-Schatz stent mounted manually on a 4.0-mm balloon. Note the characteristic waist of the balloon seen during implantation of a half stent (Fig. 162b). The result was good (Fig. 162c). The patient was discharged on coumadin and aspirin. Elective stenting in vein grafts has the additional advantage of compressing the thrombotic material commonly present in venous graft stenoses against the ves-

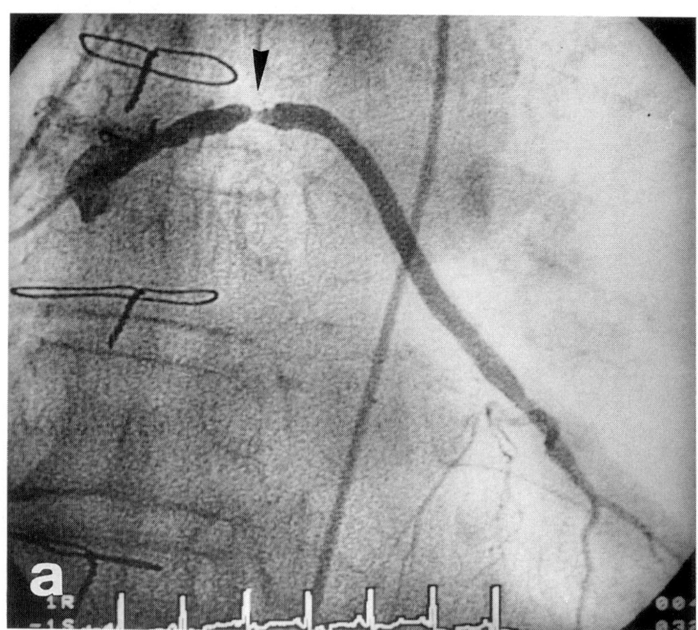

Figure 162

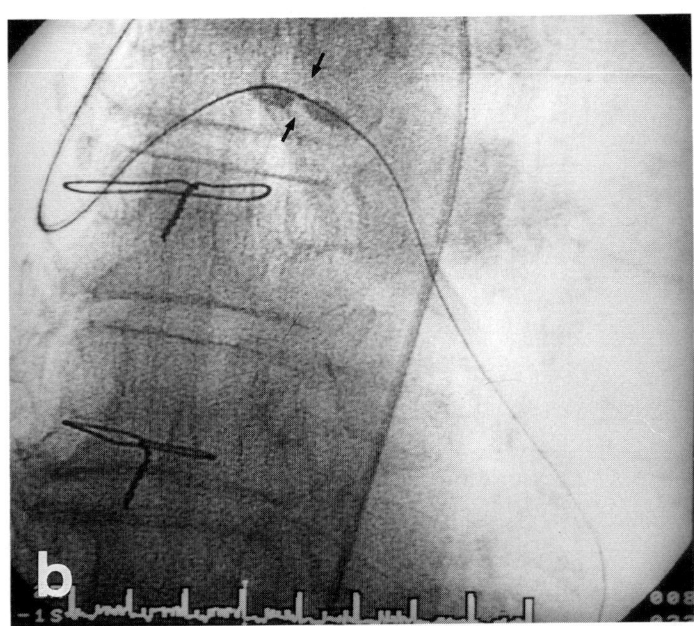

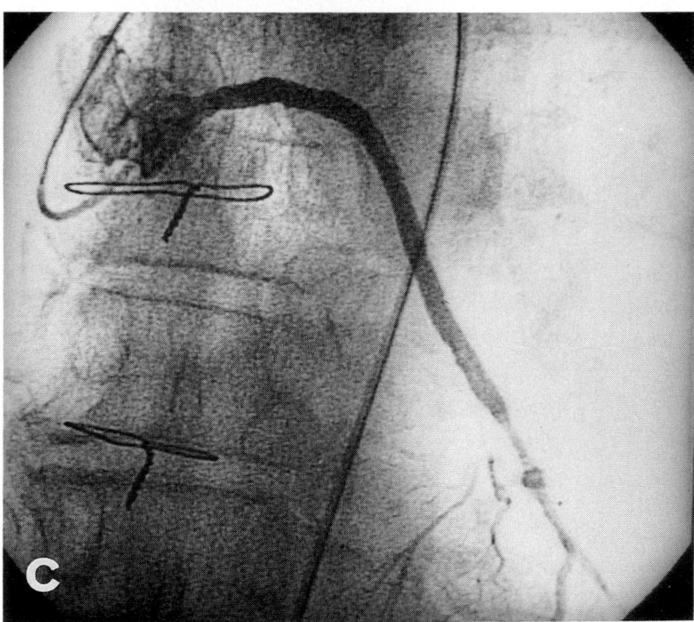

sel wall. This thrombotic materials is often responsible for the poor immediate results of balloon angioplasty. Additionally, the thrombotic material may embolize to the distal vessel following angioplasty. Stenting has the potential to prevent this problem and may result additionally in a lower restenotic rate. It is advisable, however, to predilate the lesion despite the risk of embolization of lesion fragments. An attempt to deploy a stent without predilation may fail because of the inability to pass or crack the lesion. The former faces the problems of removal of the undeployed stent with the risk of losing it during pullback. The latter may leave an incompletely expanded stent in the lesion, which portends stent thrombosis.

However, stents are not suitable for all stenosed vein grafts. Case selection is essential, and certain grafts (Fig. 68) will have poor results even with stenting and are best left alone.

7
Perspectives

In a rapidly evolving field such as PTCA, perspectives tend to be reminiscences by the time they are printed and read. Nevertheless, it is our firm belief that balloon angioplasty will remain the mainstay of PTCA for a long time. Figure 163 illustrates the recent past and the near future of PTCA. The POBA (plain old balloon angioplasty) balloon was, and will be, the largest one and the one flying highest. It will, however, all but be joined by the stent, which is gaining rapidly in size and height. CPS (cardiopulmonary support) systems will be an important asset to interventional cardiologists to keep patients with severe complications alive until surgery. Yet need for their use will fortunately remain rare (note the small size of the balloon). DCA (directional coronary atherectomy), a high flyer of the past, has lost height and size because of its poor performance in randomized trials. ELCA (excimer laser coronary angioplasty), holding a similarly promising position in the past, is going to disappear as have LBA (laser balloon angioplasty), Lastac (an argon laser system), and Rotacs (a slow-rotation angioplasty system). TEC (transluminal extraction catheter) is likely to meet the same fate. The Rotablator has still to prove its potential in randomized trials. Yet it has two niches of its own: lesions too tight to be crossed by a balloon, and stenoses too tough to be cracked by a balloon. In addition, it is easy to use and well liked by operators. Therefore, it is likely to stay.

Of the new diagnostic tools, IVUS (intravascular ultrasound) has a brighter future than angioscopy because the latter requires blood-free vessels and is hampered by a limited field of vision. Both, however, are unlikely to develop beyond research tools.

New gadgets will continue to appear on the angioplasty horizon, as are presently the laser wire for chronic occlusions, PLOSA (warm balloon), US (ultrasound) lysis, hydrolysis, and the Dispatch balloon for local drug delivery to crack the still unscathed shell of the restenosis problem. Only time will tell how big they will grow and how high they can fly. Some of these devices might never really get off the ground at all, a few may become standard equipment, but none is likely to challenge seriously the dominant role of POBA.

Hence the skill with coronary balloons, guidewires, and guiding catheters, together with knowledge about indications, pitfalls, and intelligent use of available material, will remain the basic instruments of interventional cardiologists performing PTCA. This atlas may help to develop and maintain these talents to the benefits of our patients in a field where the sun is still on the rise.

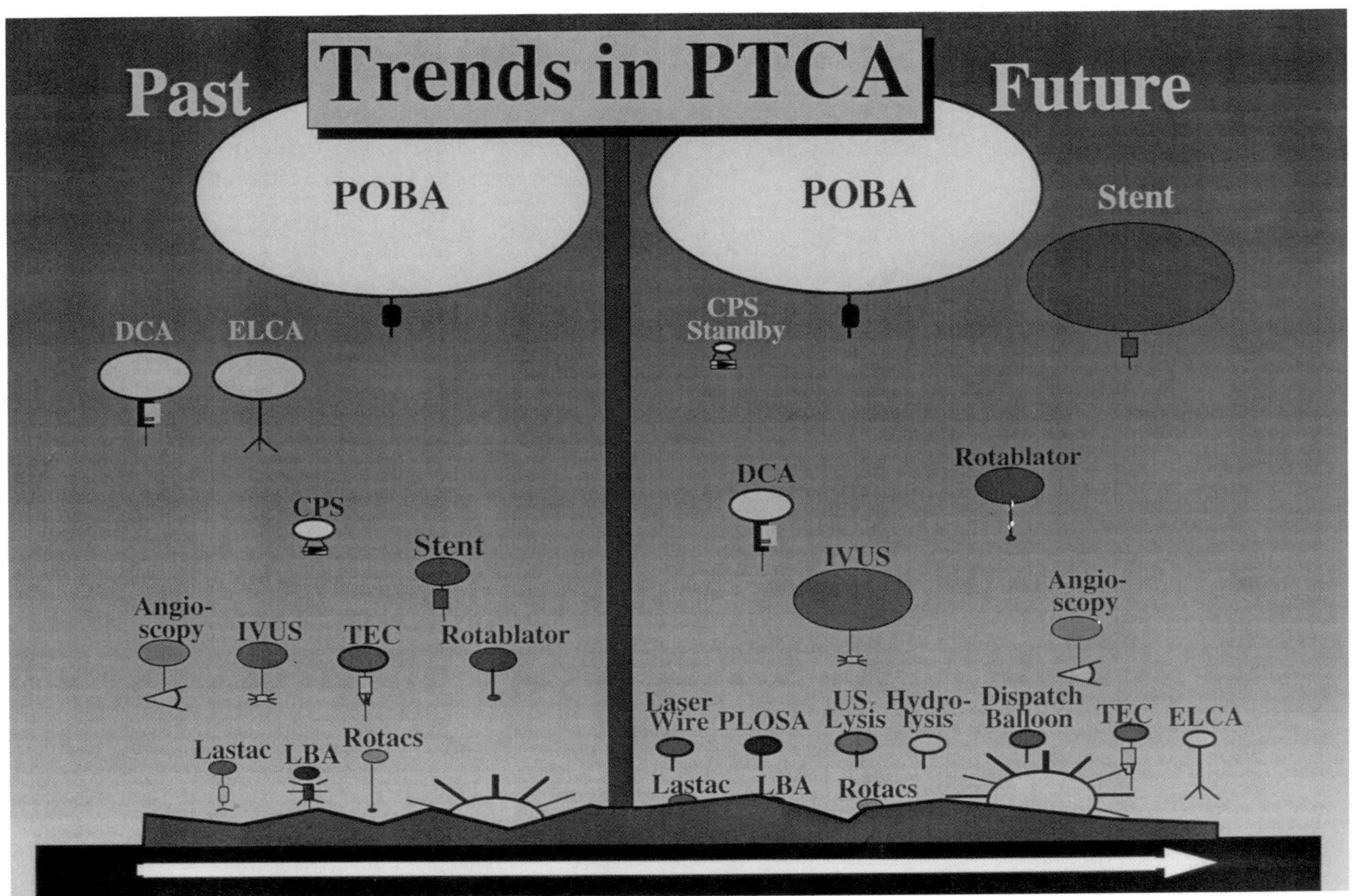
Past
Trends in PTCA
Future
POBA
POBA
Stent
CPS
Standby
DCA
ELCA
Rotablator
DCA
CPS
IVUS
Stent
Angio-
scopy
Angio-
scopy
IVUS
TEC
Rotablator
Laser
Wire
PLOSA
US.
Lysis
Hydro-
lysis
Dispatch
Balloon
TEC
ELCA
Lastac
LBA
Rotacs
Lastac
LBA
Rotacs

Figure 163

Index